M. Spitzer F. A. Uehlein G. Oepen (Eds.)

Psychopathology and Philosophy

Springer-Verlag
Berlin Heidelberg New York
London Paris Tokyo

Dr. med. Dr. phil. *Manfred Spitzer*
Klinikum der Albert-Ludwigs-Universität,
Abtl. für Allgem. Psychiatrie mit Poliklinik,
Hauptstraße 5,
D-7800 Freiburg i. Br.

Professor Dr. *Friedrich A. Uehlein*
Philosophisches Seminar II der
Albert-Ludwigs-Universität,
Wertmannplatz,
D-7800 Freiburg i. Br.

Priv.-Doz. Dr. *Godehard Oepen*
Klinikum der Albert-Ludwigs-Universität,
Abtl. für Allgem. Psychiatrie mit Poliklinik,
Hauptstraße 5,
D-7800 Freiburg i. Br.

ISBN-13:978-3-540-50357-6 e-ISBN-13:978-3-642-74133-3
DOI: 10.1007/978-3-642-74133-3

2125/3130-543210 – Printed on acid-free paper

Preface

> *"Psychopathology should make clear what we know, how we know, and what we do not know."*
> *"If you think you could eliminate philosophy, and regard it as something irrelevant it will overwhelm you in some obscure disguise. This is the point where that bulk of bad philosophy in psychopathological studies originates."*
>
> KARL JASPERS

Since the publication of KARL JASPERS' *General Psychopathology* in 1913 at least, it has become obvious that a psychopathologist cannot do without philosophical reflection. If he wants to say anything about disorders of perception and thought, or of the experiencing I, to name the subjects of this book, he must know those disorders and the problems related to them. The phenomena and problems in question are not at all simply empirical (which is to say that they concern the structure and function of the organs of sense or the central nervous system), but conceptual. We have already formed some notions and prejudices concerning those subjects - perception, e.g., is considered to be "a projection from the outside into the inward", thinking "a kind of inward talk", the I refers to "reflecting upon me by myself", etc. Unless we think about these ideas critically, we shall fail in describing disorders of experience, thought, and action. A training that would meet this demand is not only wanting in the course of study, but even a psychiatrist starting work at hospital generally finds very little time and occasion to reflect on the conceptual basis of the notions which he uses to describe the disturbances that he finds every day. This is all the more the case in a decade where "objectification" by means of "markers" and "scores" sets the fashion. In brief: although the psychiatrist, by definition, has to deal with disorders of the *mental* and therefore cannot do without systematic thought concerning his very subject, this reflection upon the mental is at present underrated.

The conditions for such systematic thought have fundamentally changed over the last decades: nowadays not only phenomenology, as in the first half of the century, is at our disposal as a conceptual framework for theories about the mental. The Continental-European *philosophy of subjectivity* and the Anglo-American *philosophy of mind* have added further conceptual instruments which, however, have not yet been widely used to deal with psychopathological problems. This volume shows some attempts in that direction.

In Freiburg there has been a long tradition of contacts between philosophy and psychiatry. They were cherished especially under the former directors of the psychiatric hospital, KURT BERINGER and HANNS RUFFIN. These contacts have thinned out, however, over the last few years. To bring this tradition back to new life, so to speak, a symposium on the subject of *Psychopathology and Philosophy* was held in Freiburg on July 15-16, 1988. This volume contains the papers that were delivered at this symposium. We are well aware that these contributions are provisional attempts rather than final thoughts. But even so or all the more, this volume may stimulate further thoughts.

Thus this book is meant for all those who have become sensitive, who have felt the provocation and a sense of uncertainty in the contact with mentally disturbed patients, and who instead of clinging to dogmatic tenets or taking refuge in the alleged objectivity of biology or statistics, take up the challenge to critical reflection, which always has to be done anew. Moreover, those who are interested in a systematic study of this subject area will find valuable data and stimulating suggestions for their own considerations.

We thank the following firms for financial aid: Janssen GmbH, Neuss; Farmitalia GmbH, Freiburg; Tropon GmbH, Cologne; Gry Pharma GmbH, Kirchzarten; Smith Kline Dauelsberg GmbH, Munich; Wyeth GmbH, Münster; and Organon GmbH, Oberschleißheim. The printing was generously supported by ratiopharm GmbH, Neu-Ulm. We wish to acknowledge our indebtedness to the helping hands of Brigitte Brand, Renate Campos, Christiane Landmann, cand. phil. Ulrike Selz, Dr. med. Beatrix Spitzer, and B. Thanner. We should like to mention especially Prof. Dr. Klaus Jakobi, who made it possible for the symposium to be held at the Philosophisches Seminar II der Universität Freiburg.

Freiburg, late summer 1988

M. Spitzer
F.A. Uehlein
G. Oepen

Vorwort

"In der Psychopathologie sollte klar werden, was man weiß, wie man es weiß und was man nicht weiß."
"Wer meint, die Philosophie ausschalten und sie als belanglos beiseite lassen zu können, wird von ihr in ungeklärter Gestalt überwältigt: So entsteht jene Masse schlechter Philosophie in den psychopathologischen Studien."

KARL JASPERS

Spätestens seit dem Erscheinen der *Allgemeinen Psychopathologie* von KARL JASPERS im Jahre 1913 scheint es unübersehbar, daß der Psychopathologe um philosophische Reflexion nicht herumkommt: Will er zu Störungen von Wahrnehmen, Denken oder Icherleben - um die Themenschwerpunkte des vorliegenden Buches zu nennen - Aussagen machen, muß er diese Gegenstandsbereiche und die mit ihnen verbundenen Probleme kennen. Diese sind keineswegs nur empirischer Natur (etwa den Bau und die Funktion der Sinnesorgane oder des Zentralnervensystems betreffend), sondern ebenso begrifflicher Art: Wir alle haben Vorbegriffe und Vor-Urteile in bezug auf die genannten Sachgebiete - etwa: Wahrnehmen ist ein "Abbilden von außen nach innen"; Denken ist "eine Art inneres Sprechen"; "Ich" bezeichnet die "Reflexion von mir auf mich" -, die es kritisch zu reflektieren gilt, soll die Beschreibung gestörten Erlebens, Denkens und Handelns nicht von vornherein fehlgehen. Eine entsprechende Ausbildung fehlt jedoch nicht nur im Medizinstudium; auch der angehende klinisch tätige Psychiater hat in der Regel wenig Zeit und Gelegenheit zur Reflexion über die Grundlagen der Begrifflichkeit, mit der er die Störungen, denen er täglich begegnet, zu beschreiben sucht, zumal in einer Zeit, in der "Objektivierung" mittels "Scores" und "Markern" eher dem wissenschaftlichen (Mode-) Trend entspricht. Kurz: Obwohl sachlich nicht wegzudenken, da es der Psychiater nun einmal definitionsgemäß mit Störungen im Bereich des *Mentalen* zu tun hat, sind systematische Überlegungen zum Gegenstand der Psychiatrie, zum Mentalen, wenig üblich und stehen derzeit niedrig im Ansehen.

Die Voraussetzungen für derartige systematische Überlegungen haben sich in den letzten Jahrzehnten wesentlich geändert. Heute steht keineswegs nur, wie in der ersten Hälfte dieses Jahrhunderts, die Phänomenologie als begrifflicher Rahmen für Theorien des Mentalen zur Verfügung. Vielmehr sind in der eher kontinental-europäischen *Philosophie der Subjektivität* und der angloamerikanischen *Philosophy of Mind* zusätzliche begriffliche Werkzeuge entwickelt worden, deren Anwendung auf psychopathologische Fragen noch weitgehend aussteht (einige Versuche hierzu finden sich im vorliegenden Band).

Kontakte zwischen Philosophie und Psychiatrie haben in Freiburg Tradition und wurden insbesondere unter den früheren Leitern der psychiatrischen Klinik KURT BERINGER und HANNS RUFFIN gepflegt, waren jedoch in den letzten Jahren seltener geworden. Um hier gleichsam einen neuen Anfang zu machen, fand am 15. und 16. Juli 1988 in Freiburg ein internationales Symposion zum Thema *Psychopathologie und Philosophie* statt, dessen Beiträge der vorliegende Band enthält. Wir sind uns darüber im klaren, daß es sich hier eher um vorläufige Versuche als um abgeschlossene Gedanken handelt. Gerade deshalb jedoch möchte der Band vielen ein Anstoß zum Weiterdenken sein.

So richtet sich das Buch an alle, die - durch den Umgang mit psychisch Kranken sensibilisiert, provoziert oder verunsichert - weder Halt in dogmatischen Setzungen suchen, noch sich in die Scheinobjektivität von Biologie oder Statistik flüchten, sondern die Herausforderung zu immer neuer kritischer Reflexion annehmen wollen. Darüber hinaus wird der systematisch an den genannten Themenkreisen Interessierte wertvolles Datenmaterial und vielseitige Anregung für seine Überlegungen finden.

Wir danken den Firmen Janssen GmbH, Neuss, Farmitalia GmbH, Freiburg, Tropon GmbH, Köln, Gry Pharma GmbH, Kirchzarten, Smith Kline Dauelsberg GmbH, München, Wyeth GmbH, Münster, und Organon GmbH, Oberschleißheim, für die finanzielle Unterstützung des Symposions. Die Drucklegung des vorliegenden Buches wurde durch die Firma ratiopharm GmbH, Neu-Ulm, großzügig unterstützt. Herzlich bedanken möchten wir uns auch bei einigen "guten Geistern", die bei Organisation, Schreibarbeiten, Lektorat und Übersetzungen mitgeholfen haben: Brigitte Brand, Renate Campos, Christiane Landmann, cand. phil. Ulrike Selz, Dr. med. Beatrix Spitzer sowie B. Thanner. Dank gilt vor allem auch Herrn Prof. Dr. Klaus Jakobi, der die Durchführung des Symposions am Philosophischen Seminar II der Universität Freiburg möglich machte.

Freiburg, im Spätsommer 1988

M. SPITZER
F.A. UEHLEIN
G. OEPEN

Contents

Contributors

Wolfgang Blankenburg, Prof. Dr. med.
Psychiatrische Universitätsklinik
Rudolf-Bultmann-Strasse 8
3550 Marburg

Hector-Neri Castañeda, PH.D.
Mahlon Powell Prof. of Philosophy
Department of Philosophy
Indiana University
Bloomington, Indiana 47405

Hinderk M. Emrich, Prof. Dr. med.
Max-Planck-Institut für Psychiatrie
Kraepelinstrasse 10
8000 München 40

Johann Glatzel, Prof. Dr. med.
Klinikum der Universität
Langenbeckstr. 1
6500 Mainz

Anne Harrington, PH.D.
History of Science Department
Harvard University
Cambridge, Massachusetts 02138

Leopold Hermle, Dr. med.
Psychiatrische Universitätsklinik
Hauptstrasse 5
7800 Freiburg

Reiner Hess, PD Dr. med.
Zentrum für Psychologische Medizin
Von Sieboldstr. 5
3400 Göttingen

Brendan A. Maher, PH.D.
Edward C. Henderson Prof. of the Psychology of Personality
William James Hall
Harvard University
Cambridge, Massachusetts 02138

Christian Mundt, PD Dr. med.
Bezirkskrankenhaus Haar
Postfach 1111
8013 Haar bei München

Godehard Oepen, PD Dr. med.
Psychiatrische Universitätsklinik
Hauptstrasse 5
7800 Freiburg

Helmut Pape, Dr. phil.
Philosophisches Seminar II der Albert-Ludwigs-Universität
Werthmannplatz
7800 Freiburg

Manfred Spitzer, Dr. med. Dr. phil.
Psychiatrische Universitätsklinik
Hauptstrasse 5
7800 Freiburg

Friedrich A. Uehlein, Prof. Dr. phil.
Philosophische Fakultät II
Bismarckplatz
8520 Erlangen

Reiner Wiehl, Prof. Dr. phil.
Philosophisches Seminar der Universität
Marsiliusplatz 1
6900 Heidelberg 1

Introduction

Psychiatry, Philosophy, and the Problem of Description

M. Spitzer

"What does 'description' mean? Every description is interpretation!"
"The chaos of conceptual confusion is rather immense."

MARTIN HEIDEGGER (1965; 1963) on psychiatry [1]

1. Medicine, Psychiatry, and Philosophy

Philosophy and psychiatry seem, at first sight, to be totally different fields in which different people at different sites do different things using different methods on different levels of abstraction pursuing different aims. So one might wonder why psychiatry, being part of medicine, has always had a special affinity to philosophy. This can be answered historically as well as systematically. Since psychiatry has been established as a field of medicine, psychiatric literature is and has always been full of philosophical thought and direct reference to philosophy. Psychiatrists have been sometimes warned not to disregard philosophy which can be shown by quoting JASPERS who wrote that everybody inclined to eliminate or disregard philosophy will be overwhelmed by philosophy in an unpercieved way (JASPERS 1973, pp. 643-644).[2] The benefits of philosophical reasoning within psychiatry are expressed in a more recent publication on truth in psychiatry by WALLACE (1988, p. 146): "So what good is philosophy to psychiatrists anyway?... at the very least it keeps us intellectually honest, humble, logical, selfcritical, and yet questing for knowledge and influence." Furthermore, there are quite a few articles of the title "philosophy and psychiatry" and "psychiatry and philosophy" respectively, although scattered with regard to time and place of publication and diverse with regard to content (cf. BLANKENBURG 1979, EDEL 1974, HÖNIGSWALD 1929, NATANSON 1963, STRANSKY 1923, STRAUS 1963).

1 In: HEIDEGGER 1987, translated by the author, as are the other German quotations in this text.
2 SHOTTER (1975, p. 40) points to the same issue: "In 1879 by putting a taboo upon anything other than experimentation, psychology lost its independence from philosophical speculation at the very moment it declared it - for it lumbered itself with a speculative philosophy which, though long since outmoded, has remained unchanged through remaining unexamined." PELLEGRINO (1986, p. 15) cites E. STRAUSS who remarked in a quite similar way: "... psychiatry seeks philosophical comprehension whether or not the individual psychiatrists follow that impulse."

Philosophical reasoning is common in the whole field of medicine and philosophers get more and more involved in medical questions as well as medical doctors get involved in philosophical reasoning.[3] Why, however, is it psychiatry above all that is related to philosophy? The answer refers to nothing less but the essence of psychiatry, as can be shown by simply looking at psychiatric everyday-life: here questions about what is *real*, whether somebody is able to make *free* decisions, how patient and doctor can *understand* what happens in the psychic life of the patient are stated again and again; psychiatrists deal with *rationality* and *irrationality*[4] respectively, with aspects of the patient that are sometimes neglected in the rest of medicine: his way of *perceiving* and *thinking* about the world as well as his way of *experiencing himself* as thinking and perceiving, to mention only the three most important subject matters which are themes of the papers contained in the present volume and about which the psychiatrist has to make *true* statements. The concepts of *reality*, *freedom*, *understanding*, and *truth* denote, however, *principle problems of philosophy* as well as the concepts of *perception*, *thought* and the *I* (self). If one sees matters this way, the close relation between psychiatry and philosophy is nothing to wonder about because of the simple fact that they share interest in the same matters.

The several lines of thought in the field of *philosophy and psychiatry* can be roughly grouped into three subject areas:

1. Thoughts about philosophy and psychiatry may be about questions in the fields of *epistemology and philosophy of science*. There is a long-standing debate on truth, method, and the scientific status of psychiatric knowledge and we do not even attempt to give an overview of the different contributions or models of solutions in this field. Questions about the possibility of true knowledge in psychiatry and about the scientific status of statements about the mind of another person as well as about the unconscious[5] are discussed. Questions about empirism and operationalism have been filled with new life during the last years by the introduction of the Diagnostic and Statistical Manual of Mental Disorders (DSM-III). Furthermore, the discussions about the use and value of phenomenology and existential philosophy within the realm of psychiatry[6] and all questions about the scientific status and method of psychiatry belong to this field.

Digressions concerning the "ontological committments" especially with regard to the mind-body problem, and the relation between neuroscience and psychiatry respectively, seem to be inevitable. We will not go into the debate on functionalism, reductive, and eliminative materialism, epiphenomenalism etc. (cf. Spitzer 1985, Pardes 1986, George 1987), but just want to say a few words (a) to those who ask for any kind of "psycho-physical transition" and (b) to those who try to establish some kind of reductionistic "nothing-butness-theory" of the mental.

3 There is a growing interest in this field as can be shown by the two relatively recent journals *Medicine and Philosophy* and *Theoretical Medicine*. Examples of thorough inquiries have been given by Diemer 1966, Engelhardt 1986, Weizsäcker and Wyss 1957, and Wieland 1975.

4 There is good reason that different attempts to clarify the concept of rationality, which is used in the whole field of medicine (cf. Clouser and Gert 1986), are discussed in the field of psychiatry (cf. Gert and Clouser 1986, Edwards, 1986, Martin 1986, Mayo 1986, Tucker and Maxmen 1986).

5 For more recent critical contributions see Laudan 1983, Grünbaum 1984.

6 The possibility of a contribution of existential philosophy to psychiatry is still a subject of ongoing debate (cf. Chessick 1986, Hanly 1985, Heidegger 1987). Other philosophers only rarely have been "applied" to psychiatry (cf. Mittel 1968).

Ad a) There is nothing like a "transition" or "liaison" (cf. ECCLES 1981, p. 362) between mind and brain. STRAWSON (1980, 1984) has argued convincingly that the concepts of mind and body are not "logically primitive" but rather is the concept of a person. One of his conclusions is that "the concept of a person is logically prior to that of an individual consciousness. The concept of a person is not to be analysed as that of an animated body or an embodied anima" (STRAWSON 1984, p. 103). With regard to the possibility of a complete neurobiological description of mental phenomena the physicist SCHRÖDINGER in his essay on *Mind and Matter* gives the example of simple mental qualities: "Certainly there is no process within the nerves, the description of which contains qualities like yellow or sweet, the objective description of an electromagnetic wave just as little contains one of these qualities" (SCHRÖDINGER 1959, p. 68). With regard to hearing he notes "that neither the description of the physicist nor of the physiologist contains any trace of a sensation of sound. Such a description in any case necessarily ends with a statement like the following: these nerve impulses travel to a certain brain region... But nowhere we will get to the 'perceiving of sound'; our scientific view simply does not contain it ... Likewise we could analyze sensations of warmth and cold, of smell and taste" (SCHRÖDINGER 1959, p. 71). These statements not only render questions of "transition" senseless, they also shed light on the problem of reduction.

Ad b) Reductionistic arguments mostly consist of two steps: first the complex mental life is regarded as being built up from allegedly more primitive or (onto-) logically prior simple elements, and secondly these elements are conceived of as being of a physical, i.e. non-mental, status. Both steps must be questioned, the latter on grounds of what has been said above, the former on grounds of general reflections about the qualities of consciousness: wholeness and simplicity. From the perspective of artificial intelligence research, more recent variants of reductionistic thought conceive the elements (bits or programs) as "mental" but nevertheless regard complex mental life as product of the interplay of more simple entities (cf. HOFSTADTER 1980, pp. 572-573). These arguments must be questioned on the same grounds: they disregard the fact that the mental is not a sum but has certain "gestalt-" features that cannot be reduced to anything.

2. The second field in which thoughts about *philosophy and psychiatry* can be grouped (as distinct from as well as related to the first) may be summed up as *ethics*. Not only the problems of free will and self-determination in the mentally ill person but also the general discussion about values, norms, deviation, mental health and mental disorder belong to this field. It contains all questions related to psychiatry as the field of - medical and human - action.[7]

This field is also famous for misconceptions which have led to scepticism about philosophical reasoning within psychiatry in general, at least in the eyes of more clinically oriented psychiatrists. The views of LAING (who claims to base his thoughts on HEIDEGGER) and SZASZ, who regard mental illness as a way of life a person is capable to choose and regard psychiatry as nothing but a means of the social system to put pressure on persons who are not ill but just dissenting (a collection of such misconceptions nicely condensed may be found in BENEDEK 1982 and SZASZ 1982) have done not only a great deal of harm to patients.[8] These views also were a major obstacle to the necessary dialogue between clinicians and philosophers.

7 In what follows we will not go into this interesting field of theory and argument; for overviews, critical discussions, and comments see APPELBAUM 1988, LAOR 1984, the issue on *Values and Medicine* in the journal of *Theoretical Medicine* 4 (1983), RICOEUR 1974, to mention just a few.

8 KLERMAN (1987, p. 1703) describes the situation of the mentally ill in these days as follows: "Deinstitutionalization as a public policy was the result of a curious alliance of civil libertarians (often with a romantic view of schizophrenia derived from the writings of Szasz and Laing) and fiscal conservatives interested mainly in reducing the expenditures of state budgets... The 'locked door' has given way to the 'revolving door', and with a growing housing shortage in major cities, the ranks of the homeless have increased. Approximately 50% of the homeless are mentally ill and have high rates of physical illness and are subject to molestation, rape, and robbery by urban predators."

3. The third field in which philosophical and psychiatric thought are closely related is mostly referred to in a rather indirect or implicit way, despite the fact that in this field philosophy and psychiatry come together most closely: philosophical thought is relevant to the science of *psychopathology* as a science of *disturbed experience, perception, and thought* of the patient. The present volume is about this third field of relationship and may show that in this field extensive, interesting and rewarding philosophical and psychopathological research may be undertaken.

"We do not only need to know the aims, guidelines, methods and critisms of other branches of knowledge and science. We also need the realization. We have to walk the paths ourselves." The present volume endeavours to comply with this postulate of HUSSERL (1966, p. XIII). The dialogue between philosophy and psychopathology may not only be fruitful for the psychopathologist but also for the philosopher because psychopathology provides many interesting data, the interpretation of which in the framework of certain philosophical theories about perception or thought might lead to new insights for the psychiatrist and the philosopher as well. Psychopathology might contribute to and even sometimes guide the philosophy of mind. As ENGELHARDT (1986, p. 5) puts it: "It has become clear that philosophical examination of ... medicine ... has also contributed to the vitality of philosophy. It has recalled philosophy to its traditional task of providing critical understandings of major social undertakings. Philosophy as a reflection on ideas and values has a place at the core of everyday life." In its most extreme form this opinion is held by PELLEGRINO (1974) and SPICKER (1986), who compare the effect of medicine on contemporary philosophy with the effect of christian theology on the medieval philosphy. EMRICH (this volume) points to the fact that analytical philosophers sometimes construct mind-models with some deficit (in search for theoretical implications) and thus come close to the psychopathologist dealing with real mental defects. CASTAÑEDA (this volume) also clearly sees the possibility of a guiding role of psychopathology with regard to some questions within the philosophy of mind.

Instead of going through all this three fields in the following sections - the reader interested might turn to the literature listed in the footnotes above -, we want to pursue just one problem which is, nevertheless, fundamental at least to the fields one and three just mentioned - the *problem of description*. It has gained new interest since the underlying approach of the *Diagnostic and Statistical Manual of Mental Disorders, third edition* (DSM-III), which is now accepted as standard in psychiatric diagnosis (and reasoning) all over the world, has often been called - and indeed calls itself - "descriptive". What exactly is the problem of description and why needs the psychiatrist be concerned with it?

2. Jasperian Phenomenology

KARL JASPERS is still regarded as one of the most important psychiatric authors, who not only linked philosophy and psychiatry but also founded psychopathology as a science.[9] JASPERS emphasizes the necessity of philosophical reasoning within the field of psychiatry. His contribution to psychiatric theory can be shown by the fact that some of the basic principles of todays psychiatry can be traced back to his thoughts. These thoughts, however, must not remain unquestioned but should be a subject of philosophical criticism. Thus, the case of

9 See the comments on his general psychopathology by BUMKE 1914, KURT SCHNEIDER 1938 and KUNZ 1948. More recently SCHMITT (1979, 1983) has stressed the same topic.

JASPERS not only shows what philosophy has already achieved within psychiatry but also what philosophy should do. In any case, JASPERS' approach which puts the patient and his symptoms into the center of interest and not - as has been the fashion not only in the days of JASPERS - biological theories about the function of the brain (which has been labelled "brain-myths" by JASPERS), seems to be of immediate concern even today: with regard to the spread of biological psychiatry as well as empirical psychological quantification the danger cannot be overlooked that the experience of the single mentally disturbed person here and now might be neglected in search for "markers" and "scores". Roughly speaking, psychiatry thus might lose its subject, the mind, in trying to "remedicalize" itself (cf. REISER 1988).

JASPERS has called his method *phenomenology* and also speaks of *analysis* as one of his methodological rules. What does he mean? - "The task of phenomenology is to clearly bring to mind the mental states that are really experienced by the patients, to see what aspects they might have in common, to differentiate and to distinguish them and to denote them with fixed terms" (JASPERS 1973, p. 47). In a footnote, JASPERS adds: "Phenomenology for us is an empirical method." In his article *On Phenomenology as a Field of Research Within Psychopathology*[10] JASPERS tries to show the aim and method of phenomenology: as the "subjective symptoms" of mentally ill patients are not just there as the "objective symptoms" in the rest of medicine, there has to be a *method* to get something like a symptom within psychopathology, too.[11] Phenomenology is this method. As JASPERS takes it empirically, it should already be noted here that it is something very different from what HUSSERL calls Phenomenology although JASPERS refers to HUSSERL and uses his terminilogy (cf. BROECKMAN 1965).

In "everyday life we always intend something, make experience because of the intended content" and "never have reason to isolate mental phenomena, e.g. to look at a perception or an emotion per se and describe it with regard to its appearance, way of being and givenness." Phenomenology, on the contrary, is about "the mental processes that happen when we experience" (JASPERS 1963, p. 316). How, then, do we proceed in a phenomenological way?

JASPERS rightly states at first, what phenomenology is *not* and how it is *not* proceeding: (a) It is not about "personal, immediate experience which cannot be formulated in words" (JASPERS 1963, p. 316), and not about the "psychiatrist with empathy, who becomes absorbed in the patient without any concepts", because "knowledge only consists in psychological determination" (p. 317). (b) JASPERS points to negative effects that theories about brain functioning may have on the description of mental activities: "We have to disregard... traditional theories, psychological constructs and materialistic myths about brain processes" (p. 317). (c) "Phenomenology does *not* have anything to do with the *genesis* of mental phenomena (JASPERS 1963, p. 317, his italics).

"Phenomenological" for JASPERS has simply no other meaning than "free of any theory", because he wanted to get rid of the psychological and physiological theories of his time, which he thought to be at best useless and at worst obstructive in the attempt to do psychopathology. Up to now HUSSERL - and his well

10 *Die phänomenologische Forschungsrichtung in der Psychopathologie* (first published in 1912; reprinted in JASPERS 1963).

11 Obviously JASPERS does not question the underlying presupposition of a medical approach to mental illness.

known statement "to the objects itself"[12] - has often been *mis*understood (and was misunderstood that way by JASPERS) as having proposed the programme of getting rid of theories at all for the benefit of pure description.

Psychopathology as a scientific enterprise is about the concepts we use to describe mental disturbances. The question arises "how do we get to the isolation, characterization and conceptual determination of mental phenomena?" (JASPERS 1963, p. 318). We cannot get to these concepts by description because they are our tools for description. In his attempt to solve this problem, which he obviously was aware of (but, as we will see, he did not solve), JASPERS mentions the concept of analysis but he does so in two different meanings: On the one hand he just speaks of *analysis* (JASPERS 1963, p. 193) and on the other hand he speaks of *phenomenological analysis* (JASPERS 1963, p. 320). The context of these terms demonstrates that he means two different things by those two concepts.

Let us start with the concept of phenomenological analysis. JASPERS does not explicitly say what this term means, but he talks about the means of phenomenological analysis: "...at first becoming absorbed in conduct, behavior and expressive movements; secondly exploration; ... thirdly what the patient has written down" (JASPERS 1963, p. 320). By this enumeration, however, the problem of generation and legitimation of basic psychopathological concepts is not solved. What JASPERS calls "means" of phenomenological analysis is rather the *material* of such an analysis. In the context of his writings it is easy to see, that by "phenomenological analysis" JASPERS means the application of phenomenology (in his sense) to a single case. "If we try by these means to come closer to the mental life of a patient, at first we see a vast, permanently flowing chaos of changing phenomena. Our first aim must be to eliminate singularities, to bring all aspects of them to mind for our use and for others, and to give them constant terms with identical usage (JASPERS 1963, pp. 320-321). *How* to do this, JASPERS does *not* say in this context.

The meaning of the term "analysis" may best be understood by looking not only at JASPERS' reflections on the meaning of that term, but also by looking at the way JASPERS carries out such an analysis. He does so in dealing with perception and its disorders.

"We analyze perception. What does analysis mean? It does not mean that we look for the elements in perception which bring perception into being. We cannot really divide perception in these elements or find isolated elements which somehow interact and produce perception. These isolated elements are never given to us, given to us is the whole complete perception" (JASPERS 1963, p. 193).

JASPERS very clearly differentiates between *analysis* and *explanation*: we explain the genesis of a perception and the products of analysis of perception are aspects or components which are of no use in explaining the origin of a perception but may be used to legitimate a certain perception. "We may well ask for the origin of our perceptions. If we do, we *explain* them. Explanation is totally different from analysis. Explanation operates with theoretical processes which are not conscious... What analysis seperates did not originate out of the constituents that had been the results of analysis. The intended use of the resulting elements of an analysis is merely to enable the psychiatrist to *definitely characterize and securely differentiate* mental processes as they really are (JASPERS 1963, pp. 193-194, his italics).

12 See HUSSERL (1913; 1976): *General Introduction into Pure Phenomenology*. From his writings it is clear that he did not intend to abolish all kinds of theory by this statement.

Thus Jaspers has said what he means by "analysis" but the question about method, i.e. how an analysis is carried out, is not yet solved. We therefore look at what he does in his analysis of perception.

He starts as follows: "At first there is the old and familiar knowledge that each perception can be analyzed into final elements which are called sensations" (Jaspers 1963, p. 194). Jaspers says that sensations are "the most simple things in the world" (p. 205), distinguishes "primary" sensations (caused by external stimuli) and "secondary" sensations (not caused by external stimuli), and thus obviously has in mind a concept that was in fashion in German psychology of his time (i.e. the beginning of the 20th century). Next to "the group of sensations... we may mention spatial and temporal qualities as a second group of phenomenologically final elements of perception" (Jaspers 1963, p. 195). Jaspers also speaks of the intuition [Anschauung] of space and time and thus refers to Kant. A third element of perception for Jaspers are the acts, which he specifies as "ways of intending" [Weisen des Meinens].

The discrepancy between Jaspers' definition of what analysis should do and what he is really doing when analyzing is obvious: *Sensations* not only do not have the status of an "old and familiar knowledge" (the concept is rather subject to a quarrel that can be traced through centuries until today; see Gregory 1987; Spitzer 1988a,b). In mentioning sensations Jaspers simply adopts what was fashion in his time and thus does not clarify how he won these "elements". Although he did not analyze at all he pretends to have carried out an analysis as he also says that he has found sensations within perception "phenomenologically" and by "immediate observation". This contradicts to what he said about the components of perception, as they are "not given as isolated". He also would not have needed an analysis if the elements of perception had been perceivable. A further contradiction of his analysis to what he says about it can be shown in his distinction between primary and secondary sensations: this distinction is made with regard to cause and genesis, which had been explicitely excluded as analytical aspects. The second group of elements of perception - spatial and temporal qualities - is introduced by the words "we may mention". There is nothing like a reason for it, no "analysis" at all, not even a short comment. All we can say is that the second element is brought forward by an allusion to Kant (who spoke of the spatial and temporal material of intuition, whereas Jaspers speaks of the respective material of sensation). The "ways of intending" are also just mentioned and are taken from Husserls Phenomenology but are in no way the result of an analysis.

What we have indicated as problems and contradictions has not been noticed by Jaspers and most of his interpreters so far. The reason for this may be the fact that Jaspers had published his thoughts in diffrent articles under headlines that do not fit to what he says in the respective articles: in his *basic* article on method (*On Phenomenology as a Field of Research Within Psychopathology*) he speaks of "phenomenological analysis" with reference to *single cases* thus presupposing the existence of a conceptual framework which can be used for description. On the other hand, in his article on a *special* problem of psychopathology (*On the Analysis of False Perceptions*) he speaks about the *general* analysis of concepts. Jaspers thus refers to single cases when he speaks of his method in general and refers to his general method when he discusses single cases. - What is left is his emphasis on detailed description of single cases and on the necessity to clarify concepts. *How* this should be done - in other words: what the science of psychopathology consists in - he does not say.

It should be emphasized that we do *not* critizise Jaspers for making presuppositions and refering to theories. We rather criticize that he, *contrary to what he really does, maintains to proceed without presuppositions and without theories.* Furthermore, as Jaspers requires to be always conscious of one's own method and procedure, this criticism has even to be made *on two levels*.

As we have stated above, Jaspers has thought of phenomenology as a way of describing free of any theory. He *dismissed* - contrary to what he says elsewhere and contrary to what he is famous for - *philosophical* (and not only psychological and physiological!) theory as a means of psychopathological research and practice: "Phenomenology cannot gain anything by theory but only lose" (Jaspers

1963, p. 327); "he [the psychopathologist] obviously cannot learn anything from philosophy..." (JASPERS 1973, p. 6, see also pp. 624ff).

With this view - theory has to be gotten rid of because it obstructs description - JASPERS has influenced not only the phenomenological oriented German psychiatrists[13] but psychiatric thinking all over the world until today.[14]

3. Empiricism and Operationalism: DSM-III

Psychiatry is regarded to be an empirical science. What, after all, is an empirical science? - In the following section it will be shown that some current assumptions about what psychiatry is and what the psychiatrist should do are based on misconceptions about what "empirical science" really means.

The most basic assumption is that it is possible to give a purely descriptive, i.e. theory-free, account of objects and events. Such an account would lead not only to scientific explanations (see 3.1) but also to the evaluation of scientific theories (see 3.2) in the field of psychiatry.

3.1 The Hempel-Oppenheim-Scheme of Explanation

The standard of scientific explanations is often seen in the so-called *Hempel-Oppenheim-Scheme of explanation*. Thus, this scheme has been used to reconstruct psychiatric reasoning, as can be shown by the examples given by MÖLLER. One of his examples runs as follows:

> "Why has patient A a clouded consciousness?"
> The explanation to this question is concieved to be as follows:
>
> "a human being with a severe disease of the kidneys has a clouded consciousness.
> A suffers from a severe disease of the kidneys.
> ___
> A has a clouded consciousness" (MÖLLER 1976, p. 18).

All questions relevant to psychiatry thus "will find a correct answer which satisfies the search for knowledge by way of the application of the Hempel-Oppenheim-Scheme of explanation" (MÖLLER 1976, p. 18). Such a reconstruction of psychiatric reasoning seems to guarantee the status of psychiatry as a science as well as the progress of scientific knowledge in this field. This view presupposes, however, that it is possible to separate descriptions from explanations and that a scientist does not do anything but to describe and to explain.

---

13 Cf. HOPPE 1919; STRANSKY 1923 (a good example of what WALLACE calls philosophobia); the writings of BINSWANGER, in which on the one hand very detailed descriptions of some patients can be found but which on the other hand are misconceived from a theoretical point of view, may serve as a good example of the attempt, simpl to describe. HEIDEGGER (1965; 1987, p. 239) is perfectly right in commenting on BINSWANGER: "What does 'description' mean? Every description is interpretation!"

14 As further can be shown, his concepts of consciousness and of the experiencing I and its disorders therefore were to be misleading and have lead psychiatrists who have focussed their work on JASPERS - e.g. KURT SCHNEIDER and via him a considerable part of the foundations of DSM-III (see SPITZER 1987) - to basic errors.

Logical empiricism and especially HEMPELS view of the nature of empirical sciences is applied to the problem-ridden field of psychiatric classification by SCHWARTZ and WIGGINS (1986), who thus try to ground the diagnostic approach of the DSM-III on a philosophical basis.

HEMPEL himself criticized the systems of psychiatric classification that had been in use in his time especially for the reason, that descriptive and theoretical aspects of a diagnosis are not clearly separated within these systems of classification. As "theory" denotes concepts about the causes of mental disorders and "description" denotes the psychic symptoms of mental disorders, HEMPEL clearly wanted to separate the causal and symptomatic view in a system of classification of psychiatric disorders. There is no doubt that this helps to clarify concepts about mental disorders.

HEMPELS solution of the problem of description consists in *operational definitions*. These were to guarantee the "empirical import" (i.e. the connection of scientific statements with reality): "An operational definition of a term is conceived as a rule to the effect that the term is to apply to a particular case if the performance of a specified operation in that case yields a certain characteristic result" (HEMPEL 1965, cited in SCHWARTZ and WIGGINS 1986, p. 107). Terms that can be defined by operational definitions are regarded as being "purely descriptive".

The descriptive term "hard" is taken as an example (cf. SCHWARTZ and WIGGINS 1986, pp. 107-108): the term seems to be descriptive, but must have an operational definition, because it depends on the circumstances what we may call hard and what not (we may take the butter out of the fridge and say it is hard while at the same time regarding the wood of the table we are sitting at is not hard). An operational definition of "hard" according to HEMPEL consists of a process in which one material is scratched by the other thus showing which of the two materials is harder.

According to SCHWARTZ and WIGGINS (1986) the diagnostic criteria of the DSM-III represent operational definitions of descriptive terms which are to characterize mental disorders. For this reason the DSM-III meets the standard of scientific statements, i.e. DSM-III-diagnoses do have empirical import. The authors admit, however, that the diagnostic criteria have to be further developed and that there should be tests which a psychiatrist had to apply, to see whether a specific symptom is there or not:

"For example, DSM-III cites seven criteria for the diagnosis of *paranoid disorder*. The applicability of each of these criteria to patients should be testable through specific operations. Even the negative criteria, such as criterion E, 'No prominent hallucinations', should be testable through operations. And a negative result on such a test would support the application of criterion E for paranoid disorder to this particular patient. And each of the other six criteria for this disorder would also have to have its own operational definition(s)" (SCHWARTZ and WIGGINS 1986, p. 109).

According to SCHWARTZ and WIGGINS, diagnostic criteria *are* operational definitions or at least should be formulated with such an aim in mind. As it is easy to see, this approach leads to the formulation of *criteria for criteria*[15], i.e. criteria that say whether a certain criterion should be applied. But even these *sub-criteria* do not solve the problem as one can ask for criteria for these sub-criteria.

15 See SPITZER and DEGKWITZ 1986. For a discussion of the historical roots of the notion of criteria within psychiatry, see SPITZER 1987.

This issue is not a theoretical one at all. To give an example: delusions are a prominent symptom of schizophrenia and are included in the list of diagnostic criteria for this mental disorder in the DSM-III as well as the DSM-III-R. But delusions are far from being an operational definition *itself* as Schwartz and Wiggins suggest. Furthermore, there is no operational definition of a delusion but there is rather the attempt to find defining criteria, as Oltmanns (1988), for instance, tries to give seven of such defining criteria of delusions. But even these sub-criteria are in no way operational definitions as postulated by Schwartz and Wiggins. The third criterion given by Oltmanns, for instance, goes as follows: "The belief is held with firm conviction. The person's statements or behaviors are unresponsive to the presentation of evidence contrary to the belief" (Oltmanns 1988, p. 5). - What does "firm" mean? What is an "unresponsive" behavior (deluded patients do respond quite well to most of the questions we will ask them)? The second criterion reads as follows: "The belief is not shared by others" (Oltmanns 1988, p. 5). But as there is a "folie à deux" and even a "folie à douze", this criterion does not apply to all cases of delusions.

Faust and Miner in their account on the problematic scientific status of DSM-III provide another example: "...Many [psychiatrists] would claim that it is on a more specific level - in the criteria used to define the mental disorders - that the objectivity lies. It is easy to demonstrate that this is not so, no matter how 'specific' or reductionistic one attempts to be. Take the specific face of 'aggressive conduct.' Aggression is among the central elements that make up one of the diagnostic criteria for a number of disorders, e.g., intermittent explosive disorder and conduct disorder, socialized, aggressive. Identification of aggressive acts may seem simple but even direct observation does not remove complexities. For example, a psychologist, observing and coding the behavior of 5-year-olds, sees one child strike another and puts a check under the category 'aggressive behavior.' Exactly what determined this classification? Was it that the force of the child's blow exceeded a certain level; that the behavior was directed, successfully, toward another child; that there were indications, marked by accompanying verbal statements, that the act was intentional; or that other nonverbal indicators were exhibited? Obviously, 'aggressive behavior' is multidimensional, and one must consider not only which dimensions are relevant and how the dimensions are to be measured but also the context in which the behavior occurs" (Faust and Miner 1986, p. 963).

The examples clearly show that criteria are not the *deus ex machina* which they often are thought to be with regard to the problem of the adequate description of a mental disorder. Oltmanns (1988, p. 5) comments his list of seven criteria as follows: "It is not reasonable to assume, however, that all of these features are equally important... It should be noted that some of these characteristics may not be unique to delusional beliefs." As it is well known that the diagnostic criteria of the various mental disorders, as presented in the DSM-III and DSM-III-R, are not specific to any mental disorder, and as we now learn that the sub-criteria (defining a certain single criterion) are not criterion-specific as well, it seems, thus, that the more specific the description of a mental disorder tries to be (e.g. the more it goes down from the "disease" to the level of its criteria and to the level of criteria of the criteria), the more unspecific the description turns out to be.

The problem can even be extended in an even more general way: whenever one uses words for describing an object or event (or more complex things such as behavior and verbal behavior), one can ask for criteria that should be applied or fulfilledwhen using a certain descriptive term. But this *also* can be done with any criterion that is given in such a process. One might argue that there has to be an end which consists in statements that are so basic, that the question of further criteria does not arise. However, *this is just not the case*. As can be seen by the sub-criteria of Oltmanns, going down the line from criteria to sub-criteria to sub-sub-criteria might lead to more and more complex (and not simple!) issues.

The easiest way to show that the idea of criteria as being operational definitions is misleading, is to go back to the clinical practise: While sitting in front of a depressed patient who states that he has lost almost all his money, and trying to find out whether the statement is a delusion or not, one does not apply operational definitions. The point here is: Even if there was a - presumably very long - list of operational definitions by which our conclusions might be reconstructed correctly, we simply do not arrive at a conclusion that way.

One might still argue that, whether psychiatry is really done that way or not, the possibility of its empiricist respectively operationalistic reconstruction guarantees, at least in principle, its scientific status. But the empiricist approach, as a matter of fact, even proves to be - in principle, i.e. regardless of any practical difficulties - an impossible way of reconstructing psychiatric reasoning.

3.2 Basic Statements

The problem of pure description not only arises in the field of scientific explanation but also in the field of the evaluation of scientific theories: A theory is true if it corresponds to reality, false if it contradicts reality. Having accepted this seemingly simple ground of scientific reasoning, the question arises, how theory and reality can be brought together. A theory can be conceptualized as a system of sentences. Sentences, however, only can be consistent with, or contradicting to, other sentences. It is not possible to say, that a sentence contradicts an object or an event. Therefore the need of a link between theory on the one hand and reality on the other hand starts up.

For this reason empiristic philosophers conceptualized *observational statements* (*Beobachtungssätze*; M. SCHLICK) respectively *record statements* (*Protokollsätze*; O. NEURATH). These statements should serve as theory-free descriptions of reality in order to provide the possibility of a matching process between reality, represented by these statements, and theory. By virtue of this process theories ought to be evaluated.

This attempt to solve the old problem of any *correspondence theory of truth* is not as simple and unproblematic as it seems to be: in speaking of observational statements or record statements one speaks of *statements*, i.e. of language which never is free of theory. Additionally there is the imponderable necessity of a being who observes or records which leads to even more "impurities" of the seemingly pure description. To conclude: as there is no theory-free language, there are also no observational or record statements that are free of any theory. Therefore there is no possibility of comparing theories with "reality" that has been put into words, i.e. described in theory-free statements. Therefore, the question of truth with regard to scientific theories is still open.

Interestingly, POPPER's concept of *basic statements (Basissätze)* is often mentioned in this field of argumentation (cf. HEIMANN 1972, 1979; MÖLLER 1976). However, the concept of basic sentences is useless in the field of psychiatry, as can be shown easily: as we have seen, observational or recording statements had, according to their "inventors" SCHLICK and NEURATH the function, to represent reality. POPPER, on the contrary, does not conceptualize basic sentences with regard to the question of observation or recording. In his attempt to reconstruct the process of scientific progress he does not start with reality (proceeding to the question of how it can be linked with theory) but rather he starts with theories (proceeding to the problem of how theories are then called right or wrong). Thus, his problem is not, how reality can take the form of sentences, but - on the contrary - of what kind sentences have to be in order to be able to falsify a theory. This, however, is a different question and the problem of theory-free description of reality is not POPPER's problem and especially not a problem basic statements are intended to solve. Furthermore, POPPER sees no problem in replacing "observable event" by "an event involving position and movement of macroscopic physical bodies": "... every basic statement must either be itself a statement about relative positions of physical bodies, or [that] it must be eqivalent to some basic statement of this 'mechanistic' or 'materialistic' kind" (POPPER 1968, p. 103). POPPERS basic statements are presumably suitable for the reconstruction of the process of the growth of knowledge in physical sciences. The psychiatrist, however, neither deals with spatial relations between bodies nor can his statements be reduced to statements of the respective content.

With regard to the DSM-III, FAUST and MINER (1986) are perfectly right when they say "that the methodological doctrine underlying DSM-III - strict empiricism - has not been achieved, cannot be achieved, and should not be pursued, at least in its extreme form" (FAUST and MINER 1986, p. 962). They argue, that the DSM-III rests on Baconian ideals of empiricism thus relying on the possibility of pure description. But as there are no purely descriptive observational resp. record statements, as "there are no such things as objective or irrefutable facts" (FAUST and MINER 1986, p. 964) and since "there is no such thing as pure data" (HARRE 1972, cited in FAUST and MINER 1986, p. 964), Baconian empiricism is a misconception of science.

As FAUST and MINER point out with regard to the emphasis of DSM-III on reliability, that it is misleading to strive for better measurement only regardless of the problem of understanding what one is measuring. "In the long run, there is little to be gained by attempting to measure purely understood things precisely" the authors (FAUST and MINER 1986, p. 966) state adding that KUHN has shown that scientific progress in physics did not occur on grounds of refinements of measurement.

4. Conclusion

The impossibility of pure description brings with it a corollary, that might be even more important: *If everything that we have so far regarded as "pure" data is a result of certain steps of interpretation, these steps should be the subject of thorough reasoning*. The question, why we interpret the patient's utterances in a certain way and not in another way, rarely is a subject of reflection, as can be shown.[16] We might, therefore, gain insight in a variety of symptoms in applying adequate theories to what the patient tells us. We agree with FAUST and MINER, that "minimizing inference may be superficially attractive but really has very little to offer as a systematic goal, even on the basic observational level. Observation without inference is impossible, and there is nothing minimal about the inferences characterizing much of basic observation in the paragon of science - physics. Hydrogene atoms were inferred from complex patterns of scintillations on zinc-

16 See the contribution of SPITZER on Ich-Störungen, this volume.

sulfide screens. Inferences regarding subatomic particles are even more complex and abstract. Are physicists performing bad science?" (Faust and Miner 1986, p. 966).

If minimal inference is not an aim, the control of inference surely is one. What does that mean? - In speaking of a patients hallucinations we apply a certain theory of perception, and in speaking of his disturbed thought we as well apply a theory of thought. It might be that the "theory behind" natural language is the best theory to be applied but that should be a subject of empirical study. As natural languages and the meaning and connotation of terms change - yesterday *the mind* was thought of as a mirror and a lamp, then as a steam engine, today more as a personal computer, and tomorrow it might be concevied as a chaotic interactive network - there must be a continuous process of criticism of what we mean by the basic terms we use to describe (disturbed) mental phenomena. Terms make sense only within a framework of a theory, and thus the psychopathologist has to reflect his theories. With respect to perception, thought, and the experiencing I - the themes of the following contributions -, philosophy has much to offer for anybody who thoroughly wants to know the theoretical horizon of these terms. There is no reason for "philosophobia" (Wallace 1988) or a "nonphilosophical or even antiphilosophical" attitude (Kroll 1986) among psychiatrists; rather any attempt of psychopathology to win better descriptions and a better understanding of (disturbed) perception, thought, and the experiencing I cannot help including philosophical reasoning about theories in order to get better ones.

Summary: Two of the most outstanding attempts to clarify psychiatric concepts and reasoning are reviewed; the "phenomenology" of Karl Jaspers as well as the "descriptive approach" of the DSM-III are thought to be a remedy against false, meaningless or vague theories in the field of psychopathology, because both emphasize pure description. It is shown, however, that the solution to the problem of bad theories is not to abolish theories at all (this is shown to be misunderstood or exaggerated empiricism), as one needs to have theories in order to have a language and to use it for description. So any attempt to get better descriptions and a better understanding of (disturbed) *perception, thought,* and *the experiencing I* can only consist in reflections on the theories we have and use, i.e.: in philosophical reasoning.

Psychiatrie, Philosophie und das Problem der Beschreibung

Zusammenfassung: Zwei der bemerkenswertesten Versuche der Kärung psychiatrischer Begrifflichkeit bzw. psychiatrischen Denkens werden untersucht: Sowohl die "Phänomenologie" im Sinne von Karl Jaspers als auch der "deskriptive Ansatz" des DSM-III sind jeweils gedacht als Mittel gegenüber falschen, bedeutungslosen oder unklaren psychopathologischen Theorien, da bei beiden die Betonung auf reiner Beschreibung liegt. Wie gezeigt wird, kann die Lösung des Problems schlechter Theorien jedoch nicht in der Abschaffung von Theorien überhaupt liegen (dieser Versuch erweist sich als falsch verstandene, übertriebene Empirie), da jede zum Zweck der Beschreibung notwendige Sprache (irgend-)eine Theorie voraussetzt. Daher muß jeder Versuch einer besseren Beschreibung, bzw. eines besseren Verstehens von *Wahrnehmung, Denken* bzw. des *erfahrenden Ich* Überlegungen mit einbeziehen, die sich auf die Theorien richten, die wir verwenden und in uns herumtragen. Solche Überlegungen aber leistet philosophisches Denken.

References

Appelbaum, P.S. (1988): The right to refuse treatment with antipsychotic medications: retrospect and prospect. Am. J. Psychiatry **145**, pp. 413-419.

Benedek, I. (1982): Freedom and Schizophrenia. Metamedicine **3**, pp. 337-341.

Binswanger, L. (1947): Ausgewählte Vorträge und Aufsätze I. Francke, Bern.

Binswanger, L. (1955): Ausgewählte Vorträge und Aufsätze II. Francke, Bern.

Blankenburg, W. (1979): Psychiatrie und Philosophie. In: Psychiatrie der Gegenwart, Bd. I/1, pp. 827-875.

Broekman, J.M. (1965): Phänomenologisches Denken in Philosophie und Psychiatrie. Confin. psychiat. **8**, pp. 165-187.

Bumke, O. (1914; 1973): Allgemeine Psychopathologie. In: Saner, H. (ed.): Karl Jaspers in der Diskussion, pp. 11-13. Piper, München.

Castañeda, H.-N. (1988): Persons Egos and I's: Their Sameness Relations (this volume).

Chessick, R.D. (1986): Heidegger for Psychotherapists. American Journal of Psychotherapy **40**, pp. 83-95.

Clouser, K.D., Gert, B. (1986): Rationality and Medicine: Introduction to the theme. The Journal of Medicine and Philosophy **11**, pp. 119-121.

Diemer, A. (1966): Zur Grundlegung einer Philosophie der Medizin. Festvortrag anläßlich des 37. Fortbildungskurses für Ärzte in Regensburg am 13. Oktober 1966.

Eccles, J.C. (1981): The Self-Conscious Mind and the Brain. In: Popper, K.R., Eccles, J.C.: The Self and Its Brain, pp. 355-376. Springer International, Berlin, Heidelberg, London, New York.

Edel, A. (1974): Psychiatry and Philosophy. In: Arieti, S.: American Handbook of Psychiatry, 2nd Ed., Vol. 1, pp. 961-975, Basic Books, New York.

Edwards, R.B. (1981): Mental Health as Rational Autonomy. The Journal of Medicine and Philosophy **6**, pp. 309-322.

Edwards, R.B. (1983): A response to "on being 'mentally healthy'". The Journal of Medicine and Philosophy **8**, pp. 199-201.

Emrich, H.M. (1988): Die Beziehung zwischen Philosophie und Psychiatrie, vom Standpunkt einer systemtheoretischen Konzeption produktiver Psychosen aus betrachtet. (this volume).

Engelhardt, H.T. jr (1986): From Philosophy and Medicine to Philosophy of Medicine. The Journal of Medicine and Philosophy **11**, pp. 3-8.

Faust, D., Miner, R.A. (1986): The empiricist and his new clothes: DSM-III in perspective. Am. J. Psychiatry **143**, pp. 962-967.

Gadamer, H.-G. (1975): Wahrheit und Methode. Mohr, Tübingen.

Gatens-Robinson, E. (1986): Clinical judgment and the rationality of the human sciences. The Journal of Medicine and Philosophy **11**, pp. 167-178.

George, M.S. (1987): Neuroscience and Psychiatry. Am. J. Psychiatry **144**, p. 1103.

Gert, B., Clouser, K.D. (1986): Rationality in medicine: an explication. The Journal of Medicine and Philosophy **11**, pp. 185-205.

Gregory, R.L. (1987): Sensation. In: Gregory, R.L. (ed.): The Oxford Companion to the Mind, pp. 700-701. Oxford University Press, Oxford, New York.

Grünbaum, A. (1984): The Foundations of Psychoanalysis. A Philosophical Critique. University of California Press, Berkeley, Los Angeles, London.

HANLY, C. (1985): Logical and Conceptual Problems of Existential Psychiatry. The Journal od Nervous and Mental Disease **173**, pp. 263-275.

HEIDEGGER, M. (1987): Zollikoner Seminare (ed. by M. Boss). Klostermann, Frankfurt a.M.

HEIMANN, H. (1972): Grundsätzliche Überlegungen zur Erfahrungswissenschaftlichen Methodik in der Psychiatrie. Nervenarzt **43**, pp. 345-350.

HEIMANN, H. (1979): Psychopathologie. In: Psychiatrie der Gegenwart, Bd. I, 2nd ed., pp. 1-42.

HÖNIGSWALD, R. (1929): Philosophie und Psychiatrie. Eine kritische Untersuchung. Archiv für Psychiatrie **87**, pp. 715-741.

HOFSTADTER, D.R. (1980): Gödel, Escher, Bach: an Eternal Golden Braid. Vintage, New York.

HOPPE, A. (1919): Zur logischen Grundlegung der Psychopathologie. Zeitschrift für Neurologie und Psychiatrie **51**, pp. 376-424.

HUSSERL, E. (1893-1917; 1966): Zur Phänomenologie des inneren Zeitbewußtseins. Husserliana, Bd. X, Nijhoff, Haag.

HUSSERL, E. (1913; 1976): Ideen zu einer reinen Phänomenologie und phänomenologischen Philosophie. Erstes Buch: Allgemeine Einführung in die reine Phänomenologie. Husserliana, Bd. III, 1, Nijhoff, Haag.

JASPERS, K. (1911; 1963): Zur Analyse der Trugwahrnehmungen. In: Gesammelte Schriften zur Psychopathologie, pp. 191-251. Springer, Berlin, Göttingen, Heidelberg.

JASPERS, K. (1911; 1963): Die Trugwahrnehmungen. In: Gesammelte Schriften zur Psychopathologie, pp. 252-313. Springer, Berlin, Göttingen, Heidelberg.

JASPERS, K. (1912; 1963): Die phänomenologische Forschungsrichtung in der Psychopathologie. In: Gesammelte Schriften zur Psychopathologie, pp. 314-328. Springer, Berlin, Göttingen, Heidelberg.

JASPERS, K. (1913; 1973): Allgemeine Psychopathologie, 9th ed. Springer, Berlin, Heidelberg, New York.

KAULBACH, F. (1968): Philosophie der Beschreibung. Köln, Graz.

KLERMAN, G.L. (1987): Future Prospects for Clinical Psychopharmacology. In: MELTZER, H.Y. (ed.): Psychopharmacology. The Third Generation of Progress, pp. 1699-1705. Raven Press, New York.

KOEHLER, K. (1984): Gibt es noch eine Seele? Thomas von Aquin und die moderne Psychiatrie. Fortschr. Neurol. Psychiat. **52**, pp. 329-337.

KROLL, J. (1979): Philosophical foundations of french and U.S. nosology. Am. J. Psychiatry **136**, pp. 1135-1138.

KUNZ, H. (1947; 1973): Allgemeine Psychopathologie. In: SANER, H. (ed.): Karl Jaspers in der Diskussion, pp. 17-20. Piper, München.

LAING, R.D. (1960): The devided Self. An Existential Study in Sanity and Madness. Tavistock, London.

LAOR, N. (1984): Common Sense Ethics and Psychiatry. Psychiatry **47**, pp. 135-150

LAUDAN, L. (ed. 1983): Mind and Medicine. Problems of Explanation and Evaluation in Psychiatry and the Biomedical Sciences. University of California Press, Berkeley, Los Angeles, London.

MARTIN, M. (1986): Defining irrational action in medical and psychiatric contexts. The Journal of Medicine and Philosophy **11**, pp. 179-184.

MAYO, D.J. (1986): The concept of rational suicide. The Journal of Medicine and Philosophy **11**, pp. 143-155.

MITTEL, N.S. (1968): The philosophy of Alfred North Whitehead: its relevance for psychiatric theory. Psychiatric Quaterly **42**, pp. 321-330.

MÖLLER, H.-J. (1976): Methodische Grundprobleme der Psychiatrie. Kohlhammer, Stuttgart, Berlin, Köln, Mainz.

NATANSON, M. (1963): Philosophische Grundfragen der Psychiatrie I, Philosophie und Psychiatrie. In: Psychiatrie der Gegenwert, Bd. I/2.

NETTLER, G. (1983): On being "mentally healthy". The Journal of Medicine and Philosophy **8**, pp. 197-198.

OLTMANNS, T.F. (1988): Approaches to the Definition and Study of Delusions. In: OLTMANNS, T.F., MAHER, B.A. (eds.): Delusional Beliefs, pp. 3-11. Wiley, New York, Chichester, Brisbane, Toronto, Singapore.

PARDES, H. (1986): Neuroscience and psychiatry: marriage or coexistence? Am. J. Psychiatry **143**, pp. 1205-1212.

PELLEGRINO, E.D. (1986): Philosophy of Medicine: Towards a Definition. The Journal of Medicine and Philosophy **11**, pp. 9-16.

PELLEGRINO, E.D., SPICKER, S.F. (1984): "Back to the origins": Erwin Straus - philosopher of medicine, philosopher in medicine. The Journal of Medicine and Philosophy **9**, pp. 3-5.

REISER, M.F. (1988): Are psychiatric educators "losing the mind"? Am. J. Psychiatry **145**, pp. 148-153.

RICOEUR, P. (1974): Psychiatry and Moral Values. In: ARIETI, S.: American Handbook of Psychiatry, 2nd Ed., Vol. 1, pp. 976-990, Basic Books, New York.

SCHMITT, W. (1979): Karl Jaspers und die Methodenfrage in der Psychiatrie. In: JANZARIK, W. (ed.): Psychopathologie als Grundlagenwissenschaft, pp. 74-82, Enke, Stuttgart.

SCHMITT, W. (1983): Die Psychopathologie von Karl Jaspers in der modernen Psychiatrie. In: PETERS, U.H. (ed.): Psychiatrie, Bd. 1, pp. 36-52, Beltz, Weinheim.

SCHNEIDER, K. (1938; 1973): 25 Jahre 'Allgemeine Psychopathologie' von Karl Jaspers. In: SANER, H. (ed.): Karl Jaspers in der Diskussion, pp. 13-16. Piper, München.

SCHRÖDINGER, E. (1959): Geist und Materie. Viehweg, Braunschweig.

SCHWARTZ, M.A., WIGGINS, O.P. (1986): Logical Empiricism and psychiatric classification. Comprehensive Psychiatry **27**, pp. 101-114.

SHELP, E.E. (ed., 1983): Values and Medicine. Theoretical Medicine 4, pp. 5-111.

SHOTTER, J. (1975): Images of Man in Psychological Research. Methuen, London.

SPICKER, S.F. (1986): Cognitive and conative issues in contemporary philosophy of medicine. The Journal of Medicine and Philosophy **11**, pp. 107-117.

SPITZER, M. (1985): Allgemeine Subjektivität und Psychopathologie. Haag & Herchen, Frankfurt a.M.

SPITZER, M. (1986): Erfahrung - Aspekte einer Begriffserklärung. Nervenarzt **57**, pp. 342-348.

SPITZER, M. (1987): Symptom and Criterion in Medicine and Psychiatry. In: WEINGARTNER, P., SCHURZ, G. (eds.): Logic, Philosophy of Science and Epistemology (Proceedings of the 11th International Wittgenstein-Symposium), pp. 183-185.

SPITZER, M. (1988a): Halluzinationen. Springer, Berlin, Heidelberg, London, Paris, Tokyo.

SPITZER, M. (1988b): Wahrnehmung. Wege und Irrwege in der Bestimmung einer grundlegenden menschlichen Fähigkeit. In: BUSSMANN, C., UEHLEIN, F.A. (eds.): Pommersfeldener Beiträge, Bd. 5, pp. 179-217, Haag & Herchen, Frankfurt a.M.

SPITZER, M. (1988c): Ichstörungen: In Search for a Theory. (this volume).

SPITZER, M., DEGKWITZ, R. (1986): Zur Diagnose des DSM-III. Nervenarzt **57**, pp. 698-704.

STRANSKY, E. (1923): Psychiatrie und Philosophie. Eine Entgegnung auf Hildebrandts Vortrag "Medizin und Philosophie". Monatsschrift für Psychiatrie und Neurologie **53**, pp. 251-262.

STRAUS, E.W. (1963): Philosophische Grundfragen der Psychiatrie II. Psychiatrie und Philosophie. In: Psychiatrie der Gegenwart, Bd. I/2, pp. 926-994.

STRAWSON, P.F. (1959; 1984): Individuals. An Essay in Descriptive Metaphysics. Methuen, London, New York.

STRAWSON, P.F. (1966; 1974; 1980): Self, Mind and Body. In: STRAWSON, P.F.: Freedom and Resentment (and other essays). Methuen, London, New York.

SZASZ, T.S. (1970): The Manufacture of Madness. Harper and Row, New York.

SZASZ, T.S. (1982): On the Legitimacy of Psychiatric Power. Metamedicine **3**, pp. 315-324.

THOMASMA, D.C. (1986): Philosophical reflections on a rational treatment plan. The Journal of Medicine and Philosophy **11**, pp. 157-165.

TUCKER, G.J., MAXMEN, J.S. (1986): "Rational" hospital psychiatry. The Journal of Medicine and Philosophy **11**, pp. 135-141.

WALLACE E.R. (1988): What is "Truth"? Some philosophical contributions to psychiatric issues. Am. J. Psychiatry **145**, pp. 137-147.

WEIZSÄCKER V., V., WYSS, D. (1957): Zwischen Medizin und Philosophie. Vandenhoeck und Ruprecht, Göttingen.

WIELAND, W. (1975): Diagnose. Überlegungen zur Medizintheorie. de Gruyter, Berlin, New York.

Part One

Disturbances of Perception and Formal Thought

Affekte als Wahrnehmungs- und Denkstörungen

R. Wiehl

1. Logik, Ethik und Psychologie als mögliche Örter für die Erörterung des Themas

Die folgenden Überlegungen zum Thema "Affekte als Wahrnehmungs- und Denkstörungen" gehen von der Voraussetzung aus, daß es sich hier um ein philosophisches Thema, zumindest auch um ein solches Thema handelt. Deswegen drängt sich zunächst die Frage auf: Inwiefern ist dies ein philosophisches Thema? Ist es überhaupt ein philosophisches Thema? Liegt es nicht näher, hier überhaupt nur den möglichen Gegenstand einer Untersuchung der Psychologie und der Psychiatrie zu sehen? Nun kann man, wo immer ein Thema für eine empirische Wissenschaft vorliegt, darin auch etwas Philosophisches entdecken, und dies umso eher, wenn die entsprechende Wissenschaft direkt mit Fragen des menschlichen Daseins zu tun hat. Emotionalität und Rationalität sind zweifellos ursprüngliche Gegenstände der Philosophie, die die Frage des Menschseins direkt berühren. Und seit es so etwas wie eine philosophische Erkenntnistheorie gibt, hat die Wahrnehmung seit altersher die Rolle eines ausgezeichneten Paradigmas gespielt. Philosophische Theorien der Wahrnehmung gibt es von der Antike bis in die Moderne, von PLATO bis HUSSERL; und jedesmal war diese philosophische Wahrnehmungstheorie niemals nur Selbstzweck. Sie war ein Paradigma, an dem sich entschied, ob und wie menschliche Wahrheitserkenntnis überhaupt möglich ist. Wenn man demnach davon ausgeht, daß hier ein *philosophisches* Thema gegeben ist, so ist damit noch nicht gesagt, in welchem Sinne wir hier von einem Thema der *Philosophie* reden können und wollen. Die empirischen Wissenschaften erwarten heute im allgemeinen von der Philosophie, soweit sie diese nicht überhaupt für überflüssig halten, allenfalls die Dienstleistung eines kritischen Beitrages zur Begriffsbildung und zur Methodologie, so wie ehemals im Mittelalter die Theologie glaubte, die Philosophie in ihre Dienste nehmen zu sollen. Eine solche Aufgabe einer Dienstleistung liegt dort umso näher, wo die Philosophie wie heute so oft, darauf verzichtet, den Spieß umzukehren und ihrerseits die ihr wichtigen Wissenschaften in den Dienst zu nehmen. Wie immer die Frage nach dem Verhältnis von Philosophie und Psychologie, bzw. Psychiatrie von den jeweils Betroffenen beurteilt werden wird - vorausgesetzt es handelt sich hier um ein Thema der Philosophie - stellt sich die Frage, wo und wie dieses ein Thema der Philosophie ist. Die Frage nach dem Wo, nach dem systematischen Ort des Themas stellt sich, sofern die Philosophie heute immer in mannigfache Teildisziplinen und Richtungen zersplittert ist, die Frage nach dem Wie, sofern vor aller Entscheidung über eine mögliche philosophische Methode der Frage nach dem Zugang zum Thema eine wichtige Rolle bei der angemessenen Erörterung zukommt. Ich möchte auf diese Fragen zunächst zwei mögliche Antworten zu geben versuchen, die sich an zwei maßgeblichen philosophischen Positionen der Neuzeit orientieren, die durch ihre Gegensätzlichkeit zumindest eine Klärung des Bereiches möglicher Antworten erwarten lassen. Ich meine die philosophischen Theorien von SPINOZA und KANT. Den Antworten, die wir diesen Theorien entnehmen können, kommt insofern paradigmatische Bedeutung zu, als diese Theorien beispielhaft gegensätzliche Positionen der neuzeitlichen Philosophie repräsentieren, nämlich die Position der Metaphysik einerseits und die der Transzendentalphilosophie andererseits. Was bedeutet es demnach, eine Antwort auf die Frage nach dem Wo und Wie unseres Themas einmal von der Metaphysik und zum anderen von der Transzendentalphilosophie zu erwarten?

KANTS Transzendentalphilosophie stellt bekanntlich eine kritische Antwort auf die Probleme der Metaphysik seiner Zeit dar. Ob diese Antwort es rechtfertigt, jene kritisierte Metaphysik damit als überwunden anzusehen oder ob diese Metaphysik ihrerseits ein Begriffspotential gegenüber der Transzendentalphilosophie bereithält - diese Frage ist hier nur im Blick auf das Thema "Affekte als Wahrnehmungs- und Denkstörungen" relevant. KANTS Antwort auf die Frage nach dem Wo und Wie der Erörterung dieses Themas läßt sich der "Transzendentalen Methodenlehre" in seiner *Kritik der reinen Vernunft* entnehmen. Danach gliedert sich die Philosophie als solche zunächst und vor allem in zwei Teile: in eine reine und in eine empirische Philosophie. Offenkundig gehört unser fragliches Thema in den Bereich der empirischen Philosophie, und zwar, sofern sowohl die Affekte wie auch die Wahrnehmungs- und Denkstörungen empirisch gegeben und insofern Gegenstände einer empirischen Erkenntnis sind. Fragen wir nun aber weiter, wo nun innerhalb einer empirischen Philosophie und auf welche Weise das genannte Thema dort abgehandelt werden soll, so hört bereits die Eindeutigkeit der Antwort auf. Denn folgt man KANTS Einteilung der empirischen Philosophie, so wird man zu dem Ergebnis kommen, daß es sich bei dem Thema "Affekte als Wahrnehmungs- und Denkstörungen" überhaupt nicht um ein einheitliches Thema handelt, daß in demselben vielmehr verschiedenartige philosophische Fragen zur Erörterung stehen, die dementsprechend an verschiedenen philosophischen Örtern innerhalb der empirischen Philosophie zu erörtern sind. Diese verschiedenen Örter sind: die angewandte allgemeine, bzw. nicht empirisch allgemeine Logik, die angewandte, bzw. empirische Moral und schließlich die empirisch allgemeine Psychologie, bzw. Anthropologie. Was die erste dieser drei Disziplinen betrifft, die allgemeine angewandte Logik, so hat KANT den Anspruch erhoben, für dieselbe einen neuen Begriff aufgestellt zu haben. Anders als die reine allgemeine Logik, die von allen empirischen Bedingungen eines möglichen Verstandesgebrauches abstrahiert, hat die angewandte allgemeine Logik mit "den Regeln des Verstandesgebrauches unter den subjektiven empirischen Bedingungen zu tun, die uns die Psychologie lehrt". Und sie handelt "von der Aufmerksamkeit, von deren Hindernis und Folgen, dem Ursprunge des Irrtums, dem Zustand des Zweifels, des Skrupels, der Überzeugung..." (KANT, KdrV, A 54, B 79). Offensichtlich bilden Wahrnehmungs- und Denkstörungen den Gegenstand einer solchen angewandten Logik, sofern es sich bei diesen Störungen um Modi des Irrtums handelt und sofern unter den verschiedenen möglichen Quellen dieser Art von Irrtümern den Affekten eine wichtige Rolle zukommt. Aber ebenso gehört die genannte Thematik in den Bereich der angewandten allgemeinen Moral, bzw. der allgemeinen Tugendlehre. Diese enthält, KANTS Begriff zufolge, im Unterschied zur reinen Moral nicht nur "die notwendigen sittlichen Gesetze eines freien Willens überhaupt", sondern sie hat es zu tun mit diesen Gesetzen "unter den Hindernissen der Gefühle, Neigungen und Leidenschaften, denen die Menschen mehr oder weniger unterworfen sind..." (KANT, KdrV, A 55, B 79). Affekte als Wahrnehmungs- und Denkstörungen - dies ist für eine solche angewandte Moral ein zentrales Thema, sofern die Affekte als Hindernisse einer wahren Erkenntnis des Guten und der sittlichen Gesetze des freien Willens gelten, einer Erkenntnis, die wie jegliche Erkenntnis auf Wahrnehmungen und Gedanken beruht.

Schließlich aber gehört unser Thema, folgt man KANTS transzendentaler Begriffseinteilung der Philosophie, speziell der empirischen Philosophie, in den Bereich der empirischen Psychologie, bzw. der Anthropologie. Auch in diesem Bereich hat KANTS "Revolution der Denkungsart" nachhaltig gewirkt. Denn die Unterscheidung zwischen einer reinen Erkenntnis a priori und einer empirischen Erfahrungserkenntnis in Philosophie und Wissenschaft veranlaßte ihn, die empirische Psychologie, die bis dahin zur Metaphysik gehört hatte, aus dieser reinen Philosophie auszugliedern und dem empirischen Teil derselben zuzuschlagen. Dabei sah KANT aber mit aller Deutlichkeit, daß diese empirische Psychologie seiner Zeit "noch nicht so reich" war, um allein ein Studium auszumachen, so daß man ihr eine Weile noch "aus ökonomischen Bewegursachen" ein "Plätzchen in der Philosophie verstatten" müsse (KANT, KdrV, A 848-849, B 876-877). Aber anders als für die angewandte Logik und für die angewandte Moral sah KANT hier schon für die empirische Psychologie die zukünftige Verselbständigung gegenüber der Philosophie voraus. Wie aber würde eine solche 'rein' empirische Wissenschaft mit dem Thema "Affekte als Wahrnehmungs- und Denkstörungen" umgehen? KANTS transzendentale Begriffseinteilung der gesamten Philosophie in einen reinen und einen empirischen Teil antizipiert grundsätzlich im philosophischen Begriffe die Verselbständigung der empirischen Wissenschaften gegenüber der Philosophie, auch wenn er bei dieser Antizipation noch an dem Genos einer empirischen Philosophie festgehalten hat und auch wenn seine Nachfolger, vor allem HEGEL, bemüht waren, die allgemeinen theoretischen Gehalte der zunehmend autonomen empirischen Wissenschaften für die Philosophie zu retten. Die andere Seite der begrifflichen Antizipation einer autonomen empirischen Wissenschaft war die durchgängige Formalisierung der gesamten 'reinen' Philosophie und ihrer Erkenntnis. Auch wenn KANT demnach das unbestreitbare Verdienst zukommt, das moderne und bis heute weithin herrschende Verhältnis von Philosophie und Wissenschaft antizipiert zu haben, so enthält diese Antizipation für eine Erörterung der Affekte als Wahrnehmungs- und Denkstörungen eine Reihe von Schönheitsfehlern. Ein solcher Schönheitsfehler liegt in der resultierenden Zweideutigkeit des Begriffes von Empirie. Eine empirische Wissenschaft wird als Teil einer empirischen Philosophie nicht unbedingt in der gleichen Weise empirisch sein wie als verselbständigte empirische Wissenschaft und Forschung. Ein zweiter Schönheitsfehler ist darin zu sehen, daß die Bereiche der angewandten Logik und der angewandten Moral nicht so eindeutig voneinander getrennt werden können, um mit Bestimmtheit die jeweilige Zuständigkeit der einen und der anderen empirischen Philosophie für die Erörterung der Affekte als Wahrnehmungs- und Denkstörungen festzulegen. KANT hat weder von der angewandten Logik noch von der angewandten Moral eine hinreichend systematische Darstellung gegeben, die uns über ein reiches Datenmaterial hinaus eine Antwort auf die Frage nach dem Wie der Erörterung unseres Themas zu geben vermöchte. Schließlich haben KANTS transzendentale Begriffseinteilungen für die Frage nach den Bedingungen einer bestimmten philosophischen Erörterung unseres Themas noch eine weitere Schwierigkeit mit sich gebracht. Denn indem der Begründer der Transzendentalphilosophie die empirische Psychologie aus den Fesseln der traditionellen Metaphysik befreit und diese empirische Disziplin in eine Anthropologie auf transzendentalphilosophischer Grundlage überführt hat, hat er zugleich Raum für eine neue Unterscheidung geschaffen, nämlich für die Unterscheidung zwischen einer physiologischen und einer pragmatischen Anthropologie.

Das Kriterium für die Unterscheidung zwischen diesen beiden Anthropologien hat KANT zugleich mitgeliefert. Die physiologische Anthropologie "geht auf die Erforschung dessen, was die Natur aus dem Menschen macht, die pragmatische auf das, was er aus freihandelndes Wesen aus sich selber macht oder machen kann und soll" (KANT, Anthropologie, S. 119). Auch diese Unterscheidung kann durchaus als wegweisend für die Entwicklung der verschiedenen Wissenschaften vom Menschen gelten. Aber sie bringt für die Erörterung des Themas von den Affekten als Wahrnehmungs- und Denkstörungen das Mißliche mit sich, daß sie die Vielzahl der Örter für eine solche Erörterung um einen weiteren solchen Ort bereichert. Dabei kommt erschwerend hinzu, daß jenes aufgeführte Unterscheidungskriterium, ungeachtet der leichten Faßlichkeit seiner Formulierung, sich in seinem konkreten Gebrauch als nicht besonders funktionstüchtig erweist, um die beiden verschiedenen Örter in ihrer wechselseitigen Lage klar gegeneinander abzugrenzen. So wollte KANT etwa die Theorie der dunklen, bzw. der unbewußten Vorstellungen in der physiologischen Anthropologie lokalisiert sehen und dies im Einklang mit der Einsicht, daß das Feld dieser Vorstellungen "unermeßlich sei" und daß uns dies "Bewunderung über unser eigenes Wesen einflößen" kann, zu sehen, daß "gleichsam auf der großen Karte unseres Gemütes nur wenig Stellen illuminiert sind" (KANT, Anthropologie, S. 135). Andererseits finden in der pragmatischen Anthropologie eine Reihe von Störungen und Krankheiten des Gemütes ausführliche Erwähnung, ungeachtet dessen, daß diese durch den freien Willen des Menschen kaum beeinflußt werden können.[1] Alle diese Schwierigkeiten, die mit der Vielzahl der Örter und der mannigfachen Überlagerung derselben für die Erörterung unseres Themas gegeben sind, sprechen nun umso nachdrücklicher für jene andere philosophische Theorie, nämlich für die Metaphysik des SPINOZA. Hier ist der Ort des Themas eindeutig bestimmt. Denn diese Metaphysik beansprucht schon allein durch ihren Titel nichts anderes zu sein als eine philosophische Ethik. Hier geht es um die grundlegende Frage nach dem Sein und Wesen des höchsten Gutes (summum bonum), um die Frage, wie der Mensch in seinem Streben dieses Gutes teilhaftig werden könne, welche Schwierigkeiten und Hindernisse einer solchen Partizipation im Wege stehen und auf welche Weise diese Schwierigkeiten und Hemmnisse überwunden werden können.[2] Dieser Vorzug einer klaren und eindeutigen Ortsbestimmung geht in jener Metaphysik Hand in Hand mit einem anderen theoretischen Vorteil. SPINOZA hat nicht nur hier und dort und bei dieser oder jener Gelegenheit Bemerkungen über das Thema "Affekte als Wahrnehmungs- und Denkstörungen" gemacht, er hat vielmehr eine ausgearbeitete Theorie des Zusammenhanges zwischen Wahrnehmungen, Affekten und Gedanken vorgelegt, die entsprechende systematische Schlußfolgerungen auf jenes Thema und für seine philosophische Erörterung gestatten.

Diese Schlußfolgerungen lassen sich in einer einzigen Folgerung zusammenfassen: Sofern die Affekte die Wahrnehmungen und Gedanken der Menschen stören, sind sie als ebensoviele Störungen oder Störquellen anzusehen, die den Menschen daran hindern, des höchsten Gutes teilhaftig zu werden; und zwar, sofern eine solche Teilhabe in der wahren Erkenntnis dieses Gutes mittels ungestörter Wahrnehmungen und Gedanken gründet, oder mit einer solchen Wahrheitserkenntnis identisch ist.[3]

Der theoretische Vorteil, den diese eindeutige metaphysische Ortsbestimmung für eine angemessene philosophische Erörterung der Affekte als Wahrnehmungs- und Denkstörungen mit sich bringt, hat nun unvermeidlich einen entsprechenden theoretischen Nachteil, der nun seinerseits wiederum zugunsten einer transzendentalen Erörterung und zugunsten ihrer verschiedenen theoretischen Örter zu argumentieren gestattet. Denn zum einen wird eine philosophische Erkenntnis, wie immer sie es mit der Metaphysik des SPINOZA hält, sich nicht ohne weiteres auf den Geltungsbereich einer mehr oder weniger allgemeinen Moral einschränken lassen wollen, um das übrige Feld des Wissens ganz den einzelnen empirischen Wissenschaften zu überlassen. Und selbst wenn die Philosophie sich auf den Bereich der Ethik beschränken lassen wollte, so könnte

---

1 Vgl. KANTs Unterscheidung der Gemütskrankheiten gegenüber den Gemütsschwächen in der Anthropologie, §§ 50-53 (S. 212-220), insbesondere in § 52 (S. 214): "Es ist schwer, eine systematische Einteilung in das zu bringen, was wesentliche und unheilbare Unordnung ist. Es hat auch wenig Nutzen, sich damit zu befassen: weil, da die Kräfte des Subjects dahin nicht mitwirken (wie es wohl bei körperlichen Krankheiten der Fall ist), und doch nur durch den eigenen Verstandesgebrauch dieser Zweck erreicht werden kann, alle Heilmethode in dieser Absicht fruchtlos ausfallen muß. Indessen fordert doch die Anthropologie, obgleich sie hierbei nur indirect pragmatisch sein kann, nämlich nur Unterlassungen zu gebieten, wenigstens einen allgemeinen Abriß dieser tiefsten, aber von der Natur herrührenden Erniedrigung der Menschheit zu versuchen." KANT teilt diese "Verrückung" in tumultarische, methodische und systematische, bzw. in Unsinnigkeit, Wahnsinn, Wahnwitz und Aberwitz.

2 Vgl. SPINOZA, *Tractatus de Emendatione Intellectus* (insbesondere S. 3-20), der im gewissen Sinne als Einleitung in die Ethik gelesen werden kann.

3 Vgl. hierzu Wiehl 1983.

sie sich nicht damit begnügen, die bestehenden moralischen Normen und Gesetze einfach zu registrieren und in ihrer empirischen Gegebenheit zu katalogisieren. Eine philosophische Ethik enthält immer auch - absichtlich oder unabsichtlich - eine kritische Bewertung der vorgefundenen moralischen Normen und Gesetze im Hinblick auf interne oder externe normative Ideale. Außerdem setzt jedes moralische Wissen, jede mögliche kritische Erörterung moralischer Werte und Normen ein theoretisches Wissen vom Menschen und von seinen durchschnittlichen Verhaltensweisen voraus. Auch in dieser Hinsicht gilt: Die philosophische Erkenntnis wird ein solches theoretisches Wissen, wo immer sein Ursprung liegen mag, nicht ungeprüft als theoretische Grundlage einer möglichen Ethik übernehmen. Sie wird vielmehr prüfen, wieweit ein solches Wissen zur Gewinnung eines menschlichen Grundwissens vom Menschen taugt. Und sie wird bei der Erörterung dieses Grundwissens Sorge tragen, daß dieses nicht unbemerkt von normativen Vorurteilen geleitet ist, die der Möglichkeit einer Ethik überhaupt widerstreiten oder aber die gesuchte Ethik bereits antizipieren. Man wird also bei der Erörterung der Affekte als Wahrnehmungs- und Denkstörungen gut daran tun, die prinzipielle Differenz zwischen Transzendentalphilosophie und Metaphysik nicht zu überfordern und sich darauf zu beschränken, die herangezogenen unterschiedlichen paradigmatischen Theorien lediglich dazu zu verwenden, relevante Begriffs- und Erkenntnisunterscheidungen für die Thematik in Spiel zu bringen. Zu diesen wichtigen theoretischen Unterscheidungen gehört nun auch diese, daß die bestimmte Differenz zwischen einer Vielzahl und einer Einzahl von Örtern keineswegs nur für das Thema als solches relevant ist, sondern für jeden der in diesem Thema thematischen Begriffe seine bestimmte Bedeutung hat. So verlangt KANTS Transzendentalphilosophie, daß Begriffe wie "Affekt" und "Leidenschaft" ihren Ort in der praktischen Philosophie und allenfalls in der Anthropologie zugewiesen erhalten, während Sinneswahrnehmung und empirisches Denken ihren ursprünglichen Ort im Bereich der theoretischen Philosophie haben und allenfalls, wie auch die Affekte und Leidenschaften, noch in der Anthropologie abgehandelt werden können. Ganz anders dagegen in SPINOZAS metaphysischer Ethik. Hier gehören Affekte, Wahrnehmungen und Gedanken in ein- und denselben philosophischen Bereich. Und wenn sie innerhalb dieses Bereiches auch an verschiedenen Orten vorkommen, so nicht deswegen, weil es sich bei ihnen um grundsätzlich unvergleichbare Gegebenheiten handelt, sondern weil in ihrer gesetzmäßigen Verbindung immer auch unterschiedliche Aspekte mitverknüpft werden.

2. Störungen als Störungen der Rationalität menschlicher Erkenntnis

Die Erörterung der Affekte als Wahrnehmungs- und Denkstörungen ist demnach in der einen der beiden exemplarischen Theorien an verschiedene philosophische Bereiche und Örter, in der anderen an einen bestimmten Bereich und nur bedingt an verschiedene Örter innerhalb desselben gebunden. Das bedeutet, daß wir es in einem Fall mit verschiedenen möglichen Themen, im anderen Fall mit einem einzigen Thema zu tun haben. Aber die Vergleichung der beiden exemplarischen philosophischen Theorien hinsichtlich der möglichen

Örter unseres Themas lehrt noch ein weiteres. Keine der beiden Theorien gibt eine Vollständigkeit der Örter und auch beide zusammengenommen nicht. So hat zwar KANTS schroffe Trennung der verschiedenen Örter eine bestimmte philosophisch-bedeutsame Frage nicht prinzipiell ausgeschlossen, nämlich die Frage, auf welche Weise theoretisches Wissen die praktische Einsicht stören, und umgekehrt, wie praktische Einsicht theoretische Erkenntnis behindern könne. Aber sie hat eine Erörterung dieser Fragen auch nicht gerade begünstigt. Von SPIZONAS Ethik läßt sich sagen, daß sie eine solche Frage, zumindest in dieser direkten und unmißverständlichen Form eigentlich überhaupt nicht stellen, geschweige denn beantworten kann; und die Frage, wie die Sinnlichkeit die rationale Erkenntnis im Gebiete der reinen Theorie stören oder beeinträchtigen könne, kann hier allenfalls in erkenntnistheoretischen Präliminarien zur Ethik thematisch werden. Wieweit nun auch immer die Differenzen zwischen KANTS Transzendentalphilosophie und SPINOZAS Ethik hin und her gewendet werden, in einem für die hier behandelte Thematik entscheidenden Punkte stimmen beide Theorien überein, nämlich in ihrem jeweiligen Vorbegriff der Störung. Eine Störung ist hier wie dort gleichbedeutend mit einer Störung der menschlichen Erkenntnis, d.i. entweder einer Störung der Erkenntnis der Wahrheit oder einer Störung der Erkenntnis des Guten oder schließlich einer Störung der Erkenntnis überhaupt oder einer Erkenntnis, die auf das Wahre und Gute gleichermaßen und in einem zugleich ausgerichtet ist. Diese grundsätzliche Gemeinsamkeit hinsichtlich des Begriffes der Störung relativiert die Differenzen zwischen Transzendentalphilosophie und Metaphysik. Sie läßt diese Differenzen als vergleichsweise zweitrangig erscheinen. Man kann sagen: Die Transzendentalphilosophie ergründet die Möglichkeiten der Störungen der menschlichen Erkenntnis durch eine Analyse der immanenten Elemente der Erkenntnis und durch die Bestimmung der Gesetzmäßigkeit der Verbindung dieser Elemente zu einer konstitutiven Erkenntnis des Wahren und Guten. Dagegen untersucht die Metaphysik die Möglichkeiten des menschlichen Verhaltens zu Gott, zu den Dingen der Welt und zu den anderen Menschen unter dem Gesichtspunkt einer Gesetzmäßigkeit der Erkenntnis, die Störungen nicht prinzipiell ausschließt. Aber die Gemeinsamkeit der beiden so heterogenen philosophischen Theorien in Sachen des Begriffes der Störung reicht noch weiter. Beide Theorien sind philosophische Theorien der Vernunft. Beide räumen der Vernünftigkeit, der Rationalität den höchsten Erkenntniswert ein. Beide anerkennen in der Vernunft das Prinzip der Wahrheit, bzw. der Wahrheitserkenntnis. Und wenn für beide Störungen in erster Linie Störungen der menschlichen Erkenntnis sind, so gilt hier wie dort, daß eine wie immer gestörte Erkenntnis das Wesen der Vernunft als Prinzip der Wahrheit nicht aufzuheben vermag.

Daß die Vernunft das unaufhebbare Prinzip der Wahrheit im Hinblick auf ungestörte und gestörte menschliche Erkenntnis ist, bedeutet nun vor allem, daß die Vernunft als solche nicht selbst die Quelle und der Ursprung einer Störung der Erkenntnis sein kann. Wo die Vernunft nun innerhalb der menschlichen Erkenntnis als eine wesentliche Komponente derselben als gestört erscheint, da kann, der Grundannahme jener Vernunftphilosophie zufolge, die Vernunft nicht selbst Ursprung und Grund ihrer eigenen Störung sein. Somit stellt sich für eine Philosophie der Vernunft die Frage nach dem Ursprung der Erkenntnisstörungen mit besonderer Dringlichkeit. Und solche Erkenntnisstörungen gibt es viele und verschiedenartige: Irrtum und Täuschung, Schlechtigkeit und Verdorbenheit. Auf der Suche nach den Quellen solcher Störungen hat sich die moderne Vernunftphilosophie ebenso wie die Logosphilosophie der Alten an der Grunddifferenz der beiden Erkenntnisquellen der Sinnlichkeit und des Verstandes, bzw. der Vernunft orientiert.[4] Wenn nun der Ursprung jeder möglichen Erkenntnisstörung nicht in der Vernunft als solcher gesucht werden kann, so bleiben nur die folgenden möglichen Entstehungsgründe übrig: Entweder muß die Sinnlichkeit selbst als solche gestört sein und dies so, daß ihre Störung sich dem Ganzen der Erkenntnis, und somit auch der Vernunft in dieser Erkenntnis mitteilt; oder aber es muß auch die Sinnlichkeit wie die Vernunft als nicht störbar angesehen werden, so daß eine mögliche Störung der Erkenntnis insgesamt und auch der Vernunft allein aus dem gestörten Verhältnis zwischen Sinnlichkeit und Vernunft herrühren kann. So hat KANT etwa eine Reihe von elementaren widersprüchlichen Vernunftgedanken über Gott, Welt und Mensch als Erkenntnisstörungen erörtert, die aus dem "unbemerkten Einfluß der Sinnlichkeit auf den Verstand" (KANT, KdrV, A294, B 350)[5] herrühren und insofern ein jeweils gestörtes Verhältnis von Sinnlichkeit und Vernunft in der theoretischen Vernunfterkenntnis anzeigen. Und dementsprechend galten ihm die Affekte und Leidenschaften teils als Störungen des sinnlichen Begehrungsvermögens, teils als Störungen des Verhältnisses dieser praktischen Sinnlichkeit zur praktischen Vernunfterkenntnis. Es ist nicht schwer zu sehen, daß die Philosophie der Vernunft in ihrer transzendentalen und in ihrer metaphysischen Gestalt das Problem der Erkenntnisstörung im Grunde nur verschiebt, indem sie es von der reinen Vernunft auf das Verhältnis der Vernunft zur Sinnlichkeit, bzw. auf die Sinnlichkeit als solche verlagert. Aber im Grunde sind die Schwierigkeiten dieser paradigmatischen Vernunftphilosophien repräsentativ für die Schwierigkeiten des philosophischen Umgangs mit dem Begriff und der Wirklichkeit der Störungen überhaupt. Man kann für diese Schwierigkeiten eine Reihe von Erklärungen beibringen, von denen aber keine wirklich hinreichend überzeugt. Erinnert man etwa an die Differenz zwischen Philosophie und Heilkunde und daran, daß der Begriff der Störung ebenso wie der der Krankheit seinen eigentlichen Ort in der Heilkunde hat, so ist dem entgegenzuhalten, daß die Philosophie sich selbst im

4 Die klassische Belegstelle für diese ontologische und gnoseologische Grunddifferenz des Platonismus ist: PLATO, *Sophistes* 246 a-c.

5 "In einem Erkenntnis, das mit den Verstandesgesetzen durchgängig zusammenstimmt, ist kein Irrtum. In einer Vorstellung der Sinne ist (weil sie gar kein Urteil enthält) auch kein Irrtum. Keine Kraft der Natur kann aber von selbst von ihren eigenen Gesetzen abweichen. Daher würden weder der Verstand für sich allein (ohne Einfluß einer anderen Ursache) noch die Sinne für sich irren... Weil wir nun außer diesen Erkenntnisquellen keine andere haben, so folgt: daß der Irrtum nur durch den unbemerkten Einfluß der Sinnlichkeit auf den Verstand bewirkt werde" (KANT, KdrV, A 293-294, B 350). In seiner Logik hat KANT darüber hinaus den Verstand "in gewissem Sinne auch zum Urheber der Irrtümer" gemacht, "sofern er nämlich aus Mangel an erforderlicher Aufmerksamkeit auf jenen Einfluß der Sinnlichkeit sich durch den hieraus entspringenden Schein verleiten läßt, bloß subjektive Bestimmungsgründe des Urteils für objektive zu halten, oder das, was nur nach Gesetzen der Sinnlichkeit wahr ist, für wahr nach seinen eigenen Gesetzen gelten zu lassen" (KANT, Logik-Jäsche, A 77-78). Darüber hinaus aber konstatiert KANT eine grundsätzliche Differenz im Verhältnis der Sinnlichkeit des Erkenntnisvermögens zum Verstand einerseits und im Verhältnis der Sinnlichkeit des Begehrungsvermögens, der Neigungen und Begierden, zur Vernunft andererseits: Während die erste niemals über den Verstand "gebieten" kann, ist in den Affekten und Leidenschaften "die Herrschaft der Vernunft" ausdrücklich ausgeschlossen (vgl Anthropologie, §§ 10 und 73, S. 145, 251).

Verlauf ihrer Geschichte oft genug an diesem Vorbild der Heilkunst gemessen hat, und dementsprechend immer wieder mit therapeutischen oder kathartischen Ansprüchen in den Bereichen der Logik und Ethik, bzw. im Bereich der menschlichen Erkenntnis überhaupt aufgetreten ist. Und selbst dann, wenn die Philosophie ausdrücklich solchen Ansprüchen entsagte, die eine Kunst und Technik erfordern, konnte sie nicht umhin, ihr Verhältnis nicht nur zu den Wissenschaften, sondern auch zu den Künsten und Techniken zu klären und sich somit, zumindest indirekt, auch mit den Problemen der Störung zu beschäftigen.

Die meisten Gründe für die philosophischen Schwierigkeiten im Umgang mit dem Problem der Störungen entspringen aus der Idee einer Philosophia perennis, welche die Dinge "unter einer gewissen Art von Ewigkeit"[6] betrachtet. Für eine solche Betrachtungsweise ist das Problem der Zerstörung unendlich drängender und gewichtiger als das Problem der bloßen Störung. Daher wird die Frage nach der Möglichkeit eines Unzerstörbaren und Ewigen hier immer die Frage nach einem Unstörbaren und Störungsanfälligen verdrängen, selbst wenn es, oder gerade weil es einen realen Zusammenhang zwischen Störbarkeit und Zerstörbarkeit gibt. Das Grundverhältnis von Sinnlichkeit und Vernunft, an dem sich die Vernunftphilosophie der Alten und der Modernen, wie gesagt, von je her orientiert hat, führt direkt in diesen Problemzusammenhang hinein. Denn das Verhältnis von Sinnlichkeit und Verstand, mögen wir es auch als ein erkenntnistheoretisches Grundverhältnis ansehen, ist dem onotologischen Grundverhältnis von Körper und Geist, Leib und Seele, zumindest verwandt, wenn es nicht sogar mit demselben identisch gesetzt wird. Dieser Verwandtschaft zufolge können die Komponenten des jeweiligen Verhältnisses in Analogie zu den Komponenten des anderen Verhältnisses begriffen werden. Nun gilt es in der philosophischen Tradition ebenso seit altersher und bis in die Neuzeit hinein, daß Körper prinzipiell teilbar und angesichts dieser Teilbarkeit auch zerstörbar sind, während Seelen und Geister als einfach und daher als unzerstörbar angesehen werden. Gewiß ist dem modernen Menschen, einem tiefgreifenden Bedürfnis nach Ewigkeit zum Trotz, der selbstverständliche Glaube an eine ewige Existenz seiner selbst oder von etwas überhaupt abhanden gekommen. Aber die Philosophie hat auch in der Moderne immer wieder den Versuch unternommen, ungeachtet der wachsenden Macht des Szientismus etwas von diesem Glauben an das Ewige im Menschen zu retten.[7] So bestand etwa für Spinoza kein Zweifel, daß die Dinge der Zerstörbarkeit unterworfen sind. Aber zugleich war er bemüht, einer unendlichen Macht der Zerstörung bestimmte Grenzen zu setzen. So versuchte er zu beweisen, daß der Grund der Zerstörung eines Dinges prinzipiell nicht in diesem Dinge selbst gelegen sein kann, sondern der Macht äußerer Ursachen entspringen muß. Und was den Menschen betrifft, so versuchte er zu beweisen, daß an seinem Körper zumindest irgend etwas unzerstörbar sein muß wie auch an seiner Seele. Von Kant wissen wir, daß er in seiner *Kritik der reinen Vernunft* die Beweise einer Unsterblichkeit der Seele, an denen sich Philosophie und Theologie immer wieder versucht hatten, als Fehl-

---

6 *Ethica ordine geometrico demonstrata*, P II, prop. 44, Corollarium II: "De natura rationis est res sub quadam aeternitatis specie percipere" (Teil II, Lehrsatz 44, Folgesatz 2: "Es liegt in der Natur der Vernunft, die Dinge unter einer gewissen Art der Ewigkeit wahrzunehmen").

7 Vgl. H. Tellenbach 1988, S. 163f.

schlüsse entlarvt und damit wesentlich zum modernen Unglauben hinsichtlich der Unsterblichkeit beigetragen hat. Aber ebenso wissen wir auch, daß er diesen "Beweis der Unmöglichkeit der Unsterblichkeitsbeweise" führte, um den menschlichen Glauben an die Unsterblichkeit der Seele für die praktische Vernunft und um der Möglichkeit der menschlichen Sittlichkeit willen zu retten. Darüber hinaus galt die Vernunft, dieser Grund einer solchen möglichen Rettung des Unsterblichkeitsglaubens, als ein "Faktum", nicht als eine empirisch-kontingente Tatsache, sondern als ein Faktum der Vernunft selbst; als ein Faktum apriori, an welchem zu zweifeln sich für die philosophische Vernunft aus Gründen der eigenen Vernunft verbot. Angesichts dieser für unzerstörbar geltenden Macht der Vernunft einerseits und angesichts der wechselweise wirkenden Zerstörungsmacht der endlichen Dinge andererseits, mußte das Problem möglicher Störungen und Störanfälligkeiten von Leib und Seele als durchaus zweitrangig erscheinen.

Die Vernachlässigung des Problems der Störungen, die sich schon in der klassischen Vernunftphilosophie des Altertums beobachten läßt, hat in der Neuzeit sich wesentlich verstärkt, und zwar insbesondere da, wo diese Philosophie sich ausdrücklich die Form der Subjektivität gegeben hat. Nicht erst KANTS Transzendentalphilosophie, schon die Methaphysik des SPINOZA ist eine spezifisch neuzeitliche Vernunftphilosophie und als solche eine Philosophie der Subjektivität. Beide stehen unter dem Einfluß der cartesischen Philosophie und des Cartesianismus. Zwar weiß diese neuzeitliche Philosophie so gut wie die Philosophie des Altertums um das Vorkommen mannigfacher seelischer und geistiger Störungen, um das Vorkommen mannigfacher Störungen des menschlichen Verhaltens, ungeachtet des Bewußtseins und der Vernunft in diesem Verhalten. Seit altersher sind zahlreiche Krankheiten der Seele und des Geistes bekannt. Aber dieses Wissen und das langsam wachsende Verständnis für diese Krankheiten hat zunächst die allgemeine Grundauffassung überhaupt nicht beeinträchtigt, daß es im Menschen eine ausgezeichnete Instanz gäbe, die sich der Macht der Zerstörung entzieht. Diese Instanz der menschlichen Subjektivität, mag sie nun Seele oder Bewußtsein, Vernunft oder Geist oder dies alles zusammen genannt worden sein, galt keineswegs nur als ein Unzerstörbares und Ewiges im Menschen, sondern darüber hinaus als eine Kraft der Bewahrung und Rettung, der Heilung und der Versöhnung, als eine absolute Gegenmacht gegenüber allen Mächten der Zerstörung. Die Faszination durch eine solche theoretische Möglichkeit war stark genug, die Philosophie immer mehr von den Problemen der Störungen des Leibes und der Seele abzulenken. Man ist versucht zu sagen: die unübersehbaren Mächte der Zerstörung in der Welt der endlichen Dinge haben die Philosophie immer stärker herausgefordert, nach einem Rettenden gegen diese Mächte zu suchen. Angesichts der Vergeblichkeit dieser Suche scheint heute in unseren Tagen mehr Raum gewonnen für die Beschäftigung mit den Fragen der Störung und mit den Möglichkeiten ihrer Aufhebung. Wenn die neuzeitliche Philosophie den Phänomenen der Störung einen nur unzureichenden Raum eingeräumt hat, so hängt dies über das Gesagte hinaus mit der Logik des Verhältnisses zwischen Störung und Zerstörung, zwischen Störunanfälligkeit und Unzerstörbarkeit irgendwie zusammen. Die Logik dieses Verhältnisses besagt: Wo eine Störung nicht mehr beseitigt, wo die

Dinge nicht wieder in die ihnen gemäße Ordnung gebracht werden können, hat das Werk der Zerstörung bereits begonnen oder es wird die Zerstörung selbst nicht mehr lange auf sich warten lassen; und umgekehrt: solange einmal eingetretene Störungen sich wieder rückgängig machen lassen, solange es möglich ist, eine gestörte Ordnung wieder in ihr ursprüngliches Gleichgewicht zurückzubringen, da ist der Prozeß der Zerstörung, wenn auch nicht für alle Zeit, so doch für eine gewisse Zeit, für eine bestimmte Dauer angehalten und ausgesetzt. Mit den Störungen und mit den Kämpfen gegen die Störungen kommt die Zeitlichkeit der endlichen Dinge ins Spiel, während der absolute Gegensatz zwischen den Mächten der Zerstörung und der unzerstörbaren Macht der Erhaltung des Seienden über alle Zeit erhaben und ein ewiger Gegensatz zu sein scheint. Die Störungen und die Auseinandersetzungen mit ihnen versetzen somit jenen absoluten Gegensatz unter die Erfahrungsbedingungen der Zeitlichkeit. Die alte und die moderne Philosophie der Vernunft muß zwangsläufig Schwierigkeiten im Umgang mit den Störungen der Dinge haben, solange sie sich im reinen, nicht-empirischen Felde des Gegensatzes zwischen jenen Mächten bewegt.

Tatsächlich haben die Phänomene der Störung und der Auseinandersetzung mit den mannigfachen Arten von Störungen eine ausgezeichnete Stellung unter den Gegebenheiten möglicher Erfahrung. Denn Störungen werden zwar nicht immer und unter allen Umständen erkannt. Manche von ihnen und vermutlich sehr viele verschwinden wieder, ohne daß ihr Vorkommen je bemerkt wurde. Wenn sie sich aber bemerkbar machen, so geschieht es in Form eines Verhaltens, welches von einem durchschnittlichen und allgemein zu erwartenden Verhalten mehr oder weniger abweicht. Was in der Erfahrung zunächst und zumeist auffällt, ist nicht das durchschnittliche, als normal geltende und allgemein erwartete, sondern das ungewöhnliche und abweichende Verhalten. Man kann in diesem auffälligen Verhalten eine gewisse Teleologie nicht verkennen, sofern dasselbe durch seine Auffälligkeit die Aufmerksamkeit auf sich zieht. Störungen, die sich auf diese Weise Ausdruck verschaffen, wirken wie öffentliche Hilferufe, auch wenn sie sich dieser besonderen Sprache nicht eigens bedienen. Zweifellos gibt es auch bedrohliche Störungen, die stumm bleiben. Doch macht eine solche Verschwiegenheit die betreffenden Störungen über ihre Bedrohlichkeit als solche hinaus zusätzlich bedrohlich. Störungen sind, wie schon mehrfach angeklungen ist, Störungen von Ordnung und können daher in gewisser Hinsicht mit Unordnung gleichgesetzt werden. Es ist diese Begriffsbestimmung der Störung, die nun die Vernunftphilosophie der Alten und der Modernen in die allergrößten Schwierigkeiten bringt. Denn die Vernunft gilt in dieser Philosophie, wie gesagt, als Grundprinzip der Wahrheit. Aber zugleich ist sie hier auch das Grundprinzip der Ordnung und der Gesetzmäßigkeit überhaupt. Aus der Vernunft entspringt die universale Gesetzmäßigkeit der Ordnung. In diesem Sinne einer allumfassenden Gesetzgebung ist die Vernunft die Retterin, die Bewahrerin von Ordnung. Im Wesen der Vernunft erscheinen Wahrheit, Ordnung und Gesetzmäßigkeit nahezu als ein- und dasselbe. Auf diese Weise aber scheint überhaupt kein Raum für mögliche Störungen, kein Raum für mögliche Unordnung übrigzubleiben. Angesichts der Auffälligkeit und Unbestreitbarkeit des Vorkommens von Unordnung befindet sich die Vernunftphilosophie in einem Dilemma: Entweder sie muß die Grenzen der Macht und des Geltungsbereiches der Vernunft anerkennen und bemüht sein, diese Grenzen zu erkennen und zu bestimmen. Oder aber sie wird den Macht- und Geltungsbereich der Vernunft auch auf die Bereiche möglicher Störungen und Unordnungen ausdehnen und auch hier eine Gesetzmäßigkeit und eine Gesetzgebung der Vernunft entdecken. In dem letzteren Falle kann von einem absoluten und absolut bestimmten Gegensatz zwischen Ordnung und Unordnung keine Rede sein. Vielmehr wird hier die Unordnung im Unterschied zur Ordnung eigentlich eine andere Ordnung, möglicherweise eine Ordnung niedrigeren Ranges sein. Die Vernunftphilosophien der Alten und der Modernen haben von jeher im Blick auf die erkenntnistheoretische Grunddifferenz von Sinnlichkeit und Vernunft zwischen diesen beiden extremen Vernunftpositionen geschwankt; und sie waren ebenso von jeher bemüht, einen Ausgleich zwischen beiden auf die eine oder andere Weise zustandezubringen, um jenem Dilemma zu entgehen.

3. Ein möglicher Konflikt zwischen Rationalität und Kausalität

Auch die neuzeitlichen Vernunftphilosophien des SPINOZA und des KANT haben sich um einen solchen Ausgleich bemüht. Dabei lassen sie, ungeachtet tiefgreifender Differenzen im Detail, eine gemeinsame Grundtendenz erkennen, die auf eine Begünstigung der zweiten, zuletzt genannten Vernunftposition hinausläuft, derzufolge nicht Ordnung gegen Unordnung, sondern eine Art von Ordnung gegen eine andere zu stehen kommt, und dies so, daß beide unterschiedlichen Ordnungen sich der einen umfassenden Gesetzgebung der Vernunft unterordnen. Wenn es in diesem wichtigen Punkte überhaupt einen Unterschied zwischen SPINOZAS Metaphysik und KANTS Transzendentalphilosophie gibt, so ist es dieser: daß jene Metaphysik zwischen einer laxeren und weniger bestimmten Vernunftordnung in der Sinneserkenntnis und einer strengeren und bestimmteren Vernunftordnung in der Verstandeserkenntnis unterscheidet.[8] Dagegen kennt KANTS Transzendentalphilosophie nur den Unterschied zwischen zwei idealtypischen Klassen von Vernunftmerkmalen, die jeweils für die Ordnungen der Sinnlichkeit und des Verstandes gültig sind.[9] Diese verschiedenen Klassen von Merkmalen konstituieren aber nicht verschiedene Grade der Vernünftigkeit, sondern machen allererst in ihrer Synthesis die Vernunftordnung in den Bedingungen einer möglichen Erfahrungserkenntnis aus. Wenn nun Störungen hier wie dort als Erkenntnisstörungen aufgefaßt werden, deren Quelle entweder in einer Störung der Sinnlichkeit als solcher oder aber in einer Störung des Verhältnisses von Sinnlichkeit und Verstand gesucht werden muß, so kehrt offenkundig das oben beschriebene Dilemma unverändert wieder. Denn ent-

8 Vgl. SPINOZA, *Ethica*, P. II, prop. 36: "Ideae inadaequatae et confusae eadem necessitate consequuntur, ac adaequatae, sive clarae, ac distinctae ideae" (Teil II, Lehrsatz 36: "Die inadäquaten und verworrenen Ideen folgen mit derselben Notwendigkeit wie die adäquaten oder klaren und deutlichen Ideen"; Ethik, S. 84).

9 Maßgeblich ist dabei vor allem die Differenz zwischen Homogenität und Inhomogenität im Verhältnis der Teile zu einem Ganzen, von denen die erste den Inbegriff aller Merkmale der Gegenstände der Anschauung, letztere den Inbegriff aller Merkmale der Gegenstände des diskursiven Verstandes ausmacht. Dies demonstriert KANT in seinem dritten bzw. vierten Raum- und Zeitargument in der transzendentalen Ästhetik, KdrV A 24-25, B 39-40 und A 31-32, B 47.

weder gelten diese Störungen vom Standpunkt einer universalen Gesetzgebung der Vernunft aus als Störungen der Ordnung der Sinnlichkeit, bzw. der Ordnung der Synthesis von Sinnlichkeit und Verstand, das heißt als entsprechende Unordnungen; oder aber es müssen diese Störungen der Sinnlichkeit, bzw. der Synthesis derselben mit dem Verstande als eine Art "dritter" Ordnung angesehen werden, die sich von den bestehenden Ordnungen ungestörter Sinnlichkeit und Verständigkeit, sowie ungestörter Synthesis zwischen beiden unterscheidet. SPINOZA und KANT haben dieses Problem der "Erkenntnisstörungen" deutlich gesehen, ohne von ihrem jeweiligen Konzept einer Vernunftphilosophie her eine befriedigende Lösung zu finden. So hat etwa KANT im Blick auf die zu seiner Zeit gültige Erkenntnistheorie der WOLFFschen Schule angemerkt, daß man zwischen undeutlichen und verworrenen Vorstellungen unterscheiden müsse, sofern die ersteren mit Notwendigkeit aus dem Verhältnis einer Sinneserkenntnis zu ihrem Gegenstande rechtmäßig entspringen, während im anderen Falle die Undeutlichkeit die Folge einer Erkenntnisverwirrung sei.[10] Ähnlich hat er im Bereich der praktischen Erkenntnis zwischen Affekten und Leidenschaften differenziert. Dabei hat er besonders betont, daß es unter den ersteren zumindest einige gebe "durch welche die Natur die Gesundheit mechanisch befördert" (KANT, Anthropologie, § 79; S. 261), während ihm die Leidenschaften als Krankheiten galten, die "mehrentheils unheilbar [sind]: weil der Kranke nicht will geheilt sein und sich der Herrschaft des Grundsatzes entzieht, durch den dies allein geschehen könnte" (KANT, Anthropologie, § 81; S. 266). Solche Leidenschaften haben den Charakter einer krankhaften Sucht, zum Beispiel Rachsucht, Herrschsucht, Ehrsucht, Habsucht. SPINOZA ist KANT auf diesem Wege der Unterscheidung zwischen einer ungestörten und einer gestörten Sinnlichkeit und Affektivität in der menschlichen Erkenntnis vorangegangen. Ähnlich wie Kant hat er angesichts einer möglichen ungestörten Sinnlichkeit und Affektivität die Quelle der Störung der menschlichen Erkenntnis nicht so sehr in der sinnlich-affektiven Erkenntnis allein als vielmehr in deren Zusammenhang mit dem Verstand gesucht.

Allerdings hat SPINOZA anders als KANT nicht terminologisch zwischen Affekten und Leidenschaften unterschieden. Statt dessen findet sich bei ihm eine Unterscheidung, die in eine ähnliche Richtung weist, nämlich die Unterscheidung zwischen einem aktiven und einem passiven affektiven Verhalten des Menschen.[11] Da für SPINOZA die menschlichen Affekte Relationen der sinnlichen Erkenntnis zu ihrem Gegenstande sind, ist die Unterscheidung zwischen einer Aktivität und einer Passivität in der Erkenntnis gleichbedeutend mit einem bestimmten Unterschied in der Art und Weise des Erkennens. Die aktive Affektivität ist eine bewußte und bestimmte, eine deutliche und adäquate Erkenntnis ihres jeweiligen Gegenstandes. Bei der passiven Affektivität handelt es sich dagegen um ein vorbewußtes und unbestimmtes, um ein undeutliches und inadäquates Vorstellen. Dabei gelten dem SPINOZA die passiven Affekte keineswegs von vornherein als pathologisch, bzw. als Störungen, sowenig wie KANT die

10 KANT, Logik-Jäsche, 42-43.

11 *Ethica*, P. III, Def. 1-3 geben die anfänglichen definitorischen Bestimmungen der Differenz zwischen aktivem und passivem affektiven Verhalten, auf welche im Grunde die ganze Affektenlehre des SPINOZA und mit ihr die Ethik aufgebaut ist.

undeutlichen Vorstellungen und die Affekte, sofern diese keine Leidenschaften sind. Um Störungen handelt es sich erst dann, wenn die Affekte sich prinzipiell der Vernunft, bzw. der vernünftigen Einsicht verweigern, wenn sie also durch die Unmöglichkeit bestimmt sind, in eine aktive Erkenntnis überzugehen. Hier nun angesichts dieser Bestimmung der affektiven Störungen als Leidenschaften (Kant) und als passive Affekte, die blind und ohne Fähigkeit zur vernünftigen Einsicht auf ihr Objekt in Liebe oder Haß fixiert sind (Spinoza), zeigt sich die Schwierigkeit, welche die Vernunftphilosophien mit der Aufklärung des Problems der Störungen haben, in besonderem Maße. Denn wie soll vom Standpunkt einer allumfassenden universalen Gesetzgebung der Vernunft her verständlich werden, daß menschliches Verhalten sich der Vernunft entziehen, sich der Vernunft verweigern kann? Wie läßt sich vernünftig erklären, wie verständlich machen, daß Vernunft abwesend ist, daß Vernunft auf die eine oder andere Weise verneint wird? Ist eine Gesetzgebung der Vernunft für die Negation, für den Ausfall von Vernunft möglich? Der Widerspruch, in den hier die Vernunft zu sich selbst gerät, ist offenkundig. Dieser Selbstwiderspruch der Vernunft kann auch als Widerspruch zwischen Vernunft und Kausalität beschrieben werden. Denn die Philosophie der Vernunft setzt die allgemeine Gesetzgebung der Vernunft mit der Kausalität gleich. Damit scheint sie angesichts des Problems der Störungen vor das Dilemma gestellt, sich zumindest in einigen Fällen entweder für die Vernunft und gegen die Kausalität, oder umgekehrt für die Kausalität und gegen die Vernunft entscheiden zu müssen. Dann muß man differenzieren zwischen zwei Realisationen der Vernunft, bzw. zwischen zwei Formen der Kausalität; zwischen einer Vernunft, deren Reich sich auf das Vernünftige und Vernunftgemäße erstreckt, und einer anderen Vernunft, deren Gesetzgebung für das Unvernünftige und Widervernünftige Gültigkeit hat, zwischen einer Kausalität, welche den Bereich der Ordnung regelt, und einer anderen Kausalität, welche allgemeine Gesetze für Störungen und Unordnungen an die Hand gibt.

3.1 Relativität und Komplementarität als Prinzipien der Störungen

Diese widersprüchlichen Verhältnisse in den Begriffen der Vernunft und der Kausalität, in denen die beiden Seiten - Vernunft und Kausalität - nicht zusammenkommen können, zeigen sich insbesondere angesichts des erkenntnistheoretischen Grundverhältnisses von Sinnlichkeit und Vernunft. Denn dieses Verhältnis ist einerseits als ein Machtverhältnis, zum anderen als ein Kausalitätsverhältnis vorgestellt. Unter dem Gesichtspunkt der Macht lassen sich zunächst zwei verschiedene Verhältnisse denken, das eine, demzufolge die Vernunft über die Sinnlichkeit ihre Macht ausübt, und das andere, in dem die Sinnlichkeit eine eigene Macht gegen die Macht der Vernunft entfaltet, sei es, daß sie sich deren Gegenmacht entzieht, sei es, daß sie sogar über die Macht der Vernunft die Oberhand gewinnt. Diese verschiedenen hier möglichen Verhältnisse von Macht und Ohnmacht lassen sich nicht ohne weiteres und unter allen Umständen mit einem allgemeinen Konzept von Kausalität in Einklang bringen. Nun lassen sich allerdings eine Reihe von Möglichkeiten denken, die es erlauben, jenen Widersprüchen im Verhältnis der Vernunft und der Kausalität zu entgehen. Aber keine dieser Denkmöglichkeiten wird eine Philosophie der Vernunft auf die Dauer befriedigen können. Eine dieser Denkmöglichkeiten ist die einer grundsätzlichen Skepsis gegenüber der Macht der Vernunft und der Gültigkeit des Kausalitätsprinzips. Ferner kann man eine strikte Trennung zwischen verschiedenen Erkenntnis- und Geltungsbereichen der Vernunft, bzw. der Kausalität zu etablieren versuchen, in Verbindung mit strengen Regeln, die Grenzüberschreitungen zwischen diesen Bereichen verbieten. Eine dritte Möglichkeit ist der Ausschluß der Störung, bzw. der Unordnung aus der Philosophie und die Verbannung dieser Gegenständlichkeit in andere Disziplinen der Erkenntnis, so etwa in die Physiologie oder Psychiatrie. Nun gibt es unter den mannigfachen Charakteren von Störungen einen Charakterzug, der in der traditionellen Vernunftphilosophie nicht die gebührende Aufmerksamkeit gefunden hat, obwohl seine Erörterung geeignet gewesen wäre, einen Ausweg aus den geschilderten Dilemmata dieser Vernunftphilosophie zu finden. Ich meine die Relativität der Störungen, die Relativität von Unordnung. Diesem Relativitätsprinzip zufolge gibt es weder die absolute Ordnung noch die absolute Unordnung im Bereich möglicher menschlicher Erfahrung. Störungen sind - wie auch das entsprechende Ungestörtsein - Störungen von etwas oder an etwas, Störungen durch etwas und mit Konsequenzen für etwas. Störungen sind immer Störungen in einer bestimmten Hinsicht. Ein lebendiger Organismus kann im Ganzen oder in diesem oder jenem seiner Teile, bzw. innerhalb eines bestimmten Zusammenhanges zwischen einigen seiner Teile, bestimmten Organen oder Organfunktionen gestört sein. Die Störung kann sich in einem eigentümlich abweichenden Verhalten zeigen. Störungen sind allgemein oder singulär und dementsprechend nach bestimmten idealtypischen Unterscheidungen zu klassifizieren und in ihrer singulären Einzigartigkeit zu beschreiben. Vor allem aber besagt das Prinzip der Relativität gegenüber den Gegensätzen des Ungestörtseins und der Störung, der Ordnung und der Unordnung: Diese scheinbar absoluten Gegensätze sind in Wahrheit lediglich Unterschiede des Mehr und Weniger. Ein Weniger an Unordnung ist ein Mehr an Ordnung, ein Weniger an Ordnung ist ein Mehr an Unordnung. Dieses Mehr und Weniger ist niemals nur ein quantitatives, sondern immer auch ein qualitatives Mehr und Weniger. Dieses qualitativ-quantitative Mehr und Weniger ist eine kategoriale Form sinnlicher Erfahrungsgegebenheiten. Sie bestimmt daher Affekte, Wahrnehmung und Gedanken als solche Gegebenheiten. Insbesondere aber bestimmt sie auch die Affekte als Wahrnehmungs- und Denkstörungen.

Das Prinzip der Relativität steht aber als Prinzip der relativen Unterscheidung zwischen einem Mehr und Weniger an Ordnung, bzw. einem Mehr und Weniger an Unordnung nicht allein. Es verbindet sich vielmehr mit einem anderen, nicht weniger grundlegenden Prinzip, welches das der Komplementarität, bzw. der Kompensation genannt werden könnte. Es kommt dabei nicht so sehr darauf an, ob es sich hier um ein einziges oder um zwei verschiedene Prinzipien handelt. Jedenfalls gilt, sofern es das absolute Ungestörtsein, die absolute Vollkommenheit und Ordnung im Bereich der endlichen Dinge nicht gibt, daß Störung und Ungestörtsein, Unordnung und Ordnung untrennbar zusammengehören. Immer ist in eine Ordnung eine gewisse Unordnung eingemischt, immer ist das Ungestörtsein eine Einbindung und Fesselung mannigfacher Störungen. In gewisser Weise ist hier das eine die Bedingung der Möglichkeit des anderen: Kein Ungestörtsein ohne die Möglichkeit der Störung, keine Störung ohne die Möglichkeit des Ungestörtseins, und ebenso hinsichtlich Ordnung und Unordnung. Auch diese Bedingungsverhältnisse sind durch die Form des Mehr und Weniger bestimmt. Stabilität, bzw. Labilität einer Ordnung hängt ab von einem Mehr und Weniger an involvierter Unordnung. Vor allem aber haben Störungen und Unordnungen diese realen Möglichkeiten: Sie können konservativ, kreativ und destruktiv sein, das heißt, sie können eine bestehende Vollkommenheit, eine bestehende Ordnung erhalten, schöpferisch umgestalten oder zerstören; zumindest können sie zur Erhaltung, zur Umgestaltung und auch zur Zerstörung beitragen. Aber angesichts dieser Möglichkeiten ergibt sich auch die Möglichkeit der wechselseitigen Kompensation. Verschiedene Störungen können innerhalb eines Gesamtzusammenhanges so zusammenwirken, daß sie sich wechselweise neutralisieren oder zu einem positiven Resultat einer bestimmten Vollkommenheit oder Ordnung verbinden. Reparaturen, bzw. Therapie, haben im allgemeinen diesen Charakter der Kompensation oder der Neutralisation. Es gibt demnach aber auch eine Fülle von Fällen der Ordnung, des Ungestörtseins, die als Summen sich wechselseitig kompensierender Störungen und Unordnungen angesehen werden können. Als sinnliche Erfahrungsgegebenheiten unterliegen die Affekte, die Wahrnehmungen und die Gedanken auch diesem Prinzip der Kompensation. Insbesondere aber sind die Störungen in diesem Erfahrungsbereich durch dieses Prinzip bestimmt. Etwas von diesen Prinzipien der Relativität und der Kompensation ist in den Morallehren der Alten über das Maß und die richtige Mitte eingefangen. Diesen Lehren zufolge ist die menschliche Vollkommenheit Findung der jeweils richtigen Mitte zwischen zwei Extremen, die - für sich genommen - als Störungen, als Wahnsinn oder auch als Zug zur Unordnung aufgefaßt werden können. So ist zum Beispiel die reine Mutwilligkeit und Tollkühnheit alluzoft destruktiv und führt zum Gegenteil des Gewollten. Daher erscheint sie auch in solchen Fällen eher als eine Art von Verrücktheit und Wahnsinn, denn als Vernunft sinnvollen Handelns. Nicht anders steht es mit den gegenteiligen Einstellungen der Ängstlichkeit und Feigheit. Auch sie sind in vielen Fällen geeignet, das Tun an der Erreichung seines Zieles zu hindern, anstatt es hierin zu befördern. Beide gegenteilige Verhaltensweisen sind nicht als schlechthin unvernünftig abzutun. Aber je mehr sie sich isolieren und in das einseitige Extrem steigern, um so mehr büßen sie den letzten Rest von Vernünftigkeit ein, um schließlich als bloße Verhaltensstörungen zu erscheinen.

3.2 Eine rationale Kritik am Prinzip der richtigen Mitte

Praktische Vernunft ist, der moralischen Lehre der Alten zufolge, demnach die Fähigkeit, mittels Klugheit diese maßlosen Extreme der Einstellung und des entsprechenden Verhaltens in Schranken zu weisen, und dies dadurch, daß man versucht, gegensätzliche Extreme zu einem vernünftigen Maß der Mitte zu verknüpfen. In dieser Verknüpfung vermögen sich die Mängel und Störungen der extremen Maßlosigkeit wechselseitig zum besten zu kompensieren. Wenn die konkrete Handlungssituation es erfordert, kann die praktische Vernunft durchaus von dem geraden Mittelkurs etwas abgehen und in die eine oder andere Richtung gegensteuern. Diese Gegensteuerung folgt gleichfalls dem Prinzip des Mehr und Weniger. In manchen Situationen ist ein Mehr an Tollkühnheit besser, in anderen ein Mehr an Ängstlichkeit. Diese moralische Lehre der Alten von der Mitte und vom rechten Maße läßt sich nun fraglos über die traditionellen Anwendungsbereiche, über die Affekten- und Tugendlehren, ja über den Bereich der Ethik hinaus anwenden. So kann man neben den Affekten auch die Wahrnehmungen und die leibgebundenen Gedanken als Ergebnisse einer psychosomatischen Aktivität ansehen, in denen ein Ausgleich, ein Gleichgewicht zwischen extremen normativen Gegebenheiten erreicht worden ist. Selbst das Grundprinzip der Moderne und der modernen Philosophie, das Prinzip der Subjektivität läßt sich aus dieser Perspektive einer Vernunft so betrachten, daß kompensatorisch die richtige Mitte zu gewinnen bemüht wird. So ist - mit KANT zu reden - "das Bewußtsein seiner selbst", dies "daß der Mensch in seiner Vorstellung das Ich haben kann", etwas, das "ihn unendlich über alle anderen auf Erden lebende Wesen [erhebt]" (KANT, Anthropologie, § 1; S. 127). Dieses Selbstbewußtsein ist Prinzip und Ursprung zweier menschlicher Verhaltensweisen von sehr elementarem Charakter, nämlich des Bemerkens (animadvertere) und des Beobachtens (observare) seiner selbst. Von dem ersteren meint KANT, "daß es notwendig ist, wenn man mit Menschen zu tun hat", von dem letzteren dagegen, daß es "leichtlich zu Schwärmerei und Wahnsinn hinführt" (KANT, Anthropologie, § 4; S. 132). Hier glaubt er nicht nachdrücklich genug warnen zu können: Denn die "Ausspähung und gleichsam studierte Abfassung einer inneren Geschichte des unwillkürlichen Laufs seiner Gedanken und Gefühle [sei] ... der gerade Weg..., in Kopfverwirrung vermeinter höherer Eingebungen und, ohne unser Zuthun, wer weiß woher auf uns einfließenden Kräfte, in Illuminatism und Terrorism zu gerathen" (KANT, Anthropologie, § 4; S. 133). Noch deutlicher scheint der Gegensatz zwischen logischem Egoismus und Borniertheit die Aufgabe anzuzeigen, durch praktische Vernunft eine richtige Mitte zwischen Gegensätzen zu finden. So ist der logische Egoist einer, der es "für unnöthig [hält], sein Urtheil auch am Verstande anderer zu prüfen; gleich als ob er dieses Probiersteins (criterium veritatis externum) gar nicht bedürfe" (KANT, Anthropologie, §. 2; S. 128). Dagegen wird im Gegensatz zu einem solchen "Selbstdenker" derjenige, "welcher nicht selbst denken, wenn gleich viel lernen kann, ...ein beschränkter Kopf (borniert) genannt" (KANT, Anthropologie, § 6; S. 138). Man ist versucht, in Kants Begriff der Weisheit die Vorstellung einer richtigen Mitte zwischen den Extremen eines logischen Egoismus und einer Borniertheit zu suchen, sofern es von dieser Weisheit heißt: "Die Vorschrift, dazu zu gelangen, enthält drei dahin führende Maximen: 1) Selbstdenken, 2) sich (in Mittheilung mit Menschen) an die Stelle des anderen zu denken, 3) jederzeit mit sich selbst einstimmig zu denken" (KANT, Anthropologie, § 43; S. 200). Es liegt nicht allzufern, von diesen Maximen die beiden erstgenannten so miteinander verbunden vorzustellen, daß eine vernünftige Mitte der Klugheit und Weisheit zustandekommt, in der die einseitigen Extreme des logischen Egoismus und der Borniertheit in ihre Schranken gewiesen und wechselseitig kompensiert sind.

Auch in SPINOZAS metaphysischer Ethik finden sich zahlreiche offene und versteckte Hinweise, die sich wie Reminiszenzen der alten Morallehren des Maßes und der richtigen Mitte lesen lassen. Hierher gehört zum Beispiel die ausdrückliche "Definition" der "entgegengesetzten Affekte", von denen es heißt, daß sie "den Menschen nach verschiedenen Richtungen hinziehen, wenn sie auch zu derselben Gattung gehören, wie Schwelgerei und Habgier, die Arten der Liebe sind, und nicht ihrer Natur nach, sondern durch Zufall entgegengesetzt sind" (SPINOZA, Ethik, P. IV, Def. 5; S. 191). Auch hier kann man sich zunächst eine Maxime vorstellen, welche im menschlichen Tun die richtige Mitte zwischen den Extremen, also zum Beispiel zwischen den Extremen von Ausschweifung und Geiz zu finden verlangt. Um so erstaunlicher muß es aber dann erscheinen, daß bei genauerem Hinsehen weder bei SPINOZA noch bei KANT von einer ausdrücklichen Rückkehr zur Ethik der Alten die Rede sein kann. In KANTS Bestimmung der drei Maximen der Weisheit findet sich kein Hinweis, der diese Tugend als Mitte aufzufassen verlangt, noch werden logischer Egoismus und Borniertheit als extreme Gegensätze unvernünftiger Gedankeneinstellungen bezeichnet. Ebensowenig verfolgt SPINOZA mit seiner Definition der entgegengesetzten Affekte den Zweck, die Idee eines Mittelweges zwischen Extremen zu empfehlen. Hier geht es vielmehr um den Beweis einer allgemeinen Gesetzgebung bestimmter Gattungen der Affekte, wie zum Beispiel der Gattung "Liebe", die eine allgemeine Gesetzgebung der Natur ist, während die Gegensätzlichkeit von Affekten als eine kontingente Erscheinung betrachtet werden muß. In der Tat gibt es für die metaphysische Ethik des einen und für die transzendentale praktische Philosophie des anderen gleichermaßen gute Gründe, die eine Rückkehr zur alten Lehre vom rechten Maß verbieten. Beide, SPINOZA und KANT, haben in den Morallehren der Alten zuviel Pragmatie und Empirie, zuviel Rhetorik und Dialektik gesehen. Sie haben dies 'zuviel' als einen theoretischen Mangel aufgefaßt, als einen Mangel unzureichender philosophischer Grundlegung. Für beide war die Vorstellung der richtigen Mitte irreführend angesichts des neuzeitlichen wissenschaftlichen Gebrauches des Begriffes des Maßes. Beide haben sich ausdrücklich dagegen gewandt, das Positive vom Negativen her, das heißt, die Wahrheit vom Irrtum, das Gute vom Bösen her zu bestimmen. Wie schon gesagt: Das Thema "Affekte als Wahrnehmungs- und Denkstörungen" gehört nicht nur in die praktische Philosophie. Die verschiedenen Machtverhältnisse zwischen Sinnlichkeit und Vernunft, Macht und Ohnmacht der einen und der anderen Komponente in diesem Verhältnis haben eine theoretische und eine praktische Seite sowie einen Aspekt diesseits und jenseits der Unterscheidung von Theorie und Praxis. Da Affekte, Wahrnehmungen und Gedanken in dieses Grundverhältnis von Sinnlichkeit und Vernunft, von Leib und Seele, eingebettet sind, finden wir in ihnen die entsprechenden unterschiedlichen Machtverhältnisse wieder; und zwar sowohl in jeder einzelnen dieser psychosomatischen Gegebenheiten, als auch in jedem einzelnen so oder so bestimmten Zusammenhang zwischen diesen. So finden sich solche Machtverhältnisse zwischen Sinnlichkeit und Vernunft in den jeweiligen einzelnen Affekten als solchen, aber auch dort, wo diese Affekte lediglich als bestimmte Tönungen oder Modifikationen von Wahrnehmungen und Gedanken angesehen werden, also in den Wahrnehmungen und Gedanken. Nicht anders steht es mit diesen. Auch sie können rein als solche wie auch hinsichtlich der Affekte als deren spezifische Erkenntnistätigkeiten betrachtet werden. Schließlich finden sich jene Machtverhältnisse aber auch dort, wo die drei psychosomatischen Gegebenheiten nicht wechselweise als Modifikationen, sondern als gegeneinander relativ selbständig und in kausalen Relationen zueinander stehend bestimmt sind.

3.3 Die Vieldeutigkeit der Natur im gestörten Ich

Dabei ist, wie gesagt, für die traditionellen Vernunftphilosophien metaphysischer und transzendentaler Spielart eine gewisse Ohnmacht der Vernunft, bzw. eine entsprechende Macht und Übermacht der Sinnlichkeit der eigentliche Anlaß für gestörte und pathologische Verhältnisse im Ganzen einer Erkenntnis, die durch sinnliche und rationale Komponenten konstituiert wird. Diese Ohnmacht der Vernunft und Übermacht der Sinnlichkeit und Leiblichkeit schlägt sich nun keineswegs nur in Störungen der Affekte, der Wahrnehmungen und Gedanken nieder, sofern diese von der Sinnlichkeit beherrscht werden. Vielmehr greifen diese Störungen auf die rationalen Komponenten in jenen psychosomatischen Gegebenheiten über, ja sie greifen schließlich über das ganze hier thematische Verhältnis zwischen Affekten, Wahrnehmungnen und Gedanken hinaus. Wenn die neuzeitliche Philosophie der Vernunft das Prinzip der Subjektivität ins Spiel bringt, so auch und insbesondere hinsichtlich dieses psychosomatischen Grundverhältnisses. Es gibt danach konkrete reale Zusammenhänge zwischen Affekten, Wahrnehmungen und Gedanken nur unter der Bedingung einer möglichen Einheit des Bewußtseins, des Selbstbewußtseins, des Ich, der Person etc. Insofern besteht aber auch immer ein Zusammenhang zwischen Störungen psychosomatischer Gegebenheiten einerseits und Störungen der Subjektivität andererseits. Diese Störungen färben gewissermaßen aufeinander ab. Im einzelnen sind Störungen der Affekte, der Wahrnehmungen und der Gedanken Störungen der Subjektivität selbst, sei es in Form von Störungen des Bewußtseins, des Selbstbewußtseins, des Ich, oder des Geistes, der Person etc. Sie können aber auch solche Störungen verursachen, so wie umgekehrt Störungen der Subjektivität Ursachen der Störungen im Bereich der Affekte, der Wahrnehmungen und der Gedanken sein können. Was hier Ursache, was Wirkung des jeweils anderen ist, hängt von größeren lebensgeschichtlichen Zusammenhängen ab. Kant nennt als ein Beispiel für krankhafte Leidenschaft die Rachsucht. Diese wird das Wahrnehmungs- und Denkvermögen nicht unberührt lassen, sondern ganz ihrer Sucht unterwerfen und dementsprechend verändern. So finden wir in der Wahrnehmung und im Denken des Rachsüchtigen eine Form von Vernünftigkeit oder Klugheit, die Arglist, die man als eine Perversion der Klugheit ansehen muß. Aber in einem rachsüchtigen, arglistigen Menschen ist offenkundig auch die Subjektivität, das Selbstbewußtsein und Ich, tiefgreifend gestört. Auch der logische Egoismus und die Borniertheit gehören zu den menschlichen Unvollkommenheiten, welche die Subjektivität, - das Bewußtsein und Selbstbewußtsein - nicht unberührt lassen, und dies um so weniger, je stärker das entsprechende Verhalten gestört ist. Das gleiche läßt sich von den Störungen der Aufmerksamkeit und des Gedächtnisses, der Antizipationskraft und des Realitätssinnes sagen. Auch hier sind die Störungen oft durch Affekte und Leidenschaften verursacht und ziehen über kurz oder lang die Subjektivität insgesamt in Mitleidenschaft. Wann und aus welchen Anlässen es hier zu bleibenden Störungen der Subjektivität kommt, ist eine offene Frage. Ist umgekehrt die Subjektivität in ihrem Bewußtsein oder Selbstbewußtsein oder am Ende sogar in ihrem Ich nachhaltig gestört, so werden zwangsläufig die Affekte, die Wahrnehmungen und Gedanken und der Zusammenhang zwischen diesen teils mehr, teils weniger gestört sein.

Die Differenz zwischen Vollkommenheit und Störung, zwischen Ordnung und Unordnung setzt, wie relativ auch immer, bestimmte Werte und Normen voraus, hinsichtlich derer von einer solchen Differenz überhaupt die Rede sein kann. Vom Standpunkt einer Philosophie der Vernunft aus verweisen diese Werte und Normen auf vorauszusetzende Grundwerte und Grundnormen. Neben der Vernunft als solcher spielt die Natur die Rolle eines solchen Grundwertes, bzw. einer Grundnorm. Dabei erweisen sich diese beiden Bestimmungen der Vernunft und der Natur als eigentümlich ineinander verschränkt. Sie sind in gewisser Weise ein- und dasselbe, in anderer Hinsicht sind sie es nicht. Sie sind miteinander identisch, sofern die Vernunft als der Inbegriff aller Gesetze der Natur, und die Natur selbst als umfassende Gesetzmäßigkeit des Verhaltens natürlicher Dinge angesehen wird. Sie sind nicht identisch, sofern der Vernunft eine wie immer beschaffene Sinnlichkeit gegenüber tritt, in der es zwar Vernunft geben mag, die aber nicht in der Vernünftigkeit selbst aufgeht. So rechnen wir nicht nur die Vernunft, sondern auch die Affekte, Wahrnehmungen und Gedanken als jeweils sinnliche Gegebenheiten zu den "natürlichen Dingen", wie auch die Modi der Subjektivität - Bewußtsein, Selbstbewußtsein, Ich, bzw. Geist. Schließlich und vor allem ist der Mensch, was immer er als Mensch darüber hinaus sein mag, in seiner psychosomatischen Grundverfassung, in seiner Affektivität und Rationalität ein natürliches Ding (ens naturale). Dank der Nicht-Identität von Natur und Vernunft gibt es das Unnatürliche und das Unvernünftige, das Widernatürliche und Widervernünftige, und zwar das eine und das andere in unzähligen Spielarten der Negation. In diesen Negationen negieren sich Natur und Vernunft im Gegensatz zu ihrer Übereinstimmung. Hier aber ist nun daran zu erinnern, daß der Begriff der Natur nicht eindeutig ist, zumindest nicht, wenn wir von der Natur des Menschen und der Menschenwelt, von einem natürlichen oder unnatürlichen, wenn nicht widernatürlichen Verhalten sprechen. Auch wenn die Grenzen zwischen den verschiedenen möglichen Bedeutungen von "Natur" nicht eindeutig zu ziehen sind und sich diese Bedeutungen in verschiedener Weise überlagern, so lassen sich doch zumindest folgende Begriffe einer Natur unterscheiden: 1. Die Natur, sofern der Mensch in seinen Fähigkeiten und Verhaltensweisen als ein Naturwesen unter anderen angesehen wird, der mit diesen in einer gemeinsamen naturgeschichtlichen Entwicklung vorkommt; 2. die Natur, als Inbegriff aller sozialen und kulturellen Leistungen des Menschen, die ihm wie eine Natur an sich gegenübertreten, und zwar unter Absehung von den spezifischen Differenzen zwischen den Gesellschaften und Kulturen. Man kann diesen zweiten Begriff einer Natur im Unterschied zur ersten, materialen Natur die formale Natur des Menschen nennen.

Daneben gibt es eine dritte Natur in Form der Durchschnittlichkeit menschlicher Seins- und Verhaltensweisen. Solche Durchschnittlichkeit gibt es in der ersten und in der zweiten Natur, so wie es hier und dort Abweichungen von diesem Durchschnitt gibt, Abweichungen nach oben und nach unten, als Unter- und Überdurchschnittlichkeit. Schließlich ist von dieser dritten Natur eine vierte zu unterscheiden, Natur als Alltäglichkeit.[12] Alltäglichkeit fällt nicht mit Durchschnittlichkeit zusammen. Alltäglichkeit gibt es nur in der zweiten Natur, sofern alle menschlichen Gesellschaften und Kulturen die Differenz zwischen dem Alltäglichen und dem Unalltäglichen kennen. Aber innerhalb des Alltäglichen gibt es ebenso Druchschnittlichkeit und Undurchschnittlichkeit wie innerhalb des Unalltäglichen.

Diese vier Naturen können nun nach den bisherigen Feststellungen als vernünftig, aber auch als unvernünftig angesehen werden. Sofern es sich bei den Affekten, Wahrnehmungen und Gedanken um "natürliche Gegenstände" handelt, sind sie als solche wie auch hinsichtlich möglicher Störungen in ihren Zusammenhängen nach dieser vierfachen Bedeutung von Natur zu unterscheiden. Die Konsequenzen einer solchen vierfachen Unterscheidung bedürfen nunmehr einer ausführlichen Ausarbeitung. Die erste dieser Konsequenzen ist, daß durch diese Unterscheidung der Rahmen der überlieferten neuzeitlichen Vernunftphilosophie endgültig gesprengt wird.

Zusammenfassung: Die vorliegende Abhandlung versucht in Auseinandersetzung mit der Ethik des SPINOZA und der Transzendentalphilosophie KANTS als zwei paradigmatischen Vernunftphilosophien, Prinzipien einer Theorie der Rationalität hinsichtlich der Affekte, Wahrnehmungen und Gedanken zu entwickeln. In dieser Perspektive werden die Affekte als Denk- und Wahrnehmungsstörungen thematisiert unter den Aspekten (1) der möglichen Örter einer Erörterung in Logik, Ethik und Psychologie; (2) der Störungen als Störungen der Rationalität menschlicher Erkenntnis in den klassischen Vernunfttheorien; (3) bezüglich eines möglichen Konfliktes zwischen Rationalität und Kausalität. Es ergeben sich hieraus Relativität und Komplementarität als Prinzipien der Störungen. Für Relatives und Komplementäres läßt sich, über eine rationale Kritik hinaus, das Prinzip der richtigen Mitte fruchtbar machen. Die Relativität von Vollkommenheit und Störung, Ordnung und Unordnung wird an bestimmten Normen und Werten erst differenzierbar. Als solche Normen erweisen sich Vernunft und Natur. Mit einer Überlegung zur Vieldeutigkeit der Natur im gestörten Ich wird das Thema für weitergehende Ausarbeitungen eröffnet.

12 Die von M. HEIDEGGER in der Philosophie unseres Jahrhunderts ausgearbeitete Theorie der Alltäglichkeit hat zwar das Verdienst, gegenüber den traditionellen Bedeutungen von Natur die vierte Bedeutung thematisch gemacht zu haben. Damit aber ist zugleich ihre eigene Unzulänglichkeit beschrieben. Es fehlt in dieser Theorie der Alltäglichkeit ein hinreichend deutlicher Verweis auf die formale Natur. Außerdem bleibt das Verhältnis von Alltäglichkeit und Durchschnittlichkeit ganz ungeklärt. Auf die Schwierigkeiten der "Ausarbeitung der Idee eines 'natürlichen Weltbegriffes'" verweist HEIDEGGER selbst (vgl. *Sein und Zeit*, S. 52).

Affects as Disturbances of Perception and Thought

Summary: Dealing with two paradigmatic philosophies of reason, SPINOZA's Ethics and KANT's Transcendental Philosophy, an attempt is made to develop principles of a theory of rationality with regard to emotions, perceptions, and thoughts. In this perspective emotions are discussed as disturbances of thought and perception in respect to (1) possible places of such a discussion within logic, ethics, and psychology; (2) the disturbances being disturbances of the rationality of human knowledge within the classical theories of reason; (3) a possible conflict between rationality and causality. This reveales relativity and complementarity as principles of the disturbances. The dimensions of relative and complementary things, of the more or less of order and disorder, perfection and disturbance can be ordered by the principle of the right mean. Relativity and more or less presuppose a certain standard of value: reason and nature. The discussion of the ambiguity of nature in the disturbed I opens up the subject for further elaboration.

Literatur

HEIDEGGER, M. (1979): Sein und Zeit, 15. Aufl. Niemeyer, Tübingen.

KANT, I. (1781; 1787; 1911): Kritik der reinen Vernunft (KdrV). Gesammelte Schriften, herausgegeben von der Königlich Preußischen Akademie der Wissenschaften, Bde. III und IV, Berlin.

KANT, I. (1789; 1917): Anthropologie in pragmatischer Hinsicht. Gesammelte Schriften, herausgegeben von der Königlich Preußischen Akademie der Wissenschaften, Bd. VII., Berlin.

KANT, I. (1800; 1923): Logik. Hg. von G.B. JÄSCHE. Gesammelte Schriften, herausgegeben von der Königlich Preußischen Akademie der Wissenschaften, Bd. IX, Berlin.

PLATO (1900ff): Opera. Ed. I. BURNET, Oxford.

PLATO (1967): Sophistes. Hg. von R. WIEHL. Meiner, Hamburg.

SPINOZA, B. DE (1924): Opera. Im Auftrag der Heidelberger Akademie der Wissenschaften herausgegeben von C. GEBHARDT. Heidelberg.

SPINOZA, B. DE (1665; 1976): Die Ethik nach geometrischer Methode dargestellt. Meiner, Hamburg.

SPINOZA, B. DE (1662, 1663; 1977): Abhandlung über die Verbesserung des Verstandes. Meiner, Hamburg.

TELLENBACH, H. (1988): Subjekt und Person in der Medizin. Neue Hefte für Philosophie 27/28, S. 135-165.

WIEHL, R. (1983): Die Vernunft in der menschlichen Unvernunft. Das Problem der Rationalität in Spinozas Affektenlehre. Vandenhoeck-Rupprecht, Hamburg.

"Feelings" of Conviction: On the Relation of Affect and Thought Disorder

G. Oepen, A. Harrington, M. Spitzer, M. Fünfgeld

1. Introducing the Problem: Thought Disorder and Affect

Although usually associated with psychotic illness such as schizophrenia, the phenomena of formal and contentual thought disorder are actually rather common even among individuals not normally considered to be disturbed. BLEULER complained about the "autistic-undisciplined way of thought" (autistisch-undiszipliniertes Denken) of his fellow scientists, and MAHER has more recently stressed the point that "deluded patients are like normal people - including scientists - who seem extremely resistant to giving up their preferred theories even in the face of damningly negative evidence" (MAHER 1988, p. 22)

Not only delusional, but also technically formal thought disorders have their place in everyday life. Self-interruptions, word-finding difficulty, confusion, perseveration and incoherence - familiar to every psychiatrist - are also familiar in common situations associated with emotional stress: oral examinations, declarations of love, legal interrogations, lecturing. FREUD (1901, 1917) was the first to demonstrate convincingly that the kind of mistake and the context in which it occurs may sometimes tell us something about the material responsible for the affective arousal.

The fact that both formal and delusional thought disorders appear in otherwise normal and healthy people, coupled with the fact that delusions have also been formally identified in pathological conditions of all kinds (from paranoid schizophrenia to 20 neurological syndromes, 16 metabolic and endocrine disorders, and a very large number of syndromes associated with alcohol and other forms of substance abuse; cf. MAHER and ROSS 1984), raises some doubts about the usual assumption that some underlying breakdown of cognitive/brain functioning is always or necessarily the immediate cause of a thought disorder. MAHER (1988) has in fact argued that many delusions are much more likely to be secondary, reactive - and fully comprehensible - responses to some personal situation associated with bodily disabilities, unaccustomed sensory or motor experiences, or both. MAHER makes no claims to comprehensiveness, however, and leaves open the possibility that other noncognitive primary influences, yet to be defined, may also be important, both in delusional states and in the outbreak of formal thought disorders.

Drawing on the results of extensive experimental studies with paranoid schizophrenics, this paper proposes to consider the possibility that one of these noncognitive factors may in fact be arousal associated with emotional stress. Bleuler long ago argued that the affective state is primary in human experience, setting the frame for both thought and action: every individual's affective frame is, so to say, "filled up" with the logical argumentation we call thinking (Bleuler 1926). If Bleuler is at all right, it begins to look as if it makes little sense to study thinking disorders in isolation from their affective context.

Indeed this basic proposition, as we have stated it, is hardly new: the last 120 years of psychiatric thinking have seen considerable speculation about the role of affect in the genesis of formal and, above all, on contentual thought disorders (delusions). We are at once enriched and hindered by this historical heritage, for at least some of the problems we encounter in clarifying our ideas on this theme have historical roots. Only by making ourselves conscious of certain contradictions and instances of question-begging that have cropped up in the past, can we perhaps avoid falling victim to similar failures ourselves when we go on to interprete our own experimental data.

We will here more or less leave aside the history of thought on the relation between affect and simple formal thought disorders (cf. Jackson 1880, Freud 1901) in order to concentrate briefly on the more problematic history of thinking about the relation between affect and contentual thought disorders (delusions). In the psychiatric literature of the past 120 years, two main lines of thought can be isolated.

The first of these has its intellectual roots in the word of Hagen who, in 1870, had declared that delusions suffered by patients "grow and develop rapidly" under the influence of emotional stress. He has explained the fact that many delusional patients show no obvious manifestations of disturbed affectivity, writing: "The disturbed affect may not be recognized, not only because patients are able to control themselves or because doctors do not always investigate this possibility closely enough, but also - as a third reason - because the severity of the delusion itself may tend to mask or distract from the disturbed affect" (Hagen 1870, p. 62).

Hagen's argument for a clear causal link between emotional disorder and delusional thinking has founded a tradition in European psychiatry that was to be carried on by such distinguished psychiatrists as Kraepelin, Specht (whose book *On pathological affect in chronic paranoia* was published in 1901), and E. Bleuler. The latter was to elaborate on an hypothesis earlier formulated by Kraepelin, which held that delusions are a secondary consequence of primary disorders of reasoning ("die intellectuellen Verarbeitung von Vorstellungen"), and that these disorders are in turn often influenced by emotions and mood (thus extending the link between affect and delusion over two stages of breakdown) (Kraepelin 1889, p.109). As Bleuler saw it, disturbed affect first acts to create delusions by weakening mental associations [Schaltschwaeche], and thereby logical connections between ideas. "If these logical connections are weakened, the influence of affectivity is [further] increased" (BLEULER 1911, p. 814).

In recent years, the classic KRAEPELIN-BLEULER model of a one-way causal relationship between affect, formal thought disorder and delusions has been freshly challenged. AVENARIUS (1978, p.61) has suggested that some patients with delusions of grandeur in fact use thought confusion and incoherence (formal thought disorder) as a tactic to avoid having to confront the dissonance between their delusions and the considerably more drab reality of their lives. NEALE, in a recent article, has proposed that certain manic episodes (involving disturbances of affect and formal thought) have the defensive function of "keeping distressing cognitions and currently distressing life events out of consciousness" (NEALE 1988, p. 147). In other words, a dynamic interactive relationship is envisioned between potentially paranoid (or at any rate highly distressing) ideas and perceptions of life events, formal thought disorders and manic pathological affect.

Notwithstanding the eminence of the above-described school of thought which follow HAGEN, SPECHT and BLEULER's emphasis on the importance of affective disorder in delusioned thinking (cf. WEINSCHENK 1965), it remains a fact that "many leading psychiatrists deny that delusional persons show any excessive affect or any more than was present before the delusions appeared" (ARTHUR 1964, p. 110). The nay-sayers on this theme can be traced back historically to KARL JASPERS, who was the first to introduce the distinction between primary and secondary delusions. The former would be characterized by the impossibilty of deriving them from other disorders, especially affective disorders. KURT SCHNEIDER built on the JASPERS dipartite model by speaking of true delusional beliefs [echte Wahnideen] and delusion-like beliefs [wahnaehnliche Ideen]. A delusion that could be traced back to disturbed affect or mood was to be considered, not a true delusion, but simply a delusion-like belief.

Although the point of view proposed by JASPERS and SCHNEIDER is not generally considered acceptable today (cf. WINTERS and NEALE 1983), it is still useful in illuminating the historical roots of certain current diagnositic habits: the modern distinction between thought disorders accompanied by mood-congruence vs. those accompanied by mood-incongruence is nothing more than a reformulation of the Jasperain concept of primary vs. secondary delusions and that Schneiderian one of true delusions vs. delusion-like ideas. The DSM-III-R (p. 402) defines mood-incongruent psychotic features as follows: "Delusions or hallucinations whose content is not consistent with either a depressed or a manic [presenting] mood." The seemingly straightforward or objective-sounding terms "congruence" and "consistency" may be misleading: in fact, we are dealing with a hermeneutically-derived judgement (what sort of mood is "appropriate" or "consistent" with what delusional belief?), and not very far from the sort of distinctions JASPERS and SCHNEIDER were trying to make.

The history of thought concerning the relation between affect and delusion thus unearths a spectrum of hypotheses ranging from the view that every delusion is ultimately caused by a primary underlying affective disorder to theories that exclude by definition any causal role for affect in the rise of (true) delusions. Given such a stalemate situation, it would seem reasonable to see what might be gained by attempting to supplement classical clinical observation and theorizing with new experimental data relevant to the subject.

2. Concept and Design of Experiment

The design of our experimental study on the interaction of affect and cognition took its starting point from the unexpected results of an earlier experimental study of cognitive defects in paranoid schizophrenic patients (OEPEN et al. 1985). In a divided visual field study requiring recognition of randomly presented letters in both visual fields, we were struck by unexpected fluctuations in the performance levels of our patients. Also striking was the fact that these fluctuations were differentially distributed between the two visual fields. Interviews with the patients afterwards then unearthed a pattern of increased anxiety, acoustic hallucinations and emotional tension that correlated with those episodes where performance had deteriorated. This discovery sensitized us to the recognition of similar interference patterns in normal clinical life: thus we were able to use our experimental findings to account for the way in which a certain schizophrenic patient became notably more incoherent and confused in his thinking when recounting emotionally-loaded biographical details (in this case, loss of a girlfriend) than when the conversation focused on more neutral topics.

Coming from this background, our goal was to devise a test that could control and measure the way in which heightened emotional levels might interact with changing cognitive performance levels, thus reproducing (to be sure, in simplified model form) the sorts of spontaneously occurring fluctuations we had already observed. We were also interested in tracking down the significance of those earlier-noted asymmetries in performance disturbance; i.e. in explaining the fact that anxiety or emotional stress seemed to work differentially on performance levels in the two visual fields. Accordingly, we designed a tachistoscopic divided visual field study that combined introduction of a pseudo-random emotional stimulator with a lexical and nonverbal (face/nonface) decision task. We were especially interested in possible relations between the degree of paranoid symptomatology, thought disorder and performance patterns in the left and right visual fields. The combination of verbal and nonverbal decision tasks with targetting to the two visual fields was predicated upon two assumptions: first, that tachistoscopic divided visual field techniques are in a position to cast reliable light on cerebral hemisphere functional asymmetries; and second, that left hemisphere processes are more specialized for all language-related tasks, whereas the right hemisphere is more specialized for nonverbal, visual-perceptual skills such as face recognition (for a survey see SPRINGER and DEUTSCH 1986, HEILMANN und SATZ 1983). In other words, using verbal (word/nonword) and nonverbal (face/nonface) decision tasks in conjunction with tachistocopic targetting methods offered us a means of selectively engaging one or the other hemisphere (relatively speaking) in an experimentally controllable manner. We were then able selectively to manipulate that engagement with the further introduction of experimental emotional stimulators (cf. OEPEN et al. 1988a).

2.1 Subjects and Methods

50 right-handed male acute schizophrenic inpatients (ICD 9: 295.1 and 295.3; fulfilling the RDC-criteria for acute schizophrenia); and 30 age, sex and handedness matched controls (inpatients of the surgical ward of the Dermatological Department without central nervous system pathology) participated with informed consent in the study. Psychopathology for all 3 groups was assessed using the Brief Psychiatric Rating Scale, BPRS (Overall and Gorham 1976) and the Self Rating Paranoid-Depressivitäts-Skala; PDS (von Zerssen 1976). Each group was required to perform a lexical decision task with German function words and pronouncable nonsense words, which were presented simultaneously on each side of a fixation point within 1-3 degrees excentricity. Exposure time was 120 ms. The subjects had to press a lever ipsilateral to the target stimulus (word) with their index fingers as fast as possible. Each one consisted of 36 cards: 12 targets in the left visual field, 12 in the right visual field and 12 bilateral non-targets. Two runs were shown without experimental interference. In the third, 3 "emotional stimulators" (a provocative review of a nude, a drawing of a spider, and the Rorschach inkblot No. 10) were each shown additionally, each once in each hemifield. The full experimental sequence thus consisted of 2 runs without emotional stimuli, followed by a "stimulator" run, both for the word and the face task. Stimulus presentation was pseudorandom as to visual field, pairing of stimulators with targets or non-targets, and place of insertion between the regular test items as used in runs 1 and 2. The percentage of correct responses as well as reaction times were calculated by MANOVA. A significance level of $p = .05$ was adopted.

As supplement to this main experiment, right and left distal motoric hand-functions (movements with the strongest contralateral hemispheric control) were compared in paranoid schizophrenic patients versus normal controls. Three paper and pencil tasks were used: running through a maze; dotting circles; and dotting squares as fast as possible (Steingrueber 1971). The time required for the completion of the task was measured.

3. Results

3.1 Impact of Emotional Stimulators on Visual Field Testing

In the first runs without emotional stimulators, schizophrenics and controls displayed the expected patterns of perceptual asymmetry in the word task with better performance of the left hemisphere in the right visual field. However, schizophrenic patients performed at a considerably lower absolute level. In the trials with added emotional stimuli, controls showed a pronounced bilateral improvement, especially in the visual hemifield dominant for the task (right visual field); i.e. the degree of task-specific hemifield asymmetry increased in these subjects. Schizophrenic patients, in contrast, showed a general deterioration in left visual field performance, simultaneous with marked improvement in right visual field performance.

Reaction time results of correct responses were calculated from runs both with and without emotional stimulation and revealed distinctly different reactivity patterns for the left and the right visual field in the schizophrenic and control groups. In schizophrenics, right visual field reaction times improved without significant changes in left visual field, whereas controls showed a bilateral improvement more pronounced in the left visual field. MANOVA revealed a significant difference between schizophrenic patients and controls ($F(1.94) = 5.22$, $p = .025$).

3.2 Correlation of Test Results with Psychopathology

In schizophrenics, the BPRS-subscale "thought disorder" was significantly correlated with correct answers in the word test in the left visual field ($p = .058$). In other words, it turns out that active right hemisphere contribution in language related tasks is formally correlated with thought disorder in schizophrenia. Within the schizophrenic group, the interaction "paranoid vs. nonparanoid" x "left visual field vs. right visual field" was significant (F (1,38) = 6.22; p = .017). In other words, the subgroup of paranoid schizophrenic patients (dichotomized at the median of PDSP-scale) showed a marked advantage of the left visual field, or evidence of greater right-hemisphere activity, over nonparanoid schizophrenic patients, even in tasks normally associated with right visual field or left hemisphere dominance (i.e. word task). No significant differences were found between schizophrenics with positive versus negative symptomatology, or between hebephrenics versus paranoid-hallucinatory patients.

3.3 Results of Testing for Motoric Asymmetries

The paper and pencil tracking tasks revealed significantly larger motoric left-right differences in schizophrenic patients than in controls (p = .001). While the BPRS-subscale "thought disorder" correlated negatively with the motor performance of both hands (left hand -.4301, p = .032, right hand -.5057, p = with left hand motor performance (-.4139, p = .040). After successful neuroleptic treatment, these correlations disappeared. Analysing the total frequency of lever pressing in the tachistoscopic task, taking together correct and false answers of the right and left hand, schizophrenics showed a prevailing tendency of left hand lever pressing, whereas controls pressed the lever more often with the right hand. As both groups were righthanders and could not be separated statistically using a questionnaire (Oldfield 1971) and the Hand-Dominanz-Test (Steingrüber 1971), one may conclude that only controls showed the expected preponderance of right hand use. Looking only at false positive answers, this becomes still clearer: whereas controls showed an equal frequency of false positive reactions with their right and left hand, schizophrenics showed more false positive reactions with their left hand than with their right hand. Both observations point to an increased motoric activity of the left hand in the schizophrenic group, a consequence of the presumed more activated right hemisphere.

4. Discussion

4.1 Thought Disorder, Affect and the Right Hemisphere

The correlation of the BPRS-subscale (contentual) thought disorder and the PDS-subscale paranoid symptoms with right-hemisphere performance in the left visual field points to a specific link between right hemispheric activation and thought disorder. In other words, the diagnosis of thought disorder in schizophrenic patients seems to be positively correlated with the extent of the right hemisphere's contribution to language-related tasks.

The sudden release of left-hemisphere competence during the emotional trials argues against the wide-spread assumption of an underlying language-related, left-hemisphere bound cognitive impairment as a basis for schizophrenic thought disorder (Flor-Henry 1983). Regarding the assumption of a relative predominance of the right hemisphere for affective processes, this finding also suggests that the higher the degree of affective stress suffered by a patient, the more probable it is that thought disorder will occur. In this context, it is interesting that Mathew et al. (1988) reported finding a significant correlation between "suspiciousness" and "unusual thought content" (BPRS) on the one hand, and heightened posterior right hemispheric blood flow on the other.

As the notion of "affect" is conceptually crucial to our argument, a few comments at this juncture are in order: "Affect" is not a homogenous quality, and the notion of "more or less" affectivity is necessarily a simplifying one. In speaking of "affect" or "affective stress" above, we often, though not always, had in mind "anxiety". Yet one might rightly wonder whether it is the affective experience of anxiety that is truly causally critical here, or rather the high level of physiological arousal associated with this affective state. Further investigations on a broader statistical basis and with other kind of stimulants (perhaps using chemical drugs like amphetamines: cf. HERMLE et al.1988) are needed to decide on this issue.

4.2 The Neuroleptic Effect

Our experiments have further shown (OEPEN et al. 1988a,b) that neurochemical stabilization of a morbidly irritable right hemisphere makes it possible for the schizophrenic brain to respond positively to a form of emotional stimulation that had earlier resulted in performance deterioration. Changes were especially marked for the right-hemispheric face-test: This performance improvement in the laboratory was associated with an improved clinical picture, as assessed above all (for our purposes) in a sharp drop in scores testing for thought disorder. In short, our findings indicate a clear relationshipship between biochemically-induced stabilization of the right hemisphere and reduction in severity of thought disorder. This is naturally what one would expect if it is really so (as our findings indicate) that a hyperactive right hemisphere is critical to the genesis of this disorder.

4.3 Delusions and Brain Laterality: A 2-Stage Developmental Model

In a recent article on delusions HEMSLEY and GARETY (1986, p. 51) note that "it appears to be essential to distinguish between the establishment and maintenance of belief systems". Indeed, our data have inspired us to speculate on the possibility of deriving a neuropsychological model of delusion formation and maintenance, one in which initial ("right-hemispheric") affective responses to a situation are then buttressed and solidified through the further working out of narrative details - a secondary contribution of left hemispheric language mechanisms.

This point might be illustrated by the case history of a patient - a lonely widow living under isolated circumstances - who developed a first-time paranoid-hallucinatory psychosis with strong delusional beliefs of being influenced by the neighbors: she explained how they were molesting her with radioactive rays that manipulated her, above all, genitally. In conversation with the patient, it proved possible to show her how one might distinguish between her nonverbal experience (ill-defined sensations of genital itching and warmth) and her explanation thereof (the neighbors molesting her with rays). After an hour's interview, she was prepared to concede that her feelings, while undoubtedly real, had perhaps less to do with her neighbors' ill-will and more with her admitted loneliness and longing for sexual contact.

More direct neurological support for our laterality model of delusion formation comes from the well-known split-brain patient case reported by GAZZANIGA and LEDOUX (1978). The patient began by using his (right-hemisphere controlled) left hand to select a picture of a snow shovel, which he matched to a picture of a winter landscape flashed to his (right hemisphere controlled) left visual field (as the task demanded). His (left-hemisphere controlled) right visual field had at the same time been shown a picture of a chicken claw, and his right hand matched that to a picture of a chicken. Asked to explain his left hand selection (the shovel), he confabulated a plausible "left hemisphere" story ("chickens make a lot of mess, and you need a shovel to clean out the chicken coop") consistent with the material "seen" by the (verbal-conscious) left hemisphere.

Although the above described 2-stage laterality model of delusional formation and maintenance finds support in both clinical and experimental data, we would still stress that we recognise that it is a highly over-simplified model from a neurophysiological point of view (emotional convictions are not "in" the right hemisphere and verbal qualifications are not "in" the left). At the same time, we are convinced that such a model - even if it is wrong in many details - has heuristic value, offering us a "space" in which to conceptualize stages in a difficult and obscure psychological process, and challenging us to begin to think seriously as to how these processes might be more precisely "mapped" onto the brain. At best, then what we are presenting here represents the first rough outline of a robust neuropsychological approach to understanding delusions; at worst, we are volunteering a "useful fiction" that could serve ultimately to stimulate better, neurophysiologically more sophisticated models of the phenomena under discussion.

4.4 Formal Thought Disorder, Delusions, and Affect

With regard to the relation of formal thought disorder, affective disturbances and delusions, our model points to disturbed affect as a *cause* and *not* a *consequence* of formal thought and contentual thought disorder. Furthermore, what AVENARIUS describes as a "need for getting confused" in deluded patients who are confronted with reality should be explained in terms of a raised affective level of these patients during confrontation, which leads to formal thought disorder.

4.5 Delusions, "Felt Significance", and the Right Hemisphere

We are intrigued by the fact that the laterality model of delusion formation sketched above seems to suggest a neuropsychological framework for interpreting MAHER's phenomenological description of delusional patients: hypervigilant, closely scanning the environment, and finding great significance in coincidences. Indeed, sensitivity to coincidence represents one of the most basic characteristics of the delusional condition. MAHER speaks of "neuropathological activation of brain centers responsible for mediating the experience of significance. The coincidence is detected in the course of a very close scrutiny of the environment, which, in turn, was provoked by the need to discover the basis of felt significance (MAHER 1988, p. 30). This "felt significance" seems, then, to be a critical trigger for the development of delusional thinking. As such, it is not itself a cognitive quality, but rather pre-cognitive, and may be associated with vigilance or undirected attentiveness.

According to our own model, this pre-cognitive - or, if one will, affective "feeling of significance - needs to be understood as a "right-hemisphere" experience which causally precedes the "left-hemisphere" verbal explanation thereof. Is there in fact any reason to believe that such experiences of "felt significance" are asymmetrically moderated in the brain? We propose a cautious "yes".

To begin, there exists in the literature evidence that the right hemisphere is generally dominant for attentional and affective processes (cf. e.g. HEILMAN and SATZ 1983, GESCHWIND 1982), but this fact alone would not justify the argument we wish to make. More concrete evidence for a right hemisphere role in the pathological processes here under discussion may be found in studies of temporal lobe epilepsy associated with so-called "dreamy states". Two points are important here:

(1) In its simplest form, the "dreamy state" experience is phenomenologically often quite similar to Maher's description of the experience of "felt significance". Patients typically experience a disorienting sense of déjà vu or jamais vu; things "feel" strangely familiar or strangely unfamiliar, and there is often also a powerful "tip-of-the-tongue"-like experience without any clear content - a strong "feeling" of being on the verge of remembering something important.

(2) There is evidence dating back to the 19th-century that this experience is associated with discharges in the right temporal lobe.

HUGHLINGS JACKSON in 1880 was the first to notice the association between the dreamy state and epileptic convulsions of right hemispheric origin. He himself was inclined, however, to see the state itself, not as a product of the right hemisphere, but as a a product of the non-afflicted left hemisphere, reacting sympathetically to the violent activity levels of its twin (JACKSON 1880-81). Others, however, disagreed. Thus both CRICHTON-BROWNE (1895) and ARNOLD PICK (1903) made reference to the primary role of the right side of the brain in the production of "dreamy state" phenomena, finding support for their argument in the frequent association of the latter with various left-sided disorders of sensation. More recently, WILDER PENFIELD, using electrical stimulation techniques on the exposed brains of conscious epileptics, was able to provide more direct experimental evidence for the argument. He found that, when he stimulated the temporal lobes, he was able to elicit certain subjective signals whose function seemed to be "to interpret the relationship of the individual to his immediate environment: Examples of such signals are: these things are 'familiar' or 'frightening', they are 'coming nearer' or 'going away'; and so on" (PENFIELD 1975, p. 442). Although PENFIELD's interpretive signals appeared for the most part bilaterally represented, there were two notable exceptions: In the great majority of cases, visual illusions and illusions bearing on the passing of time, notably the "feeling of familiarity" or "dreamy mental states" could be evoked by stimulating the right hemisphere only (MULLAN and PENFIELD 1959, p. 283).

There is also less direct, but nevertheless suggestive evidence for a relationship between nonverbal *significance*-generating mechanisms and right-hemisphere processing. The deluded patient's "search for significance" may, for example, be usefully compared to the schizophrenic, possibly right-hemispheric tendency to "physiognomize" the environment.[1] While phenomenologically quite different, one may speculate that the underlying processes giving rise to both experiences may be based on a similar principle: a semi-uncontrolled "over-readiness" by preconscious systems in the brain to generate "meaningfull hypotheses" out of ambiguous perceptual "data" (cf. GREGEORY 1973, EMRICH, this volume).

5. Conclusion

The following contribution has aimed to look at how far one might attack the problem of the relationship between affect and thought disorder from an experimental basis; thus moving beyond the largely semantic and descriptive-clinical levels of argument that have tended to dominate the historical debate to date. As is doubtless clear, our results do not leave us with any final solution to the problem, but do encourage us to believe that we are slowly moving into a position to ask better questions - questions which may, in turn, suggest new empirical approaches. On the one hand, we are encouraged to believe, given our results, that affective experience can - even if it need not always - directly trigger delusional thinking, the latter then being understood as the accounting "hypothesis" explaining the feeling. On the other hand, we are still lacking sophisticated means of modelling how qualitatively different forms of "affect" might interact differently with the formation and maintenance of a delusion. We also need to develop better ways of thinking about affective experience along the parameter of time: JASPERS, SCHNEIDER and their followers may be right when they point out (as counter-argument to the KRAEPELIN-BLEULER theory of affect in thought-disorders) that paranoid patients do not show a stable disturbance of affect over time. This does not mean that the affect-thought-disorder theory is fundamentally flawed, but rather that one might need to begin thinking of affect/thought-disorder interaction as an instable, dynamic phenomenon. According to our own model, such dynamic instability could be neurologically explained in terms of the experimentally demonstrated instability of right hemisphere functioning and interhemispheric balance in paranoid schizophrenic patients.

Summary: The long-standing historical debate on the relationship between affect and thought disorder is here reexamined in the light of new experimental findings on lateralized cognitive performance in paranoid schizophrenics, both with and without the addition of experimentally controlled emotional stimulation. On runs without emotional stimulations, a correlation was found between

1 For a critical discussion cf. HARRINGTON et al., this volume.

the BPRS-subscale "thought disorder", the PDS-subscale "paranoid symptoms", and right hemisphere performance in a lexical decision task. In other words, it seems that a diagnosis of thought disorder in schizophrenia is positively correlated with the extend of the right hemisphere's contribution to language related tasks. On runs with emotional stimulation, a breakdown in right hemisphere performance was found, coupled with a release of left hemisphere cognitive capacity. This suggests that the right, not the left hemisphere is primarily disordered in schizophrenia, in contrast to what is normally claimed in the literature. These findings are incorporated into a neuropsychological two stage model of delusion formation and maintenance in schizophrenia, which stresses the prime role of right hemisphere affective responses to novel or inexplicable experiences, and the secondary contribution of presumably left hemispheric narrative or language processes. MAHER's theory of delusions - especially his discussion of the problem of "felt significance" - is reexamined in light of our model, where evidence is offered suggesting a link between the "felt significance" phenomenon and certain right hemispheric temporolimbic systems.

"Gefühle" der Überzeugung. Zur Beziehung zwischen Affektivität und Denkstörungen

Zusammenfassung: Experimentelle Befunde der Störung asymmetrisch lateralisierter kognitiver Leistungen der Hirnhemisphären (in einer tachistoskopischen Studie) werfen neues Licht auf historische und zeitgenössische Hypothesen zum Zusammenhang von Affekt und Denkstörungen. So fand sich bei akuten paranoid-halluzinatorischen Schizophrenen eine signifikante Korrelation der BPRS-Subskala "Denkstörungen" und der PDS-Subskala "paranoide Symptome" mit der rechtshemisphärischen Leistung in einer lexikalischen Unterscheidungsaufgabe. Dies deutet auf eine Abhängigkeit der klinisch diagnostizierten Denkstörungen vom Ausmaß einer rechtshemisphärischen Beteiligung bei sprachlichen Leistungen hin. In Untersuchungsdurchgängen mit zusätzlichen emotionalen Bildern fand sich ein Zusammenbruch der rechtshemisphärischen Leistungen, bei gleichzeitiger Deblockierung linkshemisphärischer Verarbeitung. Dies stützt die Vermutung, daß bei Schizophrenie die rechte Hemisphäre (nicht die linke) *primär* gestört ist, im Gegensatz zur häufig berichteten Annahme einer primären linkshemisphärischen Dysfunktion. Diese Befunde sind unter anderem Grundlage eines neuropsychologischen Zweistufenmodells von Entstehung und Aufrechterhaltung wahnhafter Denkstörungen bei Schizophrenen. Eine Betonung liegt hierbei auf der besonderen Rolle rechtshemisphärisch-affektiver Reaktionen auf unerwartet neue oder unerklärliche Erfahrungen und der sekundären Beteiligung "linkshemisphärisch"-erklärender bzw. sprachlicher Prozesse. MAHERS Wahntheorie - speziell seine Diskussion der "gefühlsmäßigen Überzeugung" - wird anhand dieses Modells diskutiert. Hierbei neu gesehene Aspekte weisen auf einen Zusammenhang zwischen dem "gefühlsmäßigen Überzeugtsein" von bestimmten Bedeutungszusammenhängen und temporolimbischen Regionen der rechten Hemisphäre hin.

References

AMERICAN PSYCHIATRIC ASSOCIATION (1987): Diagnostic and statistical manual of mental disorders (3rd ed., revised) (DSM-III-R). American Psychiatric Association, Washington, DC.

ARTHUR, A.Z. (1964): Theories and explanations of delusions: A review. The American Journal of Psychiatry **121**, pp. 105-115.

AVENARIUS, R. (1978): Der Größenwahn. Springer, Berlin, Heidelberg, New York.

BERZE, J. (1903): Das Primärsymptom der Paranoia. Marhold, Halle.

BLEULER, E. (1911): Dementia praecox. Deuticke, Leipzig, Wien.

BLEULER, E. (1926): Affektivität, Suggestibilität und Paranoia. Marhold, Halle.

CRICHTON-BROWNE, J. (1895): The Cavendish Lecture on Dreamy Mental States. Bailliere, Tindall & Co., London.

EMRICH, H.M. (1988): Die Beziehung zwischen Philosophie und Psychiatrie vom Standpunkt einer systemtheoretischen Konzeption produktiver Psychosen aus betrachtet. (In diesem Band).

FLOR-HENRY, P. (1983): Cerebral basis of psychopathology. John Wright, Boston.

FREUD, S. (1901/1978): Zur Psychopathologie des Alltagslebens. Gesammelte Werke IV, S. Fischer, Frankfurt.

FREUD, S. (1917/1978): Vorlesungen zur Einführung in die Psychoanalyse, II.-VI. Vorlesung: Die Fehlleistungen. Gesammelte Werke XI, pp. 18-76, S. Fischer, Frankfurt.

GAZZANIGA, M.S., LEDOUX, J.E. (1978): The integrated mind. Plenum Press, New York.

GESCHWIND, N. (1982): Hemishperic specialization: biological foundations. In: KATSUKI, S., TSUBAKI, T., TOYOKURA, Y. (eds.): Neurology, pp. 3-10. Excerpta medica, Elsevier, Amsterdam, Oxford, Princeton.

GRUHLE, H.W. (1932): Die Psychopathologie (der Schizophrenie). In. Bumke, O. (ed.): Handbuch der Geisteskrankheiten, Bd.IX (Die Schizophrenie), pp. 135 - 210, Springer, Berlin.

HAGEN, F.W. (1870): Studien auf dem Gebiete der ärztlichen Seelenheilkunde. Besold, Erlangen.

HARRINGTON A. (1987): Medicine, Mind and the Double Brain: A Study in Nineteenth-Century Thought. Princeton University Press, Princeton, N.J.

HARRINGTON A., OEPEN, G., SPITZER, M., HERMLE, L. (1988): Zur Psychopathologie und Neuropsychologie der Wahrnehmung von Gesichtern. (In diesem Band).

HEILMANN, K.M., SATZ, P. (1983): Neuropsychology of human emotion. Guilford Press, New York.

HEMSLEY. D.R., GARETY, P.A. (1986): The formation and maintenance of delusions: A bayesian analysis. British Journal of Psychiatry **149**, pp. 51-56.

JACKSON, H. (1880-81): On right or left-sided spasm at the onset of epileptic paroxysms, and on crude sensations, warnings, and elaborate mental stateS. Brain **3**, S. 192-205.

JASPERS, K. (1913/1973): Allgemeine Psychopathologie [General Psychopathology]. Springer, Berlin.

KRAEPELIN, E. (1889): Psychiatrie. Abel, Leipzig.

MAHER, B.A. (1988): Anomalous experience and delusional thinking: The logic of explanations. In: OLTMANNS, T.S., MAHER, B.A. (Eds.): Delusional beliefs, pp. 15-33. Wiley, New York, Chichester, Brisbane, Toronto, Singapore.

MAHER, B.A., ROSS, J.S. (1984): Delusions. In: ADAMS, H.E., SUTKER, P.B. (eds.): Comprehensive handbook of psychopathology. Plenum Press, New York.

MATHEW, R.J., WILSON, W.H. TANT, S.R., ROBINSON, L. PRAKSAH, R. (1988): Abnormal resting regional cerebral Blood flow patterns and their correlates in schizophrenia. Archives of general psychiatry **45**, pp. 542-549.

MULLAN, S., PENFIELD, W. (1959): Illusions of comparative interpretation and emotion. Archives of Neurology and Psychiatry **81**, pp. 269-284.

NEALE, J.M. (1988): Defensive functions of manic episodeS. In: OLTMANNS, T.S., MAHER, B.A. (Eds.): Delusional beliefs, pp. 138-156. Wiley, New York, Chichester, Brisbane, Toronto, Singapore.

OEPEN, G., HUBER, E., ZIMMERMANN, P., HERMLE, L., BIRG, W. (1985): Impairment of intra- and interhemispheric function in schizophrenia. In: Proceedings of the 6th South-East European Neuropsychiatric Conference, Halkidiki/Greece, pp. 573-587.

OEPEN, G. FÜNFGELD, M., HÖLL, T., ZIMMERMAN, P., LANDIS, T., REGARD, M. (1987): Schizophrenia - an emotional hypersensitivity of the right cerebral hemisphere. International Journal of Psychophysiology **5**, pp. 261-64.

OEPEN, G., FÜNFGELD, M., HÖLL, T., ZIMMERMAN, P., LANDIS, T., HERMLE, L. (1988a): Rechtshemisphärische Überaktivität und emotionale Irritabilität bei akuter Schizophrenie. In: OEPEN, G. (Hg.): Psychiatrie des rechten und linken Gehirns, pp. 53-64. Deutscher Ärzte-Verlag, Köln.

OEPEN, G., HARRINGTON, A., FÜNFGELD, M., SCHULTE, M., LANDIS, T. (1988b): Emotion and the dynamics of hemisphere functioning in schizophrenia and depression. Biological Psychiatry [submitted].

OLDFIELD, R.C. (1971): The assessment and analysis of handedness: The Edinburgh inventory. Neuropsychologia **9**, pp. 97-113.

OVERALL, J.E., GORHAM, D.R. (1976): BPRS: Brief Psychiatric Rating Scale. In: GUY, W. (ed.): ECDEU Assessment Manual for Psychopharmacology, pp. 157-169. Rev. Ed. Rockville.

PENFIELD, W. (1975): The mind and the brain. In: WORDON, F.G., SWAZEY, J.P., ADELMAN, G. (eds.): The Neurosciences: Paths of discovery. MIT Press, Cambridge, Mass.

PICK, A. (1903): On "dreamy mental states" as a permanent condition in epilepticS. Brain **26**, pp. 242-251.

SCHNEIDER, K. (1949): Zum Begriff des Wahns. Fortschr. Neurol. Psychiatr. **17**, pp. 26-31.

SPECHT, G. (1901): Über den pathologischen Affekt in der chronischen Paranoia - Ein Beitrag zur Lehre von der Wahnentwicklung. Festschrift, Erlangen.

SPRINGER, S.P., DEUTSCH, G. (1987): Linkes - rechtes Gehirn: Funktionelle Asymmetrien. Spektrum der Wissenschaft, Verlagsgesellschaft Heidelberg.

STEINGRUEBER, H.J. (1971): Zur Messung der Händigkeit. Zschr. für experimentelle und angewandte Psychologie **18**, pp. 337-357.

WEINSCHENK, C. (1965): Über die Wirksamkeit der pathologischen Affektivität bei der Wahnentstehung der endogenen Psychose. Schweizer Archiv f. Neurol. Neurochirurg. u. Psychiat. **95**, pp. 91-119.

WINTERS, K.C. , NEALE, J.M. (1983): Delusions and delusional thinking in psychotics: A review of the literature. Clinical Psychology Review **3**, pp. 227-253.

ZERSSEN, D. VON (1976): Paranoid-Depressions-Skala (PDS). Klinische Selbstbeurteilungsskalen aus dem Münchner Psychiatrischen Informationssystem. München.

Die Beziehung zwischen Philosophie und Psychiatrie, vom Standpunkt einer systemtheoretischen Konzeption produktiver Psychosen aus betrachtet

H.M. Emrich

"Nachdem ich gesehen habe, mit welcher Geistesklarheit und logischen Folgerichtigkeit gewisse Verrückte (systematisch Delirierende) vor sich und den übrigen Menschen ihre Wahnvorstellungen rechtfertigen, habe ich für immer die sichere Gewißheit der Geistesklarheit meiner Geistesklarheit verloren."

FERNANDO PESSOA

1. Einleitung

Eine Bestimmung der Beziehung zwischen Philosophie und Psychiatrie muß je nach dem Standpunkt, der innerhalb der beiden Disziplinen eingenommen wird, sehr verschieden ausfallen. Das breite Spektrum möglicher Philosophien ist jedem geläufig, und auch in der Psychiatrie gibt es eine große Breite möglicher Positionen, ausgehend von phänomenologischen Standpunkten im Sinne von JASPERS und (in ganz anderer Weise) BINSWANGER, über psychoanalytische Betrachtungen bis hin zum Reduktionismus der modernen biologischen Psychiatrie. In Abwandlung eines Wortes von FICHTE könnte man davon sprechen, daß je nachdem, was für eine Psychiatrie man wähle, dies zeige, was für ein Mensch man sei. Der wesentliche Punkt hierbei ist aber nun nicht der, daß es etwa (nur) um eine Frage des Geschmacks oder des Charakters geht, vielmehr ist die Vorentscheidung über den Standpunkt innerhalb der Psychiatrie mit einer Vorentscheidung über das eigene Weltbild verknüpft und damit, vom Wissenschaftsbegriff her gesehen, eine auch philosophische Vorentscheidung. Psychiatrie ist ebenso wie Psychologie nicht einfach eine Naturwissenschaft unter anderen, sondern zugleich philosophische Anthropologie, sie ist stets und von vorneherein philosophisch überformt. Dabei ist die Frage, welche Psychiatrie man wählt, in der Regel eine unbewußte, vorwiegend von den innerhalb der "scientific community" gerade herrschenden Strömungen geprägte Vorentscheidung. In diesem Sinne kann man wohl davon sprechen, daß sich zwischen bestimmten Richtungen in der Psychiatrie und solchen in der Philosophie typischerweise "Liaison"-artige Beziehungen ausbilden, die dann, wenn eine solche einen besonders hohen Erklärungswert oder praktischen Wert besitzt, für einige Zeit die Theorieentwicklung und die Praxis beherrschen können. Ein typisches Beispiel ist die Verbindung eines neurophysiologisch-reduktionistischen Erklärungsmodells psychischer Instanzen mit dem hiermit sachlich schwer kompatiblen hermeneutischen Ansatz bei FREUD, eine Konzeption, die trotz oder gerade wegen ihrer inneren Widersprüchlichkeit bis heute fundamentale Durchschlagskraft bewiesen hat, weil sie zwei Grundbedürfnissen der Psychiatrie, nämlich sowohl zu "erklären", als auch zu "verstehen" (im Sinne von JASPERS) entgegenkommt. Eine andere Liaison dieser Art ist diejenige zwischen dem Existentialismus HEIDEGGERS und der ontologisierenden Psychiatrie ("Daseinsanalyse") der späten fünfziger Jahre.

Es wäre interessant, die philosophische Seite der Psychiatriegeschichte einmal systematisch zu verfolgen (die sog. "Romantische Medizin" ist z.B. voll von solchen Bezügen, etwa bei HEINROTH, VON SCHUBERT, CARUS), und der Leser mag sich angeregt fühlen, einmal seinen eigenen Standpunkt sich zu vergegenwärtigen. Die derzeit übliche Position in dieser Hinsicht ist die unreflektierte Zugehörigkeit zum Reduktionismus des "naturalistischen Projekts" (Übersicht in BIERI 1987) in der vereinfachenden Sicht, nur dieses sei "wissenschaftlich", wobei irreduzibel Seelisch-Geistiges allenfalls als kommunikationstheoretisch bzw. verhaltensbiologisch bestimmbar erscheint (cf. z.B. BATESON 1985).

KANT (1782) äußert sich zum Verhältnis zwischen Psychologie und Naturwissenschaften in den "Metaphysischen Anfangsgründen der Naturwissenschaft" folgendermaßen: "Noch weiter aber, als selbst Chymie, muß empirische Seelenlehre jederzeit von dem Range einer eigentlich so zu nennenden Naturwissenschaft entfernt bleiben... Sie kann daher niemals etwas mehr als eine historische, und, als solche, so viel als möglich systematische Naturlehre des inneren Sinnes, d.i. eine Naturbeschreibung der Seele, aber nicht Seelenwissenschaft, ja nicht einmal psychologische Experimentallehre werden" (KANT 1782, S. 10f). Wir werden später darauf zurückkommen.

Eine Besonderheit der Psychiatrie der Gegenwart ist die in der Regel verkannte Tatsache, daß die Vielfalt psychiatrischer Richtungen als ein Beleg dafür angesehen werden kann, daß Psychiatrie in ihrer gegenwärtigen Gestalt als eher "theorieschwach" zu bezeichnen ist: Gerade der Theorienpluralismus, den wir in der heutigen Psychiatrie konstatieren müssen, spricht dafür, daß wir die *eine*, die gewissermaßen "richtige", die überzeugende Theorie (noch) nicht haben. Diese "Theorieschwäche" der Psychiatrie kann andererseits insofern aber auch als Stärke angesehen werden, als sie die gegenwärtige Forschung dazu verpflichtet, eine breitangelegte empirische Basis aufzubauen bzw. weiter auszubauen. Wie die meisten empirischen Wissenschaften hat sich auch die Psychiatrie der letzten 30-40 Jahre in diesem Sinne bemüht, ein möglichst vorurteilsfreies, methodisch am Modell der Naturwissenschaften orientiertes Weltbild der wissenschaftlichen und therapeutischen Arbeit zugrunde zu legen und sich somit einer Anthropologie zu verpflichten, die man am ehesten als "szientistisch" bezeichnen könnte. Diese, wenn man so will, Vorentscheidung zugunsten einer ideologiearmen Vorurteilslosigkeit bzw. einer "szientistischen Psychiatrie", hatte den wesentlichen Vorteil, daß operationalisierte Daten über Patienten mit psychischen Krankheiten verfügbar wurden, wozu die "quantitative Psychopathologie" (von Zerssen 1985), die objektivierenden Verlaufsuntersuchungen (Angst 1988) sowie die objektivierende Psychologie (Eysenck 1970) wesentliche Beiträge geleistet haben.

Wenn man das Verhältnis zwischen Psychiatrie und Philosophie *heute* zu bestimmen versucht, ist zu bedenken, daß sich die bisherigen Begegnungen als zumindest problematisch erwiesen, nachdem die psychoanalytischen Richtungen sektenartigen Charakter angenommen hatten mit der Folge, daß einerseits die naturwissenschaftliche Forschung in der Psychiatrie durch die zum Teil veralteten psychoanalytischen Konzepte behindert wurde, andererseits die psychoanalytische Arbeit in eine monopolisierende Okkupation der Hermeneutik einmündete und somit auch zu einer Behinderung eigentlich philosophisch-anthropologischer Arbeit in der Psychiatrie führte. Dogmatisch orientierte Psychoanalyse ist in diesem Sinne "mythologisch" (im positiven und zugleich negativen Sinne des Wortes); und es wird erheblicher Dynamisierungen innerhalb der Psychotherapieszene bedürfen, um die psychoanalytischen Richtungen auf den gegenwärtigen Stand der Wissenschaft zu bringen: Gerade im Hinblick auf die epochale Bedeutung der Arbeiten Freuds müssen wir sehen, daß es sich hierbei um eine durch die "dynamische Psychiatrie" der Romantik (insbesondere des Mesmerismus; cf. Ellenberger 1973) vorbereitete, historisch gebundene Leistung handelt, die nicht dogmatisiert werden darf sondern den derzeitigen wissenschaftlichen Ergebnissen angepaßt werden muß. Storr (1987, S. 87) führt hierzu in *Why psychoanalysis is not a science* aus: "Because such understanding must be derived from his own human experience, the analyst can never employ the detached, cold objectivity which is a mandatory requirement of the exact scientist." In ähnlicher Weise war die ontologisierende Psychiatrie für die Weiterentwicklung der vorwärtsdrängenden empirischen Arbeiten der Psychiatrie eher ein Hemmnis, was bei den naturwissenschaftlich-pragmatisch arbeitenden Psychiatern zu einer verständlichen vollständigen Ablehnung geführt hat.

Eine Neubegegnung zwischen Psychiatrie und Philosophie im gegenwärtigen Stadium kann dagegen als wesentlich aussichtsreicher angesehen werden, weil die psychiatrische Forschung gerade durch ihr bewußtes Absehen von den philosophischen Implikationen ihrer Arbeit im Sinne eines "szientifischen Purismus" zu vorzeigbaren Resultaten empirischer Wissenschaft geführt hat, und andererseits die philosophische gegenwärtige Diskussion sich mit Problemlagen auseinandersetzt, die mit den psychiatrischen Grundproblemen verwandt sind, so z.B. wesentlich der Frage nach dem Verhältnis von "Innenperspektive" (Selbstbewußtsein) (cf. Henrich 1982; Nagel 1986) und "Außenperspektive", einer objektivierenden Rekonstruktion des "selbstreferentiellen", selbstbewußtseinvollziehenden "Systems" im Sinne der analytischen Philosophie des Geistes (cf. Bieri 1981; Luhmann 1985). In diesem Sinne könnte man die Psychiatrie als eine Art "natürliches empirisches Forschungsgebiet der Philosophen" ansehen, wobei besonders hervorzuheben ist, daß eine Gruppe von besonders schwerkranken psychiatrischen Patienten sich häufig selbst als eine Art von "Philosophen wider Willen" auffassen, einfach deshalb, weil die von ihnen wahrgenommenen Störungen einen so erheblichen subjektiven Erklärungszwang bzw. Erklärungsdruck auf sie ausüben, daß sie aus einem üblichen naturwüchsigen (naiven, unphilosophischen) Weltbild geradezu herausgezwungen werden. Der Psychotiker ist damit gewissermaßen ein "Modell" für einen Zustand, den analytische Philosophen immer wieder bewußt herbeizuführen versuchen, indem sie das, was "Geist" ist, dadurch zu hinterfragen trachten, daß sie einige Konstitutivmomente des Mentalen gedanklich auszuschließen oder auszuklammern versuchen. Eine solche Tendenz zum "Bewußtseins-Selbstversuch" läßt sich in der gesamten abendländischen Philosophiegeschichte seit DESCARTES verfolgen (man denke beispielsweise an FICHTE, HUSSERL, WITTGENSTEIN, HUXLEY, HOFSTADTER, PUTNAM, SEARLE u.a.). Die hier vorgetragene Konzeption steht insofern in dieser philosophischen Tradition, als sie versucht, zwischen empirischen Daten und grundsätzlichen anthropologischen Überlegungen, deren Basis die Desillusionierung "wirklichkeitsschaffender Fiktionen" (WATZLAWICK 1981; PÖPPEL 1985) ist, zu vermitteln. Eine in diesem Sinne zwischen analytischer Philosophie und experimenteller, wahrnehmungspsychologisch orientierter psychiatrischer Psychoseforschung angesiedelte *Desillusionierungsanthropologie* soll im folgenden als Skizze vorgestellt werden.

2. Wahrnehmungspsychologische Untersuchungen an psychotischen Patienten

2.1 Skizze einer Systemtheorie produktiver Psychosen

Um den "Theoriedruck", unter dem die systemtheoretische Konzeption zur Erklärung produktiver Psychosen (EMRICH 1988a) entstanden ist, zu verdeutlichen, sollen zuerst kurz einige psychiatrische Tatsachen referiert werden, um die Schwierigkeiten der Problemlösungen in der Psychoseforschung darzulegen. Um mit ALEXANDER und SELESNICK (1969) zu sprechen: "Ein Rätsel ersten Ranges, das die größten Schwierigkeiten aufwirft, ist die Schizophrenie". Die Autoren sprechen zurecht von der "fast unergründlichen Natur der Krankheit", die die Behandlung ernstlich beeinträchtige. Es ist bisher weder durch histologische, elektronenmikroskopische und physiologische, noch durch biochemische und/oder molekularbiologische Methoden gelungen, einem Verständnis der Natur der Erkrankung im Sinne einer monokausalen Genese näherzukommen. Bei Verwendung aller dieser Methoden zeigt sich zwar eine erhöhte Variabilität der Befunde, keineswegs aber eine einzige beherrschende Besonderheit wie z.B. die molekularbiologisch-genetischen Befunde bei der Huntington'schen Chorea oder anderen angeborenen Stoffwechselerkrankungen. Schizophrene Psychosen lassen sich eher als "Systemschwächen" eines komplexen neurobiologischen Systems beschreiben, wobei offenbar eine interne Interaktionsstörung zwischen neuronalen Netzwerken unter besonderen Bedingungen (wie z.B. Streß) zu einer Dekompensation (in diesem Sinne einem funktionellen Systemzusammenbruch) führt. Diese konstitutionell präformierte Tendenz zur Netzwerkimbalance stellt in der vorliegenden Hypothese das neurobiologische Äquivalent der von ZUBIN und SPRING (1977) sowie NUECHTERLEIN und DAWSON (1984) vorgeschlagenen Vulnerabilitäts/Streß-Konzeption dar. Es kann davon ausgegangen werden, daß diese Systemschwäche (i.e. Netzwerkinteraktionsschwäche) sowohl durch verschiedenartige polygenetische

Erbfaktoren als auch durch ontogenetische Faktoren während der Entwicklung des ZNS und eine Fülle von ZNS-Erkrankungen (z.B. viraler Genese) bzw. auch durch toxische Einwirkungen zustande kommen kann (cf. CAZZULLO 1988). Eine psychotogene Disposition ist in diesem Sinne eine "Endstrecke", die durch vielfältige Faktoren bedingt sein kann - ja sogar beim Gesunden durch Extrembedingungen wie Reizdeprivation oder Schlafentzug ausgelöst werden kann - und die letztlich darin besteht, daß eine Netzwerkimbalance eines für die normale mentale Funktion notwendigen Gleichgewichts zwischen verschiedenen Systemen (siehe unten), (z.B. "konzeptualisierenden" und "korrigierenden" Systemen) vorliegt.

Eine Plausibilisierung dieser Annahmen kann u.a. durch neueste neurobiologische Untersuchungen von HEILIGENBERG (1987) am elektrischen Fisch gegeben werden. Aufgrund dieser Untersuchungen ist anzunehmen, daß neuronale Netzwerke im Verlauf der Evolution an ganz verschiedene funktionelle Aufgaben angepaßt werden müssen. Wegen dieser, wenn man so will, primären "Konzeptionslosigkeit" des evolutionären Prozesses, bei dem die jeweilige Adaptation an die jeweils neu erschließbaren ökologischen Nischen funktionell zu erfolgen hat, können neuronale Netzwerke als "chaotisch" charakterisiert werden, wobei für die funktionelle Anpassung das jeweils bereits vorhandene Netzwerk nicht völlig "umgestrickt" wird. Vielmehr kann gezeigt werden, daß der Evolutionsprozess zu einer Anpassung bereits vorhandener Netzwerke an neu zu bewältigende Funktionen durch Einführung neuer adaptierender bzw. korrigierender "Module" führt.

Bei einer unspezifischen Schädigung des Gesamtsystems, wie sie z.B. bei der Pathogenese einer Psychose vorliegen könnte, ist zu erwarten, daß durch diese auch die strategisch wichtigen Korrektursysteme erfaßt werden, was zu einer neuronalen Imbalance und, bei "Herausforderung des Systems" z.B. durch "Streß", zu einer Systemdekompensation führt, die sich wahrnehmungspsychologisch dann als psychotisches Erleben im Sinne von Halluzinationen und Wahnwahrnehmungen äußern kann (cf. PÖPPEL 1988).

Die diesen Überlegungen zugrunde liegende systemtheoretische Konzeption ist an neuesten wahrnehmungspsychologischen Konzepten orientiert (cf. GREGORY 1973; YELLOTT 1981; WOLF 1985,1987; HOFFMAN 1986; EMRICH 1988a). Hierbei wird angenommen, daß Wahrnehmung grundsätzlich aus dem Zusammenwirken von *drei Komponenten* (Abb. 1) resultiert: 1) einer *sensualistischen* Komponente; 2) einer *konstruktivistischen* Komponente; 3) einer *zensurierenden* Komponente. Das vorliegende Konzept besagt, daß eine besondere Interaktion zwischen diesen drei Komponenten für die biologisch sinnvolle und effiziente interne Repräsentation der äußeren Welt, wie sie bei Gesunden normalerweise vorhanden ist, notwendig ist, und daß die Pathogenese psychotischer Erkrankungen auf einer Imbalance zwischen diesen Komponenten beruht. Die "konstruktivistische Komponente" (Nr. 2) kann auch als "Phantasie-Komponente", als "hypothesengenerierende Komponente" oder als "Konzeptualisierungssystem" charakterisiert werden. Diese Konzeptualisierungs-Komponente entspricht von der neurobiologischen Forschung her der Einbeziehung der *top-down-Strategie*, die vor allem die Tatsache berücksichtigt, daß eine Datenverarbeitung von Sinnesdaten nur möglich ist auf der Basis vorher abgelaufener Konzeptualisierungen (cf. GREGORY 1973; HOFFMAN 1986). In philosophischer Hinsicht kann eine solche *konstruktivistische Komponente* auf die Philosophien von GIAMBATISTA VICO, IMMANUEL KANT, JOHANN GOTTLIEB FICHTE, FRIEDRICH HEIN-

RICH JACOBI sowie HENRI BERGSON bezogen werden. So schreibt beispielsweise JACOBI in Beilage VII des Spinoza-Büchleins: "Wir eignen uns das Universum zu, indem wir es zerreißen, und eine unseren Fähigkeiten angemessene, der wirklichen ganz unähnlichen Bilder-Idee- und Wortwelt erschaffen. Was wir auf diese Weise erschaffen, verstehen wir, insoweit es unsere Schöpfung ist, vollkommen; was sich auf diese Weise nicht erschaffen läßt, verstehen wir nicht; unser philosophischer Verstand reicht über sein eigenes Hervorbringen nicht hinaus" (JACOBI 1819, Bd. IV/2, S. 132). Im modernen Konstruktivismus, z.B. von WATZLAWICK (1985) und von VON GLASERSFELD (1985) wurde diese Grundidee aktualisiert, allerdings einseitig radikalisiert. Die *sensualistische Komponente* (Nr. 1) andererseits kann als funktioneller Begriff für die in der Neurobiologie bekannte *bottom-up-Strategie* bezeichnet werden, die in der Neurophysiologie des visuellen Systems in hervorragender Weise z.B. durch die Arbeiten von HUBEL und WIESEL (1979) belegt ist. Die *Zensor-Komponente*, die auch im oben dargestellten Sinne als *Korrektursystem* aufgefaßt werden kann, ist wahrnehmungspsychologisch besonders gut durch das Auftreten von Illusionen belegt, wobei angenommen wird, daß solche Illusionen (cf. WOLF 1987) unter Normalbedingungen biologisch sinnvoll sind und deshalb nur unter besonderen experimentellen Bedingungen beobachtet werden können. Eine Schwächung der zensorischen Komponente führt dann zur Aufhebung der vorhandenen Sinnestäuschung, was die Basis für die oben angedeutete "Desillusionierungsanthropologie" darstellt.

Abb. 1: Schema der Überlagerung von sensualistischer (1), konstruktivistischer (2) und zensurierender (3) Komponente der Wahrnehmung. Im schraffierten Bereich erfolgt eine "interne Verrechnung", deren Ergebnis in das bewußte Erleben gelangt.

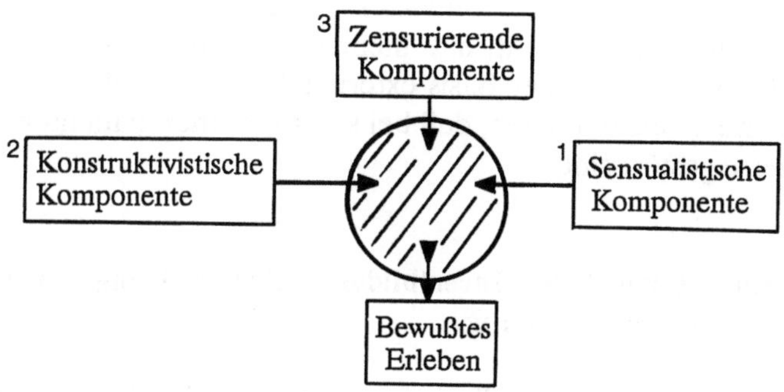

Es stellt eine hochaktuelle, derzeit noch ungelöste Frage dar, inwieweit diese Korrektur- bzw. Zensor-Komponenten als eigene neuronale Systeme im Sinne von Modulen (FODOR 1983) anzusehen sind, oder ob die zensorische Funktion dadurch zustande kommt, daß die Sinnesdatenlage mit den Konzeptualisierungen zu einer "Überlagerung" gebracht wird, wobei dann entweder die Konzeptualisierung oder die Sensorik sich durchsetzen kann. Mit konnektionistischen PDP-Modellen erarbeitete Modellierungen sprechen dafür, daß die zweite Konzeption durchaus möglich ist, was allerdings noch nicht beinhaltet, daß diese im ZNS auch in dieser Form realisiert ist (Knopf et al. 1988).

An dieser Stelle ist die Frage aufzuwerfen, welcher Art die postulierte Imbalance zwichen den drei Komponenten der Wahrnehmungsleistung sein könnte. Aufgrund der oben skizzierten Konzeption, daß eine unspezifische Schädigung des Gesamtsystems insbesondere die strategisch wichtigen Adaptations- und Korrektursysteme treffen müßte, wird vorgeschlagen, daß die wesentliche Störung, die für die Pathogenese einer produktiven psychotischen Symptomatik von Bedeutung ist, das Gleichgewicht zwischen der konstruktivistischen Komponente (Nr. 2) und dem zensurierenden System (Nr. 3) betrifft. So ist beispielsweise zu erwarten, daß eine Schwäche der Kontroll- und Korrektursysteme, die für akustische Wahrnehmung ausschlaggebend sind, zu akustischen Halluzinationen führen kann, und zwar in dem Sinne, daß das Korrektursystem durch die Aktivität des internen hypothesengenerierenden Apparates (Komponente 2) überfordert ist. In diesem Sinne ist anzunehmen, daß produktive Symptome auf einer Imbalance zwischen Konzeptualisierung und adaptiver Korrektur beruhen, so daß interne, teilweise momentan sinnlose Hypothesen bewußt wahrgenommen werden.

In diesem Zusammenhang ist auf die Beziehung zwischen Kreativität und interner Aktivität des *konstruktivistischen Systems* zu verweisen: die adaptiven Mechanismen haben die Aufgabe, das momentan biologisch Sinnvolle im Hier und Jetzt zu sichern - die hypothesengenerierenden Systeme dagegen haben die Aufgabe, innovative Lösungen und Lösungsmöglichkeiten vorzuschlagen, wobei offensichtlich unter einer Fülle solcher Vorschläge nur einige wenige Lösungen tatsächlich sinnvoll sind, somit als *kreativ* bezeichnet werden können und damit der internen *Zensur* nicht notwendigerweise verfallen. In diesem Sinne ist anzunehmen, daß Wahrnehmung kein in sich einheitlicher Prozess ist, vielmehr jede Sinneswahrnehmung im Sinne von Gregory (1973) gewissermaßen auf einer *internen Wette* in dem Sinne beruht, daß mehr oder weniger plausibel erscheinende interne Hypothesen auf der Basis externer Datensets falsifiziert werden; und in diesem Sinne ist anzunehmen, daß bei schizophrenen Patienten derartige interne *Wettprozesse* gestört sind.

2.2 Wahrnehmung binoculärer Invertbilder - ihre Störung als Indikator produktiv-psychotischer Symptomatik

Das Phänomen der Wahrnehmungsillusion sogenannter visueller Invertbilder ist eindrucksvoll in Disneyland, Kalifornien, im "Haunted Mansion" und neuerdings auch in der Schweizerhof-Passage in Bern zu beobachten. Die dort ausgestellten menschlichen Gesichtsmasken drehen sich ganz präzise beim seitlichen Auf- und Abgehen des Beobachters hin und her. Die Wahrnehmungsillusion kommt dadurch zustande, daß es sich bei diesen Gesichtsmasken um dreidimensionale Hohlmasken handelt, die durch eine interne Korrekturleistung des ZNS als "vertraute", konvexe Gesichtsabbildungen wahrgenommen werden. Da diese Wahrnehmungsrekonstruktion jeweils aus einer unterschiedlichen Perspektive erfolgt, entsteht die Illusion eines präzisen Mitdrehens der betrachteten Gesichtsmaske. Diese Wahrnehmungsillusion ist bereits seit der italienischen Renaissance bekannt, wurde von von HELMHOLTZ und MACH im 19. Jahrhundert untersucht und 1973 von GREGORY weiteren wahrnehmungspsychologischen Studien unterzogen. Experimente, die insbesondere von YELLOTT (1981) und WOLF (1985) durchgeführt wurden, zeigten, daß das menschliche Gehirn bestimmte Hypothesen über die drei-dimensionale Struktur von Objekten testet und diese mit den retinalen Sinnesdaten vergleicht. Bei Objekten mit einem hohen Vertrautheitsgrad ist es nun so, daß infolge des semantischen Gehalts des Gesehenen eine Datenkorrektur dann erfolgt, wenn das Objekt mit "überwältigender Wahrscheinlichkeit" nur in invertierter Form sinnvoll interpretiert werden kann (YELLOTT 1981, S. 120). In diesem Sinne kann das Wahrnehmen von Invertbildern als ein Indikator dafür angesehen werden, daß das oben angesprochene zensurierende System, der sogenannte *ratiomorphe Apparat* (WOLF 1985) funktionell wirksam wird.

Aufgrund der oben dargestellten wahrnehmungspsychologischen, systemtheoretisch fundierten Hypothese über die Pathogenese produktiv psychotischer Symptome ist anzunehmen, daß Patienten mit produktiven psychotischen Symptomen eine Schwäche der Komponente 3, d.h. des zensurierenden Systems, aufweisen, was im wahrnehmungspsychologischen Experiment zur Folge haben sollte, daß diese Patienten bei Testung ihrer Fähigkeit, visuelle Invertbilder semantisch bedeutungsvoller Objekte wahrzunehmen, eine Korrekturschwäche aufweisen. Die experimentelle Prüfung dieser Hypothese erfolgte unter Verwendung eines stereoskopischen Projektionssystems, das mit linear polarisiertem Licht arbeitet. Bei 28 schizophrenen Patienten, von denen 15 akut und 13 chronisch krank waren, zeigten sich im Vergleich zu 19 gesunden Kontrollprobanden erhebliche Unterschiede der Wahrnehmung stereoskopischer Invertbilder. Die gesunden Versuchspersonen waren alle in der Lage, semantisch bedeutungsvolle Objekte (menschliche Gesichter, Tiermasken, Haushaltsgegenstände, etc.) in der vertrauten Konfiguration zu sehen, auch dann, wenn durch Umkehrung der Polarisationsrichtung der Brillengläser - was zu einer rechts-links-Vertauschung der Bildinformation zwischen den beiden Augen führt - eigentlich ein Hohlobjekt hätte gesehen werden müssen (vgl. Tab. 1). Die schizophrenen, insbesondere die produktiv-psychotischen Patienten, führten diese Korrektur jedoch nur teilweise oder unvollständig aus, so daß sie zumindest partiell Hohlgesichtspartien wahrnahmen. Das Ausmaß dieser Korrekturdefizienz war von der Intensität der produktiven Symptome abhängig. Diese Befunde sind ein Beleg für die Richtigkeit der von PÖPPEL (1988) in seiner "Taxonomie des Subjektiven" vorgeschlagenen Konzeption, daß psychotische Erkrankungen durch "Störungen auf der integrativen Ebene" auftreten können. Diese Daten werden gestützt durch Befunde, die in kontrollierten Selbstversuchen der an der Studie beteiligten Ärzte erhoben wurde, daß die Einnahme von Cannabis ebenfalls zu einer Schwächung des zensurierenden Systems führt.

Der Befund einer durch Verwendung einer "psychedelischen" Droge induzierten "Zensorschwäche" unterstützt übrigens eine von ALDOUS HUXLEY in den "Pforten der Wahrnehmung" (S. 19) ausgesprochene Vermutung: "Wenn ich über mein Erlebnis nachdenke, muß ich dem Philosophen C.D. Broad in Cambridge beipflichten, 'daß wir gut daran täten, viel ernsthafter, als wir das bisher zu tun geneigt waren, die Theorie zu erwägen, die Bergson im Zusammenhang mit dem Gedächtnis und den Sinneswahrnehmungen aufstellte, daß nämlich die Funktionen des Gehirns, des Nervensystems und der Sinnesorgane hauptsächlich *eliminierend* arbeiten und keineswegs produktiv sind (...) es ist die Aufgabe des Gehirns und des Nervensystems, uns davor zu schützen, von dieser Menge größtenteils unnützen und belanglosen Wissens überwältigt und verwirrt zu werden, und sie erfüllen diese Aufgabe, indem sie den größten Teil der Informationen, die wir in jedem Augenblick aufnehmen oder an die wir uns erinnern würden, ausschließen und nur die sehr kleine und sorgfältig getroffene Auswahl übriglassen, die wahrscheinlich von praktischem Nutzen ist.' Gemäß einer solchen Theorie verfügt potentiell jeder von uns über das größtmögliche Bewußtsein. (...) Um ein biologisches Überleben zu ermöglichen, muß das größtmögliche Bewußtsein durch den Reduktionsfilter des Gehirns und des Nervensystems hindurchfließen."

Mit diesem Text erweist sich HUXLEY als ein wichtiger Vertreter der hier skizzierten *Desillusionierungsanthropologie*. Von psychiatriehistorischem Interesse ist auch die Tatsache, daß bereits H. NEUMANN im Jahre 1883 eine Theorie über die Pathogenese von Halluzinationen vorgeschlagen hat, die in wesentlichen Grundzügen der hier diskutierten Drei-Komponenten-Theorie ähnelt.

Tabelle 1: Desillusionierungs-Score "1" (cf. EMRICH et al. 1988b) für semantisch bedeutungsvolle Objekte bei Gesunden, produktiv Schizophrenen und schizophrenen Patienten ohne produktive Symptomatik.

Gesunde (n=19)	Produktive Psychosen (n=13)	nicht-produktive Psychosen (n=15)
8,7%	68,7%	14,8%

Gesunde vs. Produktive Psychosen: $p < 0,001$; Produktive Psychosen vs. nicht-produktive Psychosen: $p < 0,05$

3. Philosophisch-anthropologische Implikationen der vorliegenden systemtheoretischen Konzeption

Die Korrekturleistung des Stereosehens bei der Erzeugung visueller Invertbilder kann man mit WATZLAWICK (1981) auch als die Stabilisierung einer "wirklichkeitsschaffenden Fiktion" bezeichnen, die das zensurierende System ermöglicht. *Psychose* erscheint in diesem Sinne als ein Zustand, in dem die wirklichkeitsschaffenden Fiktionen durch mangelhaftes Funktionieren der Korrektursysteme nicht mehr in ausreichendem Maße erzeugt werden können; und somit kann der psychotische Zustand als ein Herausfallen aus der gemeinsamen, üblich gewordenen Wirklichkeitsfiktion interpretiert werden. In diesem Sinne könnte man sagen, die vorliegende desillusionierungsanthropologische Konzeption gibt nicht nur einen Hinweis auf ein Verständnis von dem, was es heißt, "psychotisch" zu sein, sondern sie enthält zusätzlich eine Komponente der Selbstinterpretation des Gesunden. Die von uns erlebte Wirklichkeit ist eine durch interne mentale, unbewußt ablaufende Prozesse überformte und korrigierte Lebenswelt (cf. PÖPPEL 1985). Die Grundzüge einer Desillusionierungsanthropologie lassen sich dementsprechend etwa folgendermaßen charakterisieren: Wir finden uns in einer Lebenswelt vor, von der wir durch mühsames, durch apriorische Erwägungen gesteuertes empirisches Ausforschen (z.B. die Untersuchung von Illusionen) herausgefunden haben, daß sie durch biologische Korrekturmechanismen, die sich in der Regel als lebenspraktisch sinnvoll erweisen, modifiziert ist und somit einen durch performative, wirklichkeitsschaffende Prozesse bedingten Charakter hat (vgl. auch das Eingangszitat von PESSOA). Diese Konzeption führt zu einer methodischen Erweiterung philosophisch-anthropologischer Forschung insofern, als es möglich ist, mit den vorliegenden lebenspraktisch wichtigen Fiktionen quantitativ zu experimentieren. Allerdings ist zu vermuten, daß eine empirische Forschung in dieser Richtung sich niemals zu einer Art "totaler Desillusionierung" vorarbeiten kann (z.B. durch Verwendung sehr aktiver psychedelischer Drogen, bzw. sehr intensiver Meditationen), weil unter solchen Bedingungen eine "psychotische" Eigenwelt erzeugt werden würde, die dem Normalbewußtsein nicht mehr im Sinne einer "intentio recta" vermittelbar wäre.

Die in der vorliegenden systemtheoretischen Skizze dargestellte Konzeption und die dabei vorgestellten experimentellen Befunde geben Hinweise auf einen experimentellen Zugang zu einer in der analytischen Philosophie derzeit besonders drängende Thematik: abzielend auf eine "Elementartheorie der Semantik" kann die Frage formuliert werden, welche Konstitutivmomente bei dem dargestellten wahrnehmungspsychologischen Paradigma dafür ausschlaggebend sind, daß das neuronale System ein Objekt als "bedeutungsvoll" im Sinne von "Vertrautheit" anerkennt und damit denjenigen Verrechnungsregeln unterwirft, die im "Desillusionierungsexperiment" eine besonders ausgeprägte Überformung durch Korrektur zeigen. Diese im Sinne von SEARLE (1987a) heute als Problem der "Intentionalität" bezeichnete Grundfrage des Verstehens der Arbeitsweise neuronaler Netzwerke spiegelt sich sprachanalytisch bereits in der Auseinandersetzung zwischen QUINE (1973) und STRAWSON (1974) wider. In *The Roots of Reference* entwickelt QUINE die Hypothese, "Meinen" könne letztlich nichts anderes bedeuten als das Meinen der eigenen mentalen Zustände. STRAWSON dagegen ist in *Logik und Linguistik* der Auffassung, daß "Bezeichnen" als Verwenden von Ausdrücken in bestimmten Situationen tatsächlich die Eindeutigkeit des intentionalen Bezuges sichert, was bedeutet, daß überhaupt von Intentionalität gesprochen werden kann.

Aufgrund der oben dargestellten Konzeption kann gesagt werden: Was bedeutungsvoll ist, was intentionalen Charakter hat, wird "gelernt": Aus lebenspraktischer Erfahrung weiß man, daß menschliche Gesichter normalerweise konvex geformt sind; und aus diesem Grunde werden Sinnesdaten, die dieser konzeptuellen Vorentscheidung widersprechen, zensiert und evtl. korrigiert. Ein Hohlmaskenmaler dagegen, der täglich mit Hohlgesichtern zu tun hat, wird im oben beschriebenen visuellen Invertbildexperiment ein scheinbar hochpathologisches Ergebnis aufweisen müssen: Er kann jederzeit Hohlmasken auf den Dias tatsächlich als solche wahrnehmen. Es ist nun möglich, durch eine Art

Elementarkomponentenanalyse der Komponenten von Bedeutung mit quantitativen Methoden zu untersuchen, welche Rolle bestimmte Formgehalte, die Beleuchtungsrichtung (RAMACHANDRAN 1988) und andere Variablen bei der Konstituierung bedeutungsvoller Wahrnehmungsgehalte spielen. Mit SEARLE (1987a, S. 87) könnte man in diesem Sinne sagen: "Die naiven Realisten hatten damit recht, daß sie materielle Gegenstände und Ereignisse als die typischen Wahrnehmungsgegenstände anerkannt haben; aber viele von ihnen haben nicht erkannt, daß der materielle Gegenstand nur deshalb der Gegenstand der visuellen Wahrnehmung sein kann, weil die Wahrnehmung einen intentionalen Gehalt hat und das visuelle Erlebnis das Vehikel des intentionalen Gehalts ist." Die vorliegende wahrnehmungspsychologische Konzeption verfolgt nun in diesem SEARLE'schen Sinne das Ziel, "das visuelle Erlebnis" als "Vehikel des intentionalen Gehalts" in Elementarkomponenten aufzulösen und diese Elementarkomponentenanalyse sowohl der weiteren philosophischen als auch der psychiatrischen Arbeit zugänglich zu machen.

Hier stellt sich die Frage, welche Rolle die bisher vorgetragene systemtheoretische Konzeption produktiv psychotischen Geschehens innerhalb einer Gesamtdarstellung einer psychiatrischen philosophischen Anthropologie spielt. Eine Systemtheorie kann im Sinne von JASPERS "erklären", wieso jemand halluziniert, wieso jemand Illusionen erlebt, etc.; sie ist aber keine Theorie über den Erlebnis*gehalt* der Halluzination/Illusion, d.h. die inhaltlich-hermeneutische Thematik, die innenperspektivische Erlebnisseite des Problems, das, wie JASPERS es nennt, "einfühlende Verstehen", bleibt als Aufgabe von der Systemtheorie unberührt und bedarf einer eigenen Zugangsweise. Das Mentale hat offenbar zwei Seiten, einen gewissermaßen durch eine "Außenrekonstruktion" einfangbaren, durch Methoden der künstlichen Intelligenz (s. unten) modellierbaren, repräsentierbaren und plausibilisierbaren Anteil und einen einer solchen Beschreibung, jedenfalls bisher, unzugänglichen. In der abschließenden Betrachtung soll deshalb auf das Verhältnis zwischen Systemtheorie und einer Theorie des "irreduzibel Mentalen" eingegangen werden.

4. Schlußbetrachtung und Ausblick: Systemtheorie und die Bedeutung des Subjektiven

Das oben bereits aufgeführte Zitat aus KANTS "Metaphysischen Anfangsgründen der Naturwissenschaft" wirft ein Licht auf die Schwierigkeiten, mit denen eine naturwissenschaftlich orientierte psychologische und psychiatrische Forschung konfrontiert ist.

Der Kontext, in dem diese Passage steht, beginnt mit einer Erörterung der naturwissenschaftlichen Bedingungen, unter denen chemische Forschung steht: "Solange also noch für die chymischen Wirkungen der Materien auf einander kein Begriff ausgefunden wird, der sich construiren läßt, d.i. kein Gesetz der Annäherung und/oder Entfernung der Theile angeben läßt, (...) so kann Chymie nichts mehr als systematische Kunst, oder Experimentallehre, niemals aber eigentliche Wissenschaft werden, weil die Prinzipien derselben nur empirisch sind und keine Darstellung a priori in der Anschauung erlauben, folglich die Grundsätze chymischer Erscheinungen ihrer Möglichkeit nach nicht im Mindesten begreiflich machen, weil sie der Anwendung der Mathematik unfähig sind" (KANT 1782, S. 10).

Diese Forderung KANTS ist inzwischen insofern erfüllt, als durch die Anwendung der Quantenmechanik auf chemische Prozesse (z.B. in der theoretischen organischen Chemie) eine mathematisierbare physikalistische Chemie entstanden ist. Auch die von KANT geäußerte Auffassung, die oben bereits zitiert wurde, daß "Seelenwissenschaft ... nicht einmal psychologische Experimentallehre werden könne" ist bereits widerlegt, und es erscheint im vorliegenden Kontext interessant, sich zu überlegen, ob in naher Zukunft eine Theorie des Mentalen möglich sein wird (etwa durch Methoden der künstlichen Intelligenz), die den KANT'schen Kriterien einer Naturwissenschaft entspricht.

J.R. SEARLE schreibt in *Intentionalität* (S. 325f) hierzu folgendes: "Mein Zugang zu geistigen Zuständen und Ereignissen war insofern vollkommen realistisch, als ich glaube, daß es tatsächlich solche Dinge wie innere geistige Phänomene gibt, die sich nicht auf etwas anderes reduzieren oder durch irgendeine Form des Umdefinierens eliminieren lassen. Es gibt tatsächlich Schmerzen, Kitzel und Jucken, Überzeugungen, Befürchtungen, Hoffnungen, Wünsche, Wahrnehmungserlebnisse, Erlebnisse des Handelns, Gedanken, Gefühle und all das übrige. (...) Niemand hat je seinen eigenen quälenden Schmerz oder seine tiefste Sorge betrachtet und kam daraufhin zu dem Schluß, daß sie nur Zustände einer Turing-Maschine seien, daß sie vollständig durch ihre Ursachen und Wirkungen definiert werden könnten oder daß man nur eine bestimmte Haltung sich selbst gegenüber einnehme, wenn man sich solche Zustände zuschreibt. Zum anderen würde niemand daran denken, andere biologische Phänomene in dieser Weise zu behandeln."

Die Auseinandersetzung zwischen dieser, das Unverlierbare des Subjektiven betonenden Haltung und der Position der künstlichen Intelligenz spiegelt sich in der Auseinandersetzung zwischen SEARLE und GREGORY in dem Buch "Mindwaves" (1987) wider. Die Details dieser Auseinandersetzung können hier nicht im einzelnen nachgezeichnet werden. Vom Standpunkt einer psychiatrischen Anthropologie aus erscheinen allerdings beide Auffassungen berechtigt: einerseits ermöglichen Modelle der künstlichen Intelligenz, wie sie z.B. vom *Konnektionismus* bereitgestellt werden (RUMELHART und MCCLELLAND 1986) eine präzisere Formulierung wahrnehmungspsychologischer systemtheoretischer Hypothesen, geben damit auch Anlaß für neue experimentelle Fragestellungen und Methoden, wie sie beispielsweise bei der oben skizzierten Elementarkomponentenanalyse von "Bedeutung" verwendet werden können. Auf der anderen Seite würde ein ärztlich tätiger Psychiater und Psychotherapeut seiner Aufgabe nicht gerecht werden können, wenn er die Achtung vor der subjektiven Eigenwelt des Patienten verlieren würde, denn nur von einer solchen Subjektivität ernstnehmenden Position aus kann eine hermeneutische Analyse des Patienten sinnvoll gestaltet werden, die somit eine komplementäre Ergänzung zur Systemtheorie darstellt.

DONALD MACKAY (1965, S. 331) formuliert die hier zugrundeliegende Doppelperspektive mit folgenden Worten: "In conclusion, may I say that what impresses me more and more is the element of irreducible mystery that attends our human condition. (...) In the end, in line with ancient wisdom, we have to face an irreducible dualism in our own nature - not, of necessity, a dualism of 'stuffs', but a dualism of aspect which no mechanistic analysis can exhaust."

Neben der hiermit zugleich aufgeworfenen ethischen Problematik stellt sich die prinzipielle Frage, inwieweit ein System sich selbst vollständig aufklären kann, d.h. es stellt sich die Frage nach der möglichen Impenetrabilität und Unexplizierbarkeit des Mentalen für es selbst hinsichtlich seiner Entstehungsweise. Es ist evident, daß eine Psychiatrie, die diese hier angesprochene Vorgängigkeit des Subjektiven vor allen Objektivationsversuchen leugnet, weil es (zumindest derzeitigen) wissenschaftlichen Methoden nicht zugänglich ist, und die damit das einfühlende Verstehen, das hermeneutische Moment, auszuklammern versucht, sich selbst aufgibt.

Zusammenfassung: Obwohl Psychiatrie grundsätzliche vorgängige philosphische Implikationen aufweist, ist die bisherige Begegnung zwischen Philosophie und Psychiatrie eher problematisch gewesen. Die derzeitige "szientistische" Psychiatrie enthält die Chance der Erarbeitung eines vorurteilsarmen empirischen Datenmaterials. Eine auf wahrnehmungspsychologischen Experimenten basierende Systemtheorie produktiver Psychosen wird vorgestellt. Diese Konzeption postuliert eine Imbalance zwischen hypothesengenerierenden und zensurierenden Systemen, die als pathogenes Moment (Vulnerabilität) angesehen wird. Ein experimenteller Beleg unter Verwendung der Wahrnehmungsillusion binoculärer Invertbilder wird dargestellt. Grundsätzliche Betrachtungen einer hier skizzierten "Desillusionierungsanthropologie" ergeben sich einerseits im Hinblick auf eine "Elementarkomponentenanalyse" von "Bedeutung", andererseits auf die unverzichtbare Relevanz des Subjektiven für die psychiatrische Theorie und Praxis.

On the Relation Between Philosophy and Psychiatry from the Point of View of a Systems-Theory Concept of Productive Psychoses

Summary: Though psychiatry contains fundamental philosophical implications, the relation between philosophy and psychiatry has, from a scientific point of view, a problematic history. The present "scientistic" psychiatry yields the chance of the accumulation of a broader empirical data basis. A concept of productive psychoses formed according to general systems theory and based on sensory-psychological experiments is presented. It is assumed that psychotogenic vulnerability results from an imbalance between conceptualizing (hypotheses generating) and censoring systems in the CNS. The hypothesis is supported by experiments using the illusion of binocular depth inversion. Fundamental considerations about a "Desillusion-Anthropology" give rise on the one hand to a discussion of a possible semantic "elementary component analysis" and, on the other, to the recognition of the undisputable autonomy of subjectivity in psychiatric theory and praxis.

Literatur

Alexander, F.G., Selesnick, S.T. (1969): Geschichte der Psychiatrie. Diana Verlag, Konstanz.

Angst, J. (1988): Risikofaktoren für den Verlauf affektiver Störungen. In: Zerssen, D. von., Möller, H.-J. (eds.): Affektive Störungen. Springer, Berlin, S. 99-110.

Bateson, G. (1985): Ökologie des Geistes. Suhrkamp, Frankfurt.

BIERI, P. (1981): Generelle Einführung. In: BIERI, P. (ed.): Analytische Philosophie des Geistes. Hain, Königstein, S. 1-28.
BIERI, P. (1987): Intentionale Systeme: Überlegungen zu Daniel Dennetts Theorie des Geistes. In: BRANDTSTÄDTER, J. (Hrsg.): Struktur und Erfahrung in der psychologischen Forschung. de Gruyter, Berlin S. 208-252.
CAZZULLO, C.L. (ed.) (1988) : Morphology and Plasticity of the Central Nervous System. MTP Press, Lancaster, (im Druck).
ELLENBERGER, H.F. (1973): Die Entdeckung des Unbewußten. Huber, Bern.
EMRICH, H.M. (1988a): Zur Entwicklung einer Systemtheorie produktiver Psychosen. Nervenarzt **59**, S. 456-464.
EMRICH, H.M., WEBER, M.M., WENDL, A., ZIHL, J. (1988b) : Impaired binocular depth inversion as an indicator of psychosis. (Submitted).
EYSENCK, H.J. (1970): The Structure of Human Personality, 3rd. ed. Methuen, London.
FODOR, J.A. (1983): The Modularity of Mind. MIT Press, Cambridge
GLASERSFELD, E. VON (1988): Konstruktion der Wirklichkeit und des Begriffs der Objektivität. In: Einführung in den Konstruktivismus (Schriften der Karl-Friedrich-von-Siemens-Stiftung, Bd. 10). Oldenbourg Verlag, München, S. 1-26.
GREGORY, R.L. (1973): The confounded eye. In: GREGORY, R.L., GOMBRICH, E.H. (eds.): Illusion in Nature and Art. Freeman, Oxford, S. 49-96.
GREGORY, R. (1987): In defence of artificial intelligence - a reply to John Searle. In: BLAKEMORE, C., GREENFIELD, S. (eds.) Mindwaves. Basil Blackwell, Oxford, S. 235-244.
HEILIGENBERG, W. (1987): Central processing of sensory information in electric fish. J. Comp. Physiol A, **161**, S. 621-631.
HENRICH, D. (1982): Selbstverhältnisse. Reclam, Stuttgart.
HOFFMAN, R.E. (1986): Verbal hallucinations and language production processes in schizophrenia. Behav. Brain Sci., **9**, S. 503-548.
HUBEL, D.H., WIESEL, T.N. (1979): Brain mechanisms of vision. Sci. Amer. **241**, S. 130-144.
HUXLEY, A. (1984): Die Pforten der Wahrnehmung, 11. Aufl. Piper, München.
JACOBI, F.H. (1819): Werke, Bd. IV/1 u. 2. (Hg.: ROTH, F., KÖPPEN, F.), G. Fleischer, Leipzig (Nachdruck: Wissenschaftliche Buchgesellschaft Darmstadt, 1980).
KANT, I. (1782): Metaphysische Anfangsgründe der Naturwissenschaft. J.F. Hartknoch, Riga.
KNOPF, H., DIRLICH, G., MCMILLAN, C., EMRICH, H.M. (1988): Konnektionistische Modellierung gestörter visueller Tiefeninversion. In: BRAUER, W. (Hrsg.): Informatik-Fachberichte. Springer, (im Druck).
LUHMANN, N. (1985): Die Autopoiesis des Bewußtseins. Soziale Welt **36**, S. 402-446.
MACKAY, D.M. (1965): A mind's eye view of the brain. In: WIENER, N., SCHADE, J.P. (eds.) Progress in Brain Research, Vol. **17**: Cybernetics of the Nervous System. Elsevier, Amsterdam, S. 321-332.
NAGEL, Th. (1986): The View from Nowhere. Oxford University Press, Oxford.
NEUMANN, H. (1883): Leitfaden der Psychiatrie für Mediciner und Juristen. Preuss & Jünger, Breslau.
NUECHTERLEIN, K.H., DAWSON, M.E. (1984): A heuristic vulnerability/stress model of schizophrenic episodes. Schizophrenia Bull. **10**, S. 300-312.
PESSOA, F. (1988): Das Buch der Unruhe. Fischer, Stuttgart.
PÖPPEL, E. (1985): Grenzen des Bewußtseins. DVA, Stuttgart.
PÖPPEL, E. (1988): Taxonomie des Subjektiven auf der Grundlage eines pragmatischen Monismus. In: BÖCKER, F. WEIG, W. (eds.): Aktuelle Kernfragen in der Psychiatrie. Springer, Berlin-Heidelberg, S. 24-36.
QUINE, W.V. (1973): The Roots of Reference. Open Court Publishing Co., La Salle, Ill.
RAMACHANDRAN, V.S. (1988): Perception of shape from shading. Nature **331**, S. 163-166.
RUMELHART, D.E., MCCLELLAND, J.L. (1986): Parallel Distributed Processing. MIT Press, Cambridge, Mass.
SEARLE, J.R. (1987a): Intentionalität. Suhrkamp, Frankfurt.
SEARLE, J. (1987b): Minds and brains without programs. In: BLAKEMORE, C., GREENFIELD, S. (eds.): Mindwaves. Basil Blackwell, Oxford, S. 209-233.
STORR, A. (1987): Why psychoanalysis is not a science. In: BLAKEMORE, C., GREENFIELD, S. (eds.): Mindwaves. Basil Blackwell, Oxford, S. 75-87.

Strawson, P.F. (1974): Logik und Linguistik. List Verlag, München.
Watzlawick, P. (1981): Die erfundene Wirklichkeit. Piper, München.
Watzlawick, P. (1985): Wirklichkeitsanpassung oder angepaßte "Wirklichkeit"? Konstruktivismus und Psychotherapie. In: Einführung in den Konstruktivismus (Schriften der Carl-Friedrich-von-Siemens-Stiftung, Bd. 10), Oldenbourg Verlag, München, S. 69-83.
Wolf, R. (1985): Binokulares Sehen, Raumverrechnung und Raumwahrnehmung. Biologie in unserer Zeit **15**, S. 161-178.
Wolf, R. (1987): Der biologische Sinn der Sinnestäuschung. Biologie in unserer Zeit **17**, S. 33-49.
Yellott, J.I. Jr. (1981): Binocular depth inversion. Sci. Amer. **245**, S. 118-125.
Zerssen, D. von (1985): Psychiatric syndromes from a clinical and a biostatistical point of view. Psychopathology **18**, S. 88-97.
Zubin, J., Spring, B. (1977): Vulnerability - A new view of schizophrenia. J. Abnorm. Psychol. **86**, S. 103-126.

Zur Psychopathologie und Neuropsychologie der Wahrnehmung von Gesichtern

A. Harrington, G. Oepen, M. Spitzer, L. Hermle

1. Einführung

Kein anderer Teil des menschlichen Körpers ist für die persönliche Identität und zwischenmenschliche Beziehungen von solch entscheidender Bedeutung wie das menschliche Gesicht. Dennoch wurde dieser Tatsache im Kontext psychotischen Erlebens bislang kaum Beachtung geschenkt. Die vorliegende Studie stellt einen ersten Versuch in diese Richtung dar, wobei drei verschiedene Störungen von Wahrnehmen und Erkennen menschlicher Gesichter bei akuter Schizophrenie und in der Meskalin-Psychose verglichen werden sollen. Diese sind: 1. Eine generelle Störung der Fähigkeit, Gesichter anderer Menschen unter emotionalem Streß oder emotionaler Stimulation zu erkennen (was wir als *affektive Prosopagnosie* bezeichnen); 2. Eine teilweise unkontrollierbare Tendenz, Gesichter in Objekten oder Strukturen der Umgebung "zu sehen", mit oder ohne deutliche affektive Begleitreaktion (dies nennen wir dann *Physiognomisierungstendenz* oder mit einem Anglismus *faces in the fire Phänomen*); und 3. Eine Störung der Wahrnehmung und/oder Ich-Identifizierung während der Betrachtung des eigenen Gesichts im Spiegel, was häufig durch Reaktionen wie allgemeines Befremden, Erschrecken, Selbstentfremdung und/oder den Eindruck gekennzeichnet ist, seinem "teuflischen Doppelgänger" zu begegnen (dies bezeichnen wir als *Spiegelphänomen*).

In der vorliegenden Studie möchten wir die genannten Sachverhalte zunächst vor allem beschreiben und dann im Rahmen eines neuropsychologischen Erklärungsansatzes kritisch diskutieren. Wir sind der Meinung, daß der neuropsychologische Erklärungsansatz in diesem Fall deutliche Vorteile über andere mögliche Ansätze aufweist, indem er in der Lage ist, kausale Beziehungen zwischen den Phänomenen aufzuzeigen, die sonst leicht übersehen werden. Andererseits sind wir weit davon entfernt, das Problem gestörten Gesichtererkennens in der Psychose dadurch zu lösen, daß die Phänomene auf ihr biologisches Substrat reduziert werden. Wir sehen keinen Grund, weshalb der gewählte neuropsychologische Ansatz nicht durch andere, mehr hermeneutische Vorgehensweisen ergänzt werden könnte.

2. Beschreibung der Phänomene

2.1 Affektive Prosopagnosie

Störungen in der Fähigkeit des Gesichtererkennens bei Schizophrenen werden nur selten spontan von den Patienten berichtet. Nichtsdestoweniger sind sie in der Psychiatrie durchaus bekannt und in neuester Zeit auch durch sorgfältige experimentelle Studien bestätigt (Berndl et al. 1988, vgl. auch Dewdney 1973). Unsere eigenen neuropsychologisch-experimentellen Befunde mit akut schizophrenen Patienten weisen darauf hin, daß diese Störungen des Gesichtererkennens zumindest teilweise situationsspezifisch moduliert sind, wobei Streß oder emotionale Stimulation die Symptome verstärken. In unserer Studie verglichen wir eine Gruppe akut schizophrener Patienten mit einer hinsichtlich Alter, Geschlecht, Händigkeit und Bildungsstand entsprechenden Kontrollgruppe in einer tachistoskopischen Versuchsanordnung (divided visual field test), wobei in beiden Gesichtsfeldern gleichzeitig eine Wortaufgabe (linkshemishpärisch) und anschließend ein nichtverbaler Test des Gesichtererkennens (rechtshemisphärisch) zu lösen waren. Unerwarteterweise fanden sich die größten Gruppenunterschiede *nicht* in der linkshemisphärischen lexikalischen Aufgabe der Unterscheidung von Funktionswörtern von Nichtwörtern (wie zunächst aufgrund der weit verbreiteten Annahme einer linkshemisphärischen Funktionsstörung bei Schizophrenen erwartet worden war), sondern in der rechtshemisphärischen Gesicht/Nichtgesicht-Erkennungsaufgabe (methodische Details finden sich bei Regard et al. 1986 sowie Oepen et al. 1987, 1988). Der hier entscheidende Befund bestand darin, daß die Fähigkeit der akut schizophrenen Patienten, Gesichter korrekt von Nichtgesichtern zu unterscheiden, im linken Gesichtsfeld (rechte Hemisphäre) dramatisch bis fast auf Zufallsniveau unter zusätzlicher emotionaler Reizung abnahm, während Kontrollpersonen unter diesen Bedingungen eine deutliche Verbesserung ihrer Fähigkeit, Gesichter zu erkennen, aufwiesen (weitere Details in Oepen et al. 1987, 1988).

Sehen wir einmal von diesen statistischen Befunden einer Gruppendifferenz im Gesichtererkennen zwischen akut schizophrenen Patienten und Kontrollpersonen unter Laborbedingungen ab, und wenden uns anderen Beobachtungen zu, die darauf hinweisen, daß es sich bei den Unterschieden zwischen Gesunden und Schizophrenen eher um quantitative als um qualitative Unterschiede handelt. Nicht selten berichten Gesunde, daß sie in Situationen emotionaler Anspannung Gesichter umstehender Personen deutlich schlechter wahrnehmen als unter gewöhnlichen Umständen. Dies könnte den experimentell demonstrierten emotionalen Einflüssen auf das Gesichtererkennen bei Schizophrenen entsprechen. Eine kleine Umfrage unter Kollegen ergab immerhin eine nicht unerhebliche Anzahl von Berichten über eine vorübergehende Unfähigkeit, bekannte Gesichter in Situationen erhöhter affektiver Spannung spontan zu erkennen. So beschrieb z.B. ein Mann die Veränderung der Gesichter von Freunden und Bekannten im Auditorium einer Schule während eines Vortrags: die Gesichter seien ihm wie "weiße Ovale" erschienen, wobei das Phänomen nach abgeklungener Spannung wieder verschwunden war. Wir bezeichnen eine solche affektiv bedingte Verschlechterung des Gesichtererkennens als *affektive*

Prosopagnosie, ohne daß wir hierbei jedoch irgendwelche Gleichsetzungen mit der auf einem neurologisch-morphologischen Defekt beruhenden "echten" Prosopagnosie herstellen möchten (siehe auch Abschnit 3.3.1).

2.2 Physiognomische Illusionen

Die Tendenz vieler akut schizophrener Patienten, ihre Umgebung zu "physiognomisieren" und überall, z.B. in der Tapete, in Wolken etc., Gesichter hineinzusehen, ist durchaus bekannt (vgl. CONRAD 1958).

Die folgende Selbstschilderung eines schizophrenen Patienten soll dies etwas erläutern:... "Da ist das blaue Band der Straße und eine schöne Frühlingsstimmung, und plötzlich bauten sich aus den Strukturen des Asphaltes in der Straße menschliche Gesichter auf. Ich bezeichne das so, obwohl es nicht ganz genau stimmt. Das Ganze vertärkt sich, plötzlich verändert sich die Wahrnehmung dieser Strukturen; die normale Wahrnehmung bricht im Grunde zusammen. Nicht völlig, ich habe den Zustand unter Kontrolle, ich sehe plötzlich Fratzen und Gesichter, nicht Gesichter in Bäumen und Büschen und, ja, so ähnliches, die Sprache ist da nicht völlig geeignet, das alles zu beschreiben, es ist irgendwie eine andere Wirklichkeit, die wir mit unserer Sprache praktisch nicht ausdrücken können ..."

Auf Bitten eines der Autoren (G.O.) schrieb der Patient dann Überlegungen über seinen Zwang, zu physiognomisieren, auf. "... die Wahrnehmung der Natur ist völlig normal und der schönen Jahreszeit entsprechend. Ich sehe die Straße, die Birken und den Parkplatz. Plötzlich bilden sich Formen im blauen Band der Straße, im Asphalt, den kleinen Kieselsteinen, an Gesichter erinnernde Gebilde, die Natur verzerrt sich, die Blätter, die Äste von den Bäumen, die Fichtennadeln werden alle fratzenhaft verzerrt. Ich kenne dies aus Erfahrung, deswegen kaufe ich dann rasch eine Tasse Kaffee am Kiosk, denn Kaffee erweitert die Gefäße, das hilft etwas, so trinke ich 2 Tassen. Meine Wahrnehmung ist dann für mehrere Stunden völlig verändert, ich sehe Fratzen in menschlichen Gesichtern, vor allem in den Frisuren und den Augenbrauen..."

Während einer durch Meskalin-Sulfat erzeugten experimentellen Psychose wiesen gesunde freiwillige Versuchspersonen die deutliche Tendenz auf, menschliche Gesichter in der Hintergrundstruktur ihrer Umgebung zu "sehen".

Eine unserer Versuchspersonen gab am Tag nach der Intoxikation u.a. folgenden Bericht: Obgleich ich mich am Abend nach 18 Uhr bis auf eine Mischung aus Kopfweh, Übelkeit und Frösteln wieder einigermaßen "normal" fühlte, bemerkte ich beim Blick in den Spiegel erneut, daß keineswegs alles vorbei war. Als ich dann gegen 20 Uhr zu Hause ein warmes Bad nahm, sah ich an den nur geringgradig unsystematisch oberflächenstrukturierten Fliesen der gegenüberliegenden Wand plötzlich das Gesicht eines Zwerges mit Bart. Beim erneuten Hinschauen sah ich an der gleichen Wand ebenfalls in Zusammenhang mit der Struktur der Fliesen das Gesicht eines Fuchses und später ebenfalls noch ein Tiergesicht. (Am anderen Tag gelang es mir nicht mehr, diese Gesichter in irgendeiner Weise aus der Strukturierung der Fliesen "herauszusehen", obgleich ich mir die Position der Gesichter auf den Fliesen genau gemerkt hatte.) Nach einem letzten Blick in den Spiegel in abgedunkeltem Raum, der erneut Masken und Fratzen, wenn auch in abgeschwächter Form und nach längerer Dauer, zeigte, legte ich mich ins Bett.

An dieser Stelle soll auch das bekannte (und durchaus gutartige) "faces in the fire-Phänomen" erwähnt werden. Es bedeutet, daß man in so unstrukturierten, wechselnden Untergründen wie Flammen oder Wolken unter bestimmten Bedingungen geneigt ist, gesichterähnliche Formen zu sehen. In Anbetracht der Tatsache, daß die psychotische Erfahrung der physiognomischen Illusionen meist mit Angst verbunden ist, muß hervorgehoben werden, daß diese nicht-psychotischen Physiognomisierungstendenzen eher in einem Zustand allgemeiner, ungerichteter Gespanntheit aufzutreten pflegen. Eine mögliche neuropsychologische Erklärung dieser beiden zunächst widersprüchlich scheinenden Bedingungen wird weiter unten diskutiert (siehe 3.2).

2.3 Das Spiegelphänomen

Das *Spiegelphänomen* besteht darin, sein eigenes Konterfei im Spiegel als dauernd wechselnd, verzerrt, grimassierend oder anderweitig "selbständig belebt" wahrzunehmen. Die fratzenhaften Verzerrungen des Spiegelbildes werden meist als bedrohlich erlebt, nur selten wohlwollend. Besonders die Augen- und Mundpartie sind betroffen. Manchmal verschwindet ein Teil des Gesichts oder, jedoch seltener, das gesamte Gesicht vollständig. Diese Eindrücke sind in keiner Weise stabil, sondern fluktuieren kontinuierlich, wobei ihr Ausdruck sich ebenfalls langsam verändert. Bei Abwendung des Blickes und erneutem Blick in den Spiegel sieht das Gesicht zunächst wieder völlig normal aus, um dann nach einer gewissen Latenzzeit erneut mit seinem Grimassieren zu beginnen. Ein solches Spiegelphänomen kann panische Ängste auslösen. Die meisten Psychiater kennen schizophrene Patienten, die ihre Spiegel verhängen, entfernen oder sogar zerschmettern, da sie ihr teuflisch verzerrtes grimassierendes Spiegelbild nicht ertragen.

Eine 32 Jahre alte akut-exazerbierte schizophrene Patientin erklärte einem von uns (M.S.), daß sie in die Klinik gekommen sei, da sie bemerke, daß alle Leute in den letzten Tagen "blind" seien. Um Erklärung gebeten, führte sie aus:

"Die Augen der Leute, die ich überall sah, waren völlig ohne Ausdruck und schienen ganz fixiert und starr zu sein. Die Gesichter sahen anders aus.

(Frage: Haben Sie irgendwelche andere Veränderungen in diesen Gesichtern oder in Ihrem eigenen Gesicht bemerkt?)

Ja, das erschreckendste für mich war der Blick in den Spiegel. Nach einem Moment werden die Augen ganz starr und leblos und das Gesicht beginnt zu grimmassieren.

Die Patientin weigerte sich, nochmals in den Spiegel zu schauen, da es viel zu erschreckend sei. Sie wies psychopathologisch außerdem Halluzinationen in allen 5 Modalitäten auf und zeigte auch deutliche Depersonalisationssymptome. Zu einem späteren Zeitpunkt berichtete die gleiche Patientin über physiognomische Illusionen, die 3 Wochen vor stationärer Aufnahme aufgetreten seien: "An einem Tag schaute ich in die Wolken und sah plötzlich verschiedenste Gesichter in den Wolken. Am Abend des gleichen Tages sah ich vom Bett aus in der Tapete plötzlich wieder Gesichter."

Die drei beschriebenen Phänomene wurden auch in der experimentellen Psychoseforschung (vgl. BERINGER 1927) beobachtet. Die folgenden Selbstschilderungen entstammen bisher unveröffentlichten Rausch-Protokollen, die in den Jahren 1929 bis 1939 im Rahmen der Untersuchungen zur Meskalin-Psychose unter KURT BERINGER entstanden, und die im folgenden als "BERINGER-Materialien" zitiert werden.

"Prof. B. gab mir einen Spiegel. Mein Spiegelbild war überraschend, ich sah mich zum ersten Male ganz lebendig als fremdes Ich entgegenkommen, das war nicht mein Spiegelbild, das war ein anderer Mensch, von dem ich aber wußte, daß ich es war, der selbständig in dem Glase lebte. Das Spiegelbild machte sogar selbständige Bewegungen, ohne daß Verzerrungen auftraten. Ganz vertieft im Anschauen meines lebendigen Bildes, hörte ich Prof. B. sagen: "Die reinste Form des Narzißmus'." Ich schämte mich sehr und gab den Spiegel sofort zurück" (BERINGER-Materialien).

Ein Proband, der im Rausch vor allem von wogenden, fließenden Bewegungen spricht, sah Entsprechendes auch auf Fotographien von Angehörigen, die in seinem Arbeitszimmer hingen. Er beschreibt zunächst, wie die Scheinbewegungen der Umgebung etwas Automatisches für ihn sind und beispielsweise durch sein Klavierspiel nicht beeinflußt werden können: "Diese Scheinbewegung hat vielmehr etwas Starres, Unabänderliches, wie automatisch Aufgezogenes, was dem lebendigen Rhythmus und Flusse der Musik sich in keiner Weise anpaßt..." Kurz danach spricht er über das Betrachten von Fotographien: "Eine ähnliche Beobachtung mache ich, als ich nachher in meinem Zimmer Fotographien meiner Angehörigen betrachte. Auch auf diesen Fotographien führen die Gesichter Scheinbewegungen aus. Es ist aber niemals so, daß diese Scheinbewegung mit der natürlicherweise in dem Gesicht vorhandenen Bewegung, etwa einem Lächeln, irgendwie zusammenklingt. Niemals erscheinen die Gesichtszüge durch die Scheinbewegung der Stirn, der Augen, der Wangen und der Lippen irgendwie belebt, vielmehr hat auch hier die Scheinbewegung etwas durchaus Automatisches, wie Aufgezogenes. Die Tatsache, daß sich die vertrauten Züge dauernd bewegen, ohne daß doch die Lebendigkeit und Bewegtheit in ihnen auch nur um das Geringste zunimmt, hat nach einiger Zeit etwas geradezu Kaltes und Trostloses, was mir fast unheimlich ist und auch noch jetzt in der Erinnerung mich unangenehm berührt.

Der gleiche Patient hatte am gleichen Abend noch beim Einschlafen folgende Erlebnisse: Wenn ich die Augen längere Zeit geschlossen habe, so sehe ich noch Andeutungen von fratzenhaften Figuren und bunten Linien, jedoch alles sehr schwach und nicht mehr beunruhigend" (BERINGER-Materialien).

Ein weitere Proband hatte die folgenden Erlebnisse: "Professor B., der später einmal kam, tat Erstaunliches: Er veränderte seine Gestalt, sein Kopf wurde anders und bevor ich recht wußte, wie und auf welche Art, stand vor mir leibhaftig und plastisch ein Golem, so nannte ich es, eine Holzfigur offensichtlich, dunkelblau und grau in den Maßen eines Riesen, mit grob geschnitztem Kopf und messerscharfer Nase, mit blockartigem Rumpf und von ungeheurem Gewicht. Durch eine menschenunmögliche Bewegung der Oberlippe teilte er mit, daß dies seine wahre Gestalt sei und nur aus dämonischer und mir unbegreifbarer Laune sei er manchmal dort tief unten in der Klinik leitend tätig.

Eine andere Versuchsperson machte folgende Angaben, die stark an die Erlebnisse der oben beschriebenen Patientin erinnern: "Die anderen Personen saßen ohne jede Beziehung zu ihrer Umgebung herum, ihre Augen blickten starr, die Gesichter waren wie Masken..."

Auch das "faces in the fire Phänomen", d.h. physiognomische Illusionen, kommen im Meskalinrausch vor: "An anderem Ort war eben noch farbiges Mauerwerk eines Brunnens. Jetzt aber blicken hundert und mehr Gesichter mich an, gelb sind sie und blau und braun, Fratzen und Masken, Köpfe und riesige Augen, lange Nasen und Arme und Beine. Hier bildet eine Faust sich und droht, es ist ein Chaos, unfaßlich, alles voller Leben und ich wende mich ab. Ein kurzer Blick zur Seite zeigt mir, dort steht ein Brunnen, sonst nichts" (BERINGER-Materialien).

In unseren eigenen Untersuchungen mit Meskalin-Sulfat wiesen 9 von 12 männlichen freiwilligen Versuchspersonen das Spiegelphänomen mehr oder weniger ausgeprägt auf. Nach Aufforderung durch den Versuchsleiter, ihr Gesicht im Spiegel zu betrachten, bemerkten die Probanden nach einer gewissen Latenzzeit, daß ihr Spiegelbild ein gewisses Eigenleben annahm, die Gesichtszüge sich maskenhaft verzerrten, obwohl Außenstehende bestätigen konnten, daß das echte Gesicht der Probanden völlig bewegungslos geblieben war. Solche Verzerrungen der Wahrnehmung des eigenen Gesichts im Spiegel wurden üblicherweise erstmals auf dem Höhepunkt der Drogenpsychose beobachtet, waren weitaus erschreckender und unerträglicher als die Verzerrungen in der

Wahrnehmung von Gesichtern Umstehender, und dauerten deutlich länger als andere halluzinatorische und illusionäre Symptome des Meskalin-Rausches.

Der letzte Proband unserer Studie wurde auch gebeten, sein eigenes Konterfei in einer Fotographie zu betrachten. Er berichtete über die gleichen bedrohlichen Verzerrungen wie während des Blicks in den Spiegel. Es scheint also so zu sein, daß weniger der Spiegel selbst als die Tatsache, sein eigenes Gesicht zu sehen, den Ausschlag gibt.

Es ist nicht völlig klar, wie verbreitet diese Erfahrung wohl ist, noch, wie weit die Erwartung der Versuchspersonen, solche Phänomene zu erleben, einen Einfluß auf ihre Wahrnehmung hatte. Immerhin ist bemerkenswert, daß bereits in den BERINGERschen Experimenten vor 60 Jahren die gleichen physiognomischen Verzerrungen beim Betrachten von Spiegelbildern und Fotographien berichtet wurden, was gegen einen solchen Erwartungseffekt spricht. Sicherlich sind jedoch weitere Experimente der Gesichterwahrnehmung unter experimentellen und natürlichen Psychose-Bedingungen sinnvoll, wobei Gesichter im Halbprofil, auf dem Kopf stehende Gesichter sowie verschiedene Zerr-Spiegel gegen Abbildungen der frontalen Ansichten von Gesichtern und normaler Spiegelbetrachtung verglichen werden sollten.

3. Diskussion

Ein Hauptanliegen dieser Studie ist, den Blick auf eine zu Unrecht vernachlässigte Dimension schizophrenen Erlebens zu lenken in der Hoffnung, daß sie andere klinisch und experimentell tätige Forscher anrege, diesen von uns aufgeworfenen und, wie wir meinen, zu Recht gemeinsam betrachteten Themen nachzugehen. Wir möchten im folgenden kein vollständiges übergreifendes Modell der Gesichtererkennung und ihrer Störung bei Gesunden und Schizophrenen entwerfen, sondern lediglich auf ein paar Punkte hinweisen, an denen sich ein solches, eventuell später zu entwickelndes Modell orientieren könnte.

3.1 Prosopagnosie und Neurobiologie des Gesichtererkennens

Das organisch bedingte Syndrom der Prosopagnosie, das mit rechtsseitigen oder bilateralen Läsionen des occipitalen Cortex einhergeht (HECAEN 1962, DAMASIO et al. 1982) bildet eine naheliegende Analogie und einen ersten Hinweis auf möglicherweise involvierte Hirnregionen und Prozesse im Rahmen der gestörten Gesichtererkennung bei Schizophrenie. Wir sind uns jedoch gleichzeitig der Gefahr bewußt, die darin besteht, in unzulässiger Weise anzunehmen, daß dadurch, daß Defizit D mit einer Läsion der Hirnstruktur S assoziiert ist, *jeder* neue Patient mit dem klinischen Defizit D *ebenfalls* eine Läsion der Hirnstruktur S aufweisen müsse, oder überhaupt irgendeine *umschriebene Läsion* für das Vorliegen dieses speziellen Defizits in jedem Fall verantwortlich sein müsse; besonders vorsichtig sollte man bei der Übertragung der Symptome von Hirnverletzten auf Phänomene bei psychiatrischen Patienten sein (vgl. MILLER 1983). Obwohl ausreichende Evidenz für die Annahme einer grundlegenden Störung des Gesichtererkennens (und übrigens auch der mimischen Expression) bei vielen Schizophrenen vorliegt - was vorsichtig in Richtung einer Analogie zur organischen Prosopagnosie gesehen werden könnte - konnten wir jedoch zeigen, daß das Ausmaß dieser Störung zusätzlich durch den Grad emotionaler Belastung moduliert wird. Das deutet darauf hin, daß wir - selbst wenn sich der Vergleich der organischen Prosopagnosie mit der dysfunktionellen dynamischen Gesichtererkennungsstörung bei Schizophrenie als fruchtbar herausstellen sollte - vorsichtigerweise nur von einer *regional lokalisierbaren Funktionsschwäche* (verantwortlich für die grundlegende Wahrnehmungsschwäche) sprechen sollten. Diese kann zusätzlich durch affektive (und andere?) Belastung verschlimmert werden (im Rahmen dynamisch-funktioneller Veränderungen im Gehirn).

Diese Hypothese fügt sich gut in die Rolle, die heute von manchen Autoren denjenigen Prozessen zugeschrieben wird, die für die Verarbeitung affektiver Gehalte zuständig sind. So nimmt Wexler (1986) an, daß derartige Verarbeitungsprozesse das verbindende Element bei der Verknüpfung jeweils aktivierter Bereiche des ZNS zu aktuellen Funktionseinheiten im Sinne Lurias darstellen. Zusätzliche emotionale Reize können somit modulierend auf die Arbeitsweise und -qualität dieser Funktionseinheiten einwirken.

Unserem eigenen Schizophrenie-Modell (Oepen et al. 1987, 1988) liegt folgende Annahme zugrunde: Aus einer zugrundeliegenden Funktionsschwäche resultiert eine pathologische Hyperaktivität rechtshemisphärischer Prozesse. Zusätzliche emotionale Reize führen zu einer Überstimulierung und damit zu einer vorübergehenden Funktionsverschlechterung rechtshemisphärischer Prozesse, mit Enthemmung der vorher unterdrückten linkshemisphärischen Funktionen.

3.2 Physiognomisierungstendenz und ungerichtete Hirnaktivität

Die obige Hypothese, die den beobachteten Zusammenbruch der Fähigkeit zur Gesichtererkennung im linken Gesichtsfeld bei Schizophrenen mit einer Hyperaktivität der für diese Funktion verantworlichen Hirngebiete (der rechten Hemisphäre) verbindet, bietet die Möglichkeit, die Tendenz Schizophrener zur Physiognomisierung der Umwelt mit der bei den gleichen Patienten beobachteten Wahrnehmungsstörung von Gesichtern in einem gemeinsamen Rahmen zu betrachten. Die hier zu diskutierende Hypothese beinhaltet, daß die physiognomischen Illusionen in gewisser Weise ein *Enthemmungsphänomen* (vgl. Cogan 1973) darstellen, bedingt durch eine Art ungerichteter vermehrter Bereitschaft der entsprechenden funktionellen Systeme. Wahrnehmungspsychologisch könnte dies folgendermaßen erklärt werden: Wenn es zutrifft, daß unser Gehirn Objekte der Umgebung dadurch erkennt, daß es Hypothesen aus den Wahrnehmungsdaten entwirft (Rock 1984, Gregory 1974, S. 352, 616), dann ist es denkbar, daß diejenigen Hirnregionen, die auch im schizophrenen Gehirn für die Wahrnehmung und Identifizierung von Gesichtern zuständig sind, bei Überaktivierung von sich aus beginnen, stereotype Hypthesen ohne entsprechende reale Objekte der Wahrnehmung zu produzieren.[1] Dieser ungerichtete

1 Wenn auch hier vom Erkennen und Hypothesenbilden durch neuronale Strukturen bzw. das Gehirn als ganzes die Rede ist, so wissen wir durchaus um die Problematik einer solchen Redeweise, die allerdings kaum vermeidlich ist, will man nicht entweder die Dinge sprachlich unnötig komplizieren oder aber durch häufigen Gebrauch

Gesichts-Generator (der nichts anderes bedeutet, als daß aus bestimmten Wahrnehmungsdaten sinnvolle Strukturen mit Bezug zum Subjekt geformt werden) ist, wie wir zeigen konnten, durch emotionale Zusatzreizung modulierbar.

Im Rahmen unserer Erörterungen meinten wir bisher, daß diese affektive Tönung am ehesten Angst oder Spannung entspräche. Es gibt jedoch Hinweise darauf, daß affektive Anspannung keineswegs eine notwendige Bedingung dieser Physiognomisierungstendenz darstellt. Wir denken hier an die Beobachtung, daß auch eine allgemeine Entspannung mit ungerichteter mentaler Aktivität eine günstige Voraussetzung für das Auftreten halbautomatischer Konstruktionen von gesichterähnlichen Formen in unstrukturiertem Material darstellen kann, wie beispielsweise beim "faces in the fire-Phänomen". Die Tatsache, daß sowohl der akut paranoid-schizophrene Patient als auch ein entspannter abendlicher Träumer in gleicher Weise eine Tendenz zur Physiognomisierung der Umgebung im Dämmerlicht oder in unruhig strukturierten Hintergründen aufweisen, könnte folgendermaßen erklärt werden: Nicht das absolute Maß an Aktivierung, sondern das Verhältnis der Aktivierung von Hypothesen generierenden Strukturen des Gehirns (die wir mit gutem Grund vorwiegend rechtshemisphärisch lokalisieren) zu Strukturen, die mit ihnen in einer inhibitorischen (quasi kontrollierenden) Wechselbeziehung stehen, ist entscheidend für das Auftreten von Physiognomisierungstendenzen. Mit anderen Worten, nicht der absolute Grad der Aktivierung rechtshemisphärischer Strukturen, sondern ihr *relatives Überwiegen* ist Grundbedingung dafür, daß sie in wenig kontrollierter Weise eigenständig tätig werden und Hypothesen produzieren, die sonst von einem kritischen Zensor am Bewußtwerden gehindert werden (vgl. hierzu auch den Beitrag von EMRICH in diesem Band).

Ein Hinweis auf die Möglichkeit willentlich erzeugter Physiognomisierungen findet sich bereits bei LEONARDO DA VINCI, der in seinen Tagebüchern (MACCURDY S. 250) u.a. folgenden Hinweis zur Kreativität des Künstlers gibt: "A way to stimulate and arouse the mind to various inventions ... if you look at any walls spotted with various stains or with a mixture of different kinds of stones, if you are about to invent some scene you will be able to see in it ... figures in quick movement, and strange expressions of faces, and outlandish costumes..."

Bei Schizophrenen ist die rechte Hemisphäre offensichtlich primär dysfunktionell und in Krisensituationen als diejenige Struktur, die mit der existentiell wichtigen automatischen Bearbeitung der Monitor-ähnlichen Wahrnehmung und emotionalen Bewertung der Umgebung betraut ist, rasch in Gefahr, überfordert zu werden und deshalb in einem dauernden, hyperfunktionellen Alarmzustand.[2] Diese kritische Überfunktion phylogenetisch älterer Wahrnehmungs- bzw. Bewertungsstrukturen ist nun nicht mehr von einer (möglicherweise ebenfalls dysfunktionellen) phylogenetsich jüngeren, sprach- und detailorientiert arbeitenden, "vernünftigen" linken Hemisphäre ausreichend kontrollierbar, und produziert daher ungezügelt strukturierte Wahrnehmungshypothesen. Letzteres

---

von Anführungszeichen beständig das Gesagte gleichsam zurücknehmen oder zumindest relativieren. Solange man um den grundsätzlich metaphorischen und vor allem vorläufigen Charakter einer solchen Redeweise weiß, halten wir sie allerdings für brauchbar, bedarf es doch dann weder der Rede von erkenntnisähnlichen Leistungen oder Quasi-Hypothesen, noch der Rede von "Hypothesen", die dem "Erkennen" dienen.

2 Vgl. hierzu GESCHWIND 1982.

bedeutet nichts anderes als eine sinnhafte Verdichtung von Informationen - und welche optische Struktur ist für uns bedeutsamer als das menschliche Gesicht, das gleich nach der Geburt als erstes erkannt wird, und dessen Ausdruck (ob Freund oder Feind) im Sinne des eigenen Überlebens rasch entziffert werden muß und oft auch mehr ausdrücken kann, als Worte sagen können? Im Rahmen dieses - bewußt spekulativen - Modells ist erklärbar, daß bei einer willkürliche Herabminderung der (linkshemisphärischen) vernünftigen "Kontrollmechanismen" durch ungerichtete entspannte Geisteshaltung ebenfalls ein relatives Dominieren der sinngebenden bzw. Hypothesen-generierenden (rechtshemisphärischen) Strukturen auftreten kann, was auch bei Gesunden (z.B. bei entspanntem Blick in ein Feuer) zur Physiognomisierung der Umgebung führen kann.

Auch wenn die besondere Bedeutung rechtshemisphärischer Prozesse aus dem oben Gesagten hervorgeht, möchten wir eine simplifizierende Überbewertung dieser Befunde im Sinne einer atomistischen Lokalisierung gesichtererkennender oder sogar allgemein sinngebender Strukturen ausschließlich in der rechte Hemisphäre vermeiden. Sicherlich sind hier nicht eindeutig lokalisierbare, sondern eher dynamisch fluktuierende, situationsbedingt verknüpfte Hirngebiete anzunehmen, ganz abgesehen von der irrigen Annahme, mit einer Lokalisierung psychologischer Funktionen sei bereits deren Wissenschaftlichkeit gesichert oder eine zusätzliche (gar "höhere") Erkenntnis gewonnen. Da das oben geschilderte *dynamische* Modell jedoch eine sinnvolle Interpretation der von uns beobachteten Phänomene zuläßt und möglicherweise auch eine Integration klinischer Daten erlaubt, ist aus rein pragmatischen Gesichtspunkten - ungeachtet dessen, ob dieses Modell nun wahr ist oder nicht - seine Anwendung zumindest vorläufig von heuristischem Wert und möglicherweise fruchtbarer Anstoß zu weiterführenden Überlegungen.

Die überraschende Stereotypie und vorhersagbare Ausgestaltung physiognomischer Wahrnehmungsveränderungen verdient besondere Beachtung. Bereits 1928 stellte KLÜVER fest, daß die durch Meskalin induzierten Halluzinationen auf eine relativ kleine Zahl einfacher Formen oder Muster zurückgeführt werden können, die er "Formkonstanten" nannte. Andere Forscher (SIEGEL 1977, 1978; KEELER 1970; für eine zusammenfassende Darstellung vgl. SPITZER 1988) stellten fest, daß diese stereotypen Grundformen in ganz ähnlicher Weise in den verschiedensten Kulturen anzutreffen sind. So sind z.B. die verzerrten Gesichter, die von schizophrenen Patienten bzw. von Teilnehmern an experimenteller Psychosenforschung mit Drogen berichtet werden, oft den grimassenhaft verzerrten Gesichtszügen ("Fratzen") sakraler Masken der verschiedensten Traditionen überraschend ähnlich (z.B. alemannische Fastnacht, Tempelwächter und Tanzmasken aus Ceylon, Thailand, Afrika und Japan, um nur einige Beispiele anzuführen). Auffällig ist dabei, daß in allen Fällen die Augen- und Mundpartie auf Kosten anderer Gesichtszüge überbetont und verzerrt sind. Dies könnte damit in Zusammenhang stehen, daß Augen und Mund für die Übermittlung affektiver Botschaften besonders wichtig und auch für die Identifizierung bekannter Gesichter entscheidende Partien sind.

Möglicherweise sind die Störungen der Wahrnehmung von Gesichtern, ähnlich wie dies heute von den Formkonstanten KLÜVERS angenommen wird, als direkter Ausdruck der Enthemmung bestimmter Neuronenverbände zu betrachten. Dafür spricht in jedem Falle das in beiden Fällen gegebene praktisch kulturunabhängige Auftreten entsprechender Täuschungsphänomene. Dies ist gleichbedeutend damit, daß Formkonstanten ebenso wie Gesichterstrukturen nicht primär gelernt werden, sondern Ausdruck einer begrenzten Anzahl fundamental-neuropsychologischer, gleichsam "fest verdrahteter" Wahrnehmungshypothesen sind, die Basis für die Wahrnehmung bzw. künstlerische Ausformung von Erlebnissen darstellen, die bei entsprechender Enthemmung statthaben. Die Eigenart des Gehirns, aus eingehenden Wahrnehmungsdaten nach bestimmten Gesetzen sinnvolle "Hypothesen" einer begrenzten Anzahl zu bilden, ist damit letztlich die Grundlage für unsere Hypothese, mit der wir die Verwandtschaft der von uns diskutierten Phänomene "affektive Prosopagnosie", "Physiognomisierungstendenz" und "Spiegelphänomen" ebenso wie deren Ähnlichkeit unter verschiedenen Bedingungen des Auftretens (endogene oder drogeninduzierte Psychosen) bzw. die interkulturelle Ähnlichkeit ritueller Masken erklären können.

3.3 Das eigene Spiegelbild, Selbstwahrnehmung und Identität

Das Spiegelphänomen ist das subtilste und am schwierigsten zu interpretierende der von uns betrachteten Phänomene, weshalb wir uns auf wenige Bemerkungen über mögliche Ansätze beschränken wollen, sein Auftreten oder seine Ausprägung zu erklären oder modifizierende Einflüsse zu erfassen. Es handelt sich hier offenbar um einen Sachverhalt, der an der Grenze zwischen pathologischer Wahrnehmung (erfaßbar in Begriffen von Hirnfunktion, Psychophysik und Wahrnehmungspsychologie) und Ich-Pathologie angesiedelt ist (welche besser durch die Persönlichkeitspsychologie bzw. hermeneutische Ansätze erfaßbar ist). Eine flexible, interdisziplinäre Analyse des Phänomens scheint uns deshalb das einzig realistische Vorgehen zu sein.

Wir haben gesehen, daß die Annahme eines (gemäß unserem Modell vorwiegend rechtshemisphärisch lokalisierten) Systems, das aus den Wahrnehmungsdaten sinnvolle Hypothesen generiert, in der Lage ist, verschiedene Phänomene zu erklären. Neben den optischen Wahrnehmungstäuschungen (Rock 1984, Gregory 1974) erklärt es die Tendenz, unter verschiedenen Umständen die Umgebung zu physiognomisieren sowie betrachtete Gesichter zu variieren und verzerren. Die hierbei stets beobachtete Latenz bis zum Auftreten der optischen Funktionsstörungen erlaubt es, diese Phänomene in älterer neuropsychologischer Terminologie als "pathologischen optischen Funktionswandel" im Sinne von Binswanger und Bay zu sehen (Bay 1953). Eine Interferenz mit (ebenfalls vorwiegend rechtshemisphärisch verarbeiteten) zusätzlichen affektiven Reizen führt erwartungsgemäß zu einer Verschlechterung solcher spezifischer, aktiver Wahrnehmungsleistungen wie des Gesichtererkennens (affektive Prosopagnosie bei sonst Gesunden sowie Verschlechterung des Gesichtererkennens bei Schizophrenen unter emotionaler Belastung).

Die Verzerrung der eigenen Gesichtszüge beim Blick in den Spiegel, wie sie bei akut Schizophrenen sowie in der Drogenpsychose beobachtet werden kann, könnte im Rahmen dieses Modells damit erklärt werden, daß dieser (rechtshemisphärische) Hypothesengenerator relativ anderen kontrollierenden Systemen hyperaktiv und unkontrolliert in überschießender Weise arbeitet und dabei besonders die sinngebenden Strukturen der Augen- und Mundpartie von wahrgenommenen Gesichtern variiert. Daß hierbei vor allem Angst und Bedrohlichkeit empfunden werden, mag neben dem allgemeinen Befremden über die unerwarteten Grimassen und der Tatsache, daß es sich um das eigene und nicht um fremde Gesichter handelt, auch damit zusammenhängen, daß die rechte Hemisphäre eher für negative als für positive Emotionen zuständig zu sein scheint (Heilmann und Satz 1983).

Einen weiteren Hinweis für die besondere Bedeutung rechtshemisphärischer Prozesse im Kontext des Spiegelphänomens könnte eine Beobachtung von Crichton-Browne (1895, S. 17) bieten: Er beschreibt einen Patienten, der sowohl durch intensives Blicken in den Spiegel als auch durch allgemeine Gedanken über sich selbst eine epileptische Dämmerattacke bzw. einen dreamy mental state (d.h. einen Temporallappenepilepsie-Anfall) auslösen konnte, wobei die gesamte Umgebung verändert erlebt wurde, mit Verlust des Gefühles für Raum und Zeit, unter starken Ängsten und der Furcht, nie mehr er selbst sein zu können. Diese Art epileptischer Anfälle treten bekannterweise besonders häufig bei rechtshemisphärischen Herden auf (vgl. Jackson 1880-81).

Es ist ermutigend, daß hermeneutisch orientierte Psychologen das Problem des Spiegelphänomens nicht völlig übersehen haben, obwohl es bisher kaum Ansätze gab, neuropsychologische Perspektiven hier zu integrieren. Eine partielle Ausnahme bildet der experimentell arbeitende Psychoanalytiker Werner Wolff (1953), der emotionale Reaktionen nichtpsychotischer freiwilliger Versuchspersonen auf verschiedene Fotographien bekannter und unbekannter Gesichter, einschließlich ihres eigenen Gesichts, testete. Den Versuchspersonen war nicht bekannt, daß die Fotographien manipuliert waren und jeweils 2 linke oder 2 rechte Gesichtshälften spiegelbildlich ergänzt zu einem neuen Gesicht kombiniert worden waren. Es stellte sich heraus, daß die Probanden ganz besondere Schwierigkeiten aufwiesen, Gesichter als ihre eigenen wiederzuerkennen, die aus ihren beiden linken Gesichtshälften kombiniert waren, und daß sie - gefragt, eine Bewertung dieser nicht erkannten Gesichter abzugeben - dazu neigten, Bemerkungen zu äußern, die Wolff als unbewußte, verdrängte Phantasien und/oder bedrohliche Formen der Selbstwahrnehmung interpretierte. Wolff selbst war aufgrund dieser Ergebnisse zu einer neuropsychologischen Interpretation dieser Befunde geneigt und nahm an, daß die rechte Seite des Gehirns besonders mit den Funktionen des Unbewußten befaßt sei und daher möglicherweise eher als die linke Hemisphäre entsprechende Inhalte zum (Gesichts-) Ausdruck bringe.

Auf den besonderen Zusammenhang zwischen dem Erkennen von Gesichtern und rechtshemisphärischen Prozessen sei an dieser Stelle nur kurz verwiesen (Christen 1985, Damasio et al. 1982, Hecaen 1962, Landis et al. 1979).

Beringer beschrieb im Rahmen seiner Studie zur Meskalin-Psychose in den zwanziger Jahren das Spiegelphänomen in Anlehnung an tiefenpsychologische Überlegungen als "Narzißmus in reinster Form" (siehe oben; vgl. auch Abely 1930).

ROSENZWEIG und SHAKOW (1937) verglichen das Verhalten von 51 schizophrenen Patienten mit dem von normalen Kontrollpersonen, wenn die jeweiligen Probanden vor einen Spiegel gesetzt wurden: Sie berichteten, daß lediglich ein einziger schizophrener Patient sich so verhielt, daß man sein Verhalten als "normal" bezeichnen konnte, und favorisierten eine Erklärung, die sich im wesentlichen auf eine instabile Ich-Identifizierung und eine dysfunktionelle Fähigkeit zur Intersubjektivität stützt (die paradoxe Erfahrung, daß uns der Spiegel zwingt, uns selbst quasi "von außerhalb" so zu erfahren, wie andere uns sehen). In jüngerer Zeit haben andere Forscher zwischen schizophrenem und präschizophrenem Spiegelverhalten unterschieden, und meinten, daß das präschizophrene Spiegelverhalten weniger als pathologisches Symptom an sich zu verstehen sei, denn als ein Versuch, mittels des Spiegels sich seiner selbst zu versichern und wieder in Kontakt mit einem zu entfliehen drohenden Ich zu treten - mit anderen Worten, eine Form von Selbsttherapie (BLANKENBURG 1983, PANKOW 1981).

Im Interesse einer Integration von neuropsychologischen mit hermeneutisch-persönlichkeitspsychologischen Ansätzen bedürfen die folgenden grundlegenden Fragen einer weiteren Klärung:

1. Inwieweit, und in welcher Form ist die visuelle Identifizierung des eigenen Gesichtes verknüpft mit der Überzeugung von der eigenen Identität? und

2. Inwieweit kann eine neuropsychologisch zu erklärende Beeinträchtigung oder Verzerrung der Fähigkeit zur Gesichtererkennung eine kritische Störung der Selbst-Identifizierung hervorrufen, und/oder inwieweit kann sie in destruktiver Weise mit der instabilen Ich-Identität und Ich-Struktur eines schizophrenen Menschen bei Konfrontation mit seinem Spiegelbild interagieren?

Wie hoffen, daß weitere klinische und experimentelle Befunde helfen werden, diese und andere offene Fragen zu klären.

Zusammenfassung: Das Erkennen von Gesichtern hat in der menschlichen Entwicklung ebenso wie in der zwischenmenschlichen Kommunikation und deren Störungen bei schweren psychiatrischen Krankheiten, wie z.B. bei Schizophrenie, eine überragende Bedeutung. Es werden drei Phänomene beschrieben, die mit einer Veränderung der Fähigkeit, Gesichter zu erkennen, verknüpft sind. Unter *affektiver Prosopagnosie* verstehen wir eine Beeinträchtigung der Fähigkeit, bekannte Gesichter unter emotionalem Streß wiederzuerkennen. Eine *Physiognomisierungstendenz* wird sowohl bei akut Schizophrenen als auch unter ungerichteter geistiger Entspannung beobachtet. Das *Spiegelphänomen* besteht in einer meist als bedrohlich erlebten Verzerrung der eigenen Gesichtszüge beim Blick in den Spiegel und wird bei akuter Schizophrenie sowie drogeninduzierter experimenteller Psychose beobachtet. Ein neuropsychologischer Ansatz erlaubt eine gemeinsame Betrachtungsweise dieser drei Phänomene. Ein umfassendes Verständnis ist jedoch erst unter Einbeziehung hermeneutischer und persönlichkeitspsychologischer Ansätze möglich, wobei dies bisher nur ansatzweise geleistet werden kann. Auf weiterführende Untersuchungsansätze wird deshalb verwiesen.

The Psychopathology and Neuropsychology of Face-Perception

Summary: Three disorders of facial recognition and perception in acute schizophrenia and mescaline-induced psychosis are described and illustrated using original clinical and experimental material: (1) "Affective prosopagnosia" or stres-related dysfunctional face recognition; (2) "physiognomization" of the environment or persistent illusions and hallucinations of nonspecific faces; and (3) the "mirror phenomenon" or the experience of inner alienation from one's reflected face which is perceived as independently alive, sinister and generally physically distorted. It is proposed that neuropsychology suggests relationships between these phenomena that might otherwise be less apparent. No final neurobiological "solution" to the problem of dysfunctional facial perception and recognition in psychosis is presented, but various insights and suggestive models from the neurosciences are discussed. Attention is also paid to the conditions under which one might need to combine neuropsychological approaches with hermeneutically-oriented analyses.

Literatur

ABELY, P. (1930): Le signe du miroir dans les psychoses et plus spécialement dans la démence précoce. Ann. med.-psych. **88** (Pt. 1) S. 28-36.

BAY, E. (1953): Disturbances of visual perception and their examination. Brain **76**, S. 515-550.

BLANKENBURG, W. (1983): Schizophrene Psychosen in der Adoleszenz. Jap. J. of Psychopathology **4**, S. 151-170; [German Version in: Bull. Inst. Med. Kumamoto University **48**, S. 33-54].

BERINGER, K. (1927): Der Meskalinrausch. Seine Geschichte und Erscheinungsweise. Monograph. Neurol. Psychiatr. H49, Springer, Berlin, Heidelberg.

BERINGER, K. (1929-1939): Rausch-Protokolle. (Unveröffentlichtes Material, Freiburg).

BERNDL, K., GRUESSER, O-J, LÜDKE, M. (1988): Untersuchungen zur Veränderung der Wahrnehmung von Gesichtern, Mimik und Gestik durch Schizophrene. In: OEPEN, G. (Hg.): Psychiatrie des rechten und linken Gehirns, S. 93-100. Deutscher Ärzte-Verlag, Köln.

CHRISTEN, L., LANDIS, T., REGARD, M. (1985): Left hemisphere functional compensation in prosopagnosia? A tachistoscopic study with unilaterally lesioned patients. Human neurobiology **4**, S. 9-14.

COGAN, D.G. (1973): Visual Hallucinations as Release Phenomena. Albrecht v. Graefes Arch. klin. exp. Ophthal. **188**, S. 139-150.

CONRAD, K. (1958) Die beginnende Schizophrenie. Thieme, Stuttgart.

CRICHTON-BROWNE, J. (1895): The Cavendish Lecture on dreamy mental states. Bailliere, Tindall & Co., London.

DAMASIO, A.R., DAMASIO, H., VAN HOESEN, G.W. (1982): Prosopagnosia: Anatomical basis and behavioral mechanisms. Neurology **32**, S. 331-341.

DEWDNEY, D. (1973): A specific distortion of the human facial percept in childhood schizophrenia. Psychiatr. Quart. **47**, S. 82-94. Cited in Berndl (1986) [see above].

FELDMANN, H. (1958): Zur phänomenologischen Strukturanalyse der Störungen des Ichbewußtseins. Archiv für Psychiatrie und Zeitschrift f.d.ges. Neurologie **198**, S. 96-102.

GESCHWIND, N. (1982): Hemisphere specialization: Biological foundations. In: Katsuki, S., Tsubaki, T., Toyokura, Y. (Hg.): Neurology, S. 3-10. Exc. Med., Amsterdam, Oxford, Princeton.

GREGORY, R.L. (1974): Concepts and Mechanisms of Perception. G. Duckworth & Co, London.

HECAEN, H., ANGELUERGUES, R. (1962): Agnosia for faces (Prosopagnosia). Archives of Neurology **7**, S. 92-100.

HEILMANN, K.M., SATZ, P. (1983): Neuropsychology of human emotion. Guilford Press, New York.

JACKSON, H. (1880-81): On right or left-sided spasm at the onset of epileptic paroxysms, and on crude sensations, warnings, and elaborate mental states. Brain **3**, S. 192-205

KEELER, M.H. (1970): Klüver's Mechanisms of Hallucinations as Illustrated by the Paintings of Max Ernst. In: KEUP, W. (Ed.): Origin and Mechanisms of Hallucinations, S. 205-208. Plenum Press, New York, London.

KLÜVER, H. (1928): Mescal. Kegan Paul, Trench, Trubner & Co., London.

LANDIS, T., ASSAL, G., PERRET, E. (1979): Opposite cerebral hemispheric superiorities for visual associative processing of emotional facial expressions and objects. Nature **278**, S. 739-740.

LEONARDO DA VINCI: Notebooks (arranged, rendered into English and introduced by E. MACCURDY), Vol. II. Reynal & Hitchcock, New York.

MILLER, L. (1983): A note on the interpretation of data derived from neuropsychological tests. Cortex **19**, S. 131-32.

OEPEN, G. FÜNFGELD, M., HÖLL, T., ZIMMERMAN, P., LANDIS, T., REGARD, M. (1987): Schizophrenia - an emotional hypersensitivity of the right cerebral hemisphere. International Journal of Psychophysiology **5**, S. 261-64.

OEPEN, G., HARRINGTON, A., FÜNFGELD, M., SCHULTE, M., LANDIS, T. (1988): Emotion and the dynamics of hemisphere functioning in schizophrenia and depression. Biological Psychiatry [submitted].

PANKOW, G. (1981): L'étre-la du schizophrène. Paris, Aubier Montaigne.

REGARD, M. AND LANDIS, T. (1986): Affective and cognitive decisions on faces in normals". In: ELLIS, H.D., JEEVES, M.A., NEWCOMBE, F., A. YOUNG (Eds.): Aspects of Face Processing, S. 363-69, Nijhoff, Dordrecht.

ROCK, I. (1984): Perception. Scientific American Bks, Inc., New York.

ROSENZWEIG, S., SHAKOW, D. (1937): Mirror behavior in schizophrenic and normal individuals. J. Nerv. Ment. Dis. **86**, S. 166-174.

SIEGEL, R.K. (1977): Hallucinations. Scientific American **237**, S. 132-140.

SIEGEL, R.K. (1978): Cocaine Hallucinations. Am. J. Psychiatry **135**, S. 309-314.

SPITZER, M. (1988): Halluzinationen. Springer, Berlin, Heidelberg, New York, London, Paris, Tokyo.

WEXLER, B.E. (1986): A model of brain function. Its implications for psychiatric research. Br. J. Psychiatry **148**, S. 357-362.

WOLFF, W. (1953): Das rechte und das linke Gesicht. Ciba-Zeitschrift **61**: Rechts-Links-Probleme. 6, S. 2044-2047.

Zur intentionalen Struktur einer schizophasischen Selbstdarstellung

Ch. Mundt

1. Einleitung

Für eine klinisch orientierte Darstellung schizophrener Sprach- und Denkstörungen vor einem philosophischen Seminar sind vor allem zwei Zielsetzungen vorstellbar:

1. Die Störung einer im Alltag als selbstverständlich erlebten psychischen Funktion läßt sie überhaupt erst als aktive Leistung und nicht als selbstverständlich gegebenes Widerfahrnis erscheinen und eröffnet damit auch Perspektiven für die Bedingungen ihres ungestörten Ablaufs.
2. Durch die Anwendung außerklinischer Methoden und Konzeptualisierungen von philosophischer Seite ist zu erhoffen, daß sie einer vertieften Interpretation zugänglich wird, die vielleicht zu einer Verbesserung psychotherapeutischer Arbeit vornehmlich im einzeltherapeutischen aber auch im sozialen Gruppensetting beitragen kann.

Für die Interpretation schizophren gestörter Sprache haben in jüngster Zeit vor allem strukturalistische Ansätze Bedeutung gewonnen, die in den sprachlichen Symbolen die Repräsentanz der Welt sehen und im Sprachgefüge eine Entsprechung zum Sinngefüge seelischer Strebungen und Bezugnahmen, insbesondere der mitmenschlichen Beziehungsstrukturen des Patienten. Ausgehend von der Lehre DE SAUSSURES und LACANS zur Struktur des Unbewußten hat LANG (1973) im deutschen Sprachraum die schizophrene Grundstörung in diesem Sinne als defiziente Wirklichkeitsrepräsentation definiert, als das Vorkommen von Fehlstellen in den Objektrepräsentanzen, die sich mit der Sprachstruktur aufgebaut haben. Mit empirisch operationalen Ansätzen haben HOLM-HADULLA (1982) und TRESS et al. (1984) charakteristische Störungen der Sinnesgestaltung von Sätzen und Satzgefügen Schizophrener beschrieben, wobei klare Abgrenzungen gegen die Texte organisch und neurotisch gestörter Patienten gelangen. HOLM-HADULLA präzisierte und operationalisierte diese für Schizophrene charakteristischen Störungen durch die Begriffe "Substitution" und "Transfer", die sich auf die Übernahme und Referenz von Begriffen von Satz zu Satz beziehen sowie durch den Begriff "Intermingling", der auf eine Vermischung von differenten Sinngehalten abzielt; Substitution und

Transfer fand er bei Schizophrenen vermindert, Intermingling vermehrt. TRESS et al. fanden die Anzahl von Bezugnahmen auf den jeweils vorhergehenden Satz in den Texten Schizophrener signifikant vermindert gegenüber Kontrollgruppen. Die Störung wird von HOLM-HADULLA auf den Konkretismus Schizophrener zurückgeführt, hinter dem er ursächlich wiederum eine Aufhebung der Zeichen-Bezeichnetes-Differenzierung mit ihrer Offenheit für Mehrdeutigkeiten sieht. Man könnte in diesem Sinne sagen, der Schizophrene hält sich im Konkretismus gewissermaßen fest an einer punktuellen Sinnsetzung ohne die dialektische Feinabstimmung der Sinnsetzung mit dem sozialen Anderen weiterzuverfolgen, ohne also die Sinnsetzung prozeßhaft offenzuhalten. TRESS sieht hingegen die unser Alltagsreden formenden und präzisierenden Verweisungszusammenhänge im gesamten Text beim Schizophrenen in Auflösung begriffen, er nennt diese Verweisungszusammenhänge in ihrer globalen Funktion der Sinnpräszisierung "Deixis". Im Licht dieser Hypothese erscheine der Konkretismus bereits als ein Abstützvorgang, eine Reaktion des Seelenlebens auf eine primäre Sinnverlorenheit des Subjekts.

2. Kasuistik

Der nun folgende Text einer schizophrenen Patientin soll die klinische Grundlage abgeben für die Diskussion dieser kommunikativen Aspekte des Sprechaktes, der hier gestört, aber auch teilweise erhalten ist und damit die Kommunikation in einer eigentümlichen Weise verändert, aber nicht ganz verunmöglicht hat. Ich bitte Sie bei der Darbietung dieses längeren Textstücks vor allem auf dessen emotional-kommunikativen Zusammenhang mit der Untersuchungssituation zu achten. Es kommt damit der Gesamtgestalt des Textes mehr Bedeutung als der Detailfunktion zu.

Der Text wurde während eines Monologs der Patientin mit ihrer Einwilligung auf Tonband aufgezeichnet. Die dreißigjährige Patientin, seit drei Jahren arbeitslos, war in die Ambulanz der Heidelberger Psychiatrischen Klinik einbestellt zur Begutachtung wegen eines von ihr verschuldeten Verkehrsunfalls. Ein Vorgutachten, das auf gezielte Fragen des Untersuchers mit knappen Antworten der Patientin aufgebaut war, hatte keine Auffälligkeiten gezeigt. Der Monolog der Patientin von etwa 6 Minuten Dauer ergab sich im zweiten Explorationsgespräch auf die Frage nach ihrem beruflichen Werdegang. Weitere detaillierte Angaben zur emotionalen Situation des Untersuchungsganges werden in der Interpretation des Textes nachgeliefert.

"1) Verfugung verstehe ich von einer Firma und sie muß chronologisch und tabellarisch geben. 2) Das ist im ersten Moment schwer für einen Mensch, daß er chronologisch und tabellarisch ist, wenn man eine Lebensbeziehung dazu hat. 3) Dann muß man erst abwarten, muß sich schon denken, das ist auch leicht, es muß eine chronologische und eine tabellarische Verfugung gehen und muß darüber arbeiten. - 4) Die Drittländer gehen ja erst in den Import und in den Export und dann über ihr Drittländer in Import dann in die Verzollung und dann ins Drittland. 5) Es können aber noch größere Abnehmer, das kann erweitert sein, daß sie vom Anfang vom älteren Bestand oder vom jüngsten Bestand oder von Überschlagsrecht von anderen Ländern und die Zusicherung über mehrere Länder noch geben können. 6) Also daß sie eine Ware abnehmen können, vielleicht über 11 Länder oder noch schlimmer, ne, noch länger. - 7) Das kann man erkennen und praktisch ganz gut zu arbeiten dort, das versteht man, was damit gemeint ist und wie man da verfugt ist, wenn man sich danach auskennt und spricht, Sprachen dazulernt und hört und sagt und paßt auf in seiner Schulung, dann versteht man das von vorne ab, ne, also das versteht man ja, damit man weiterkommt mit sich und noch da in dem Zimmer ist eingebildet und wenn es ihr einfach weh tut, daß es so ist, muß man chronologisch und tabellarisch, also nur chronologisch und tabellarisch, das paßt in die Lebenserwartung, weil man da vielleicht andere Beziehungen hat oder überhaupt keine Beziehung dazu. 8) Dann weiß es niemand, ist es gut, ist es 'ne Beziehung oder mehr. 9) Wer ein eigener Mensch werden will, denkt sich das. So muß man arbeiten und tun. Und wenn die chronologisch und tabellarisch und wirft alles Unbefindliche ein, daß man da auch Ordnung tut, daß man da auch mitkommen sollte. 10) Dann geht man halt in die Schul', daß man lernt und daß man es besteht und ist froh drum, daß man arbeitet. - 11) Ja, dann bin ich zu anderen Firmen gegangen, war angestellt. 12) Ich mein', wenn ich da jetzt etwas anderes gemacht hätte, das war mir egal, ich war angestellt, wissen Sie. 13) Ich war net angestellt in dem Sinn, aber ich kann da weit besser Bescheid, ich war doch Angestellte. 14) Und wenn die Arbeiter sind, sind die Arbeiter, aber ich war doch da angestellt und da freut man sich und wenn man was darstellt, bringt man doch was. - 15) Ja, wenn man jetzt z.B. was Ordentliches, Sauberes darstellt, wie ich, das ist 'ne Aufmunterung. 16) Dagegen wenn ich keine Hilfestellung hab', keine Darstellung hab, das ist schwer, erdrückt mich. 17) Man ist nicht freudig, es macht kein Spaß morgens aufzustehen, das macht überhaupt kein Spaß. 18) Wenn man wenigstens was darstellen würde, daß man auch was darstellt und das ist schon was Besseres. 19) Wenn man in der Firma nichts darstellt, ermuntert einem das auch net. 20) Als wenn man nur lacht und kräht und derweil nichts schafft. 21) Wenn er jetzt in der Firma was gesagt hätte, er will auch was schaffen, nimmt vielleicht den Mut heraus, weil er vielleicht die Einsicht hat, wenn er keine Einsicht hat, das ist schon schlecht. 22) Dann ist er kein akzeptierter Mensch mehr, dann muß er irgendwas allein machen. 23) Dann muß man ihn noch fragen, wie er sich das eigentlich vorstellt. 24) So weiter zu leben, wie soll ich sagen, egal, dem ist ja alles egal, da ist er ja kein Mensch. 25) Wenn es ihm nicht egal ist, spürt er erst, daß er für was gebraucht ist, daß er für sich selbst da ist, daß er aber für sich selbst sich freut und mich, ach, ha ja, steht er jetzt auf, war den ganzen Tag, wieso weg. 26) Man muß aber dabei sein, man muß mitdenken. 27) Das ist nichts, wenn man jetzt hergeht und so denkt, also, keine Darstellung hat oder man will nicht, muß man mal fragen, ob es nicht besser ist, wenn man sich mit jemand unterhält und sagt, wo hängt's denn dran, will man mal oder will man nicht. 28) Wenn aber so ein Mensch eingestellt ist davon, der hat doch keine Darstellung. 29) Dann geht es schon. 30) Hat er ein Ziel, sieht er was und kann auch was erreichen damit, aber es darf kein Zwang sein, er muß von sich selbst ausgehen, das ist in Ordnung. 31) Es ist wunderbar, da stehe ich morgens frisch und munter und den ganzen Tag frisch und munter und nicht so läppisch da, geb net so läppisch Antwort, net übergezielt, sondern genau und hinweisend, nicht überhöflich. 32) Höflich und konkret, daß der Mensch einem auch versteht, was man meint. 33) Er ist selbst Mensch und der andere ist auch selbst Mensch. 34) Vielleicht die Lebenserwartung, er überlegt morgens, am vorhergehenden Tag was eingetroffen ist. 35) Man denkt an den Tag und kann gar net aufstehen. 36) Wenn jemand nichts Läppisches denkt, sondern was Konkretes, was der andere auch versteht und das paßt vielleicht zu der Beziehung net, aber man steht auf, will mal sagen, genau steht man wieder auf, präzise kann man da net sagen, genau steht man auf. - 37) Das wär ein Vorgang von der Lebenserwartung, aber nicht von der Lebenserwartung, sondern von der Lebenserwartung und des ist ein Vorgang, des ist ein erreichbarer Vorgang, wo ein Mensch haben möchte, hat aber einen Zwischenhalt in der Lebenserwartung, aber nicht in der Lebenserwartung. - 38) Ja, das ist ein Mensch, der ist eingestellt, nur seine eigene Lebenserwartung, nicht die genaue und konkrete Lebenserwartung oder er ist ein in sich eingeschlossener Mensch, oder er hat so eine Lebenserwartung, guten Morgen, guten Abend, Wiedersehen, das ist geblumt, alles so überdreht. 39) Mehr wollt ich eigentlich net sagen." -

3. Interpretation

Ich möchte die Interpretation des Textes so aufbauen, daß ich 1. den für den Untersucher durchschimmernden Sinn des Textes beschreibe; 2. zu fassen versuche, was an dem Text eigentlich gestört ist; und 3. schließlich einige klinische Konsequenzen für den therapeutischen Umgang mit dieser Störung formuliere.

3.1 Der erschließbare Sinn des Textes

Die Patientin hinterläßt den Untersucher mit Abschluß des Textes in einer merkwürdigen Betroffenheit, die trotz aller Schwerverständlichkeit des Textes auf eine distinkte Aussage schließen läßt. Der Versuch, diese intendierte, aber nicht voll zur Ausführung gelangte Aussage zu rekonstruieren, setzt bei diesem Gefühl der Betroffenheit an. Ich erinnere am Ende des Monologs, daß vorher die Rede gewesen war von der Kontaktarmut der Patientin in Schule, Beruf und gegenwärtigem Leben, daß sie ganze Wochen verbringe, ohne mit jemandem zu sprechen; und vom Scheitern in ihrem Beruf nach hoffnungsvollen Anfängen. Dann kam die Aufforderung zu einer von Fragen losgelösten Eigendarstellung der Biographie der letzten Jahre. Liest man den Text als eine Fortsetzung dieser Kommunikation, so stellt sich zunächst ein zwar vager, aus der im Untersucher erzeugten Gefühlslage aber stellvertretend durch ihn präzisierbarer Aussagecharakter des Textes dar:

Gleich die ersten Sätze thematisieren Beruf und Ausbildung, die "Verfugung", die man mit der Firma haben müsse, und die Beziehung. Der Ausdruck "chronologisch und tabellarisch" könnte eine Umschreibung dafür sein, daß die Beziehung zur Firma und den gestellten Aufgaben präzise sein müsse. Es folgt dann eine Passage, etwa von Satz 4 bis 6, die als Demonstration eines Fachjargons angesehen werden kann und von der Patientin auch in etwas ansprüchlicher Mimik und Gestik vorgetragen wurde, ganz im Gegensatz zu ihrer sonst eher selbstverbergenden Haltung. Hierin könnte der selbstassertive Versuch einer Kompetenzdemonstrierung gesehen werden mittels eines Fachjargons, ein Vorgang der weder Psychiatern noch Philosophen ganz fremd sein wird. Und nun kommt ein Textstück, bis zu Satz 10, in dem die Patientin den Anfangsgedanken aufgreift und ausführt, wie schwer es ist, diese "Verfugung tabellarisch und chronologisch" zu erreichen, das bedeutet wohl präzise Sachkunde mit nachfolgender Kompetenz, Akzeptanz in der Firma und seelischem Wohlbefinden. Sie gibt einen Hinweis darauf, daß es ihr wehtue, wenn einer eingebildet im Zimmer sitze, - ihr Chef, Mitarbeiter, der Untersucher oder mit falschem Anspruch sie selbst, das bleibt unklar - und daß der um diese Problematik wisse, ein "eigener Mensch" werden will, d.h. wohl eigenständig werden will. Es folgt dann ein Abschnitt, in dem sie darüber spricht, daß sie als Angestellte im Gegensatz zu Arbeitern etwas dargestellt habe, aber keine Hilfestellung bekommen habe und so Freude über die erhoffte gute Selbstdarstellung nicht eingetreten sei, vielmehr tiefer Depression Platz gemacht habe. Man kann diesen Satz übrigens auch als ein Wortspiel um den Verbstamm "Stellen" lesen. Es entsteht der Eindruck, daß die Patientin hier über das Umkippen der eigenen hoffnungsvollen Bemühungen in Resignation spricht, über ein Scheitern nach anfänglichem Aufstieg. Es folgen dann von Satz 19 an bis zum Ende des Textes allgemein gehaltene Ausführungen, in denen aber die persönliche Betroffenheit stets noch ganz deutlich mitschwingt, mit denen die Patientin wieder die Notwendigkeit umschreibt, daß der Mensch mit seiner Umgebung in einen gegenseitiges Verständnis ermöglichenden Konnex komme und daß das seelische Wohlergehen, die Anerkennung, die jemand finde, damit verbunden sei. Im Sinne bereits der ersten Sätze wird dies als zentrales Problem, als "Lebenserwartung" angesprochen, vielleicht Erwartung des Lebens an den Menschen oder des Menschen an das Leben. Der Text endet abrupt mit einem Satz, der vermittelt, sie sei nun bis an die Grenze der ihr möglichen Selbstentblößung gegangen.

Ich fasse den *kommunikativen Kontext* in meiner Interpretation zusammen: Die Patientin steht in der Begutachtungssituation vor der Angst, aufgrund der Vorfälle ihre zwar autistisch-bizarre, aber freiheitliche Lebenssituation mit Eigenversorgung zu verlieren durch eine gerichtlich verfügte Krankenhauseinweisung. Es entsteht daraus zunächst eine ängstlich distanzierende Beziehung zum Untersucher, später entwickelt sich Vertrauen auf Respektierung. Nach anfangs kurzgreifenden präzisen Fragen des Untersuchers mit knappen, weitgehend unauffälligen Antworten, wird der Text durch eine Aufforderung, frei zu erzählen, angestoßen. Er stellt eine Art Kürlauf zur Selbstexplikation dar. Sein Inhalt besagt, man müsse sich einbinden lassen in den zwischenmenschlichen Kontakt, man müsse sich auch einbinden können. Nur wenn eine präzise Sinnbildung mit dem Anderen gelinge, gelinge auch die Entwicklung und Reifung der Persönlichkeit. Sonst verkümmere man und habe keine Freude an sich selbst. Die Patientin bricht ab mit der Befürchtung von Lächerlichkeit, sie schämt sich. Eine Satz-für-Satz-Interpretation des Textes erscheint möglich. Die Betroffenheit, in der die Patientin den Untersucher zurückläßt, verweist auf den emotionalen Gehalt der Botschaft: Trauer über das Scheitern, gekränkter Stolz und Ehrgeiz, notgedrungenes Sich-Bescheiden, autistisches Sich-Abgrenzen und -Schützen, das, durch die Situation provoziert, einmal aufgehoben, dann schamhaft wiederhergestellt wird.

3.2 Phänomenologie der Störungen

Nun zur Frage, was an dem Text eigentlich gestört sei. Es fällt zunächst auf, daß die Sätze, für sich genommen, häufig keinen verstehbaren Sinn ergeben, daß in großer Zahl grammatikalische Fehler und semantische Auffälligkeiten vorkommen und daß es eine Fülle von Iterationen gibt. Häufig fehlt das Prädikat im Satz. Die Patientin verwendet nur wenige Male das Wort "ich" in den Sätzen 1, 11 bis 13 und 39, für eine Biographie sicher ungewöhlich; ansonsten bewegt sie sich in allgemeinen Formulierungen mit dem Pronomen "man", das die Aussagen von ihrer Person abzieht und Allgemeingültigkeit suggeriert. Der Text steht praktisch durchgängig im Präsens, bis auf die Sätze 11 bis 13, was man von einer biographischen Darstellung nicht erwarten würde. Es ist dadurch für die biographischen Abläufe eine Unschärfe der Zeitperspektive gegeben, die in diesem Fall auch eine Unschärfe der kausalen Perspektiven mit sich bringt. Nur zweimal taucht die kausale Konjunktion "weil" auf; 19 mal immerhin die konditionale Konjunktion "wenn", allerdings nicht im konditionalen Gebrauch, sondern reihend; 12 mal das sehr unbestimmte additive "dann", sehr oft natürlich eine ganz unbestimmte Reihung mit "und" und 15 mal das ebenfalls recht unbestimmt gebrauchte "daß", "damit". Konditionale Satzverknüpfungen sind damit relativ selten, auch kommen nie verbindende, auf den vorhergehenden Satz bezugnehmende Partikel vor wie "also", "somit" oder Erläuterungen wie "damit ist gemeint, daß" etc. Wir finden damit deutlich die von Holm-Hadulla beschriebene Reduktion von Transfer und Substitution in diesem Text, ohne sie allerdings hier an einem Kontrolltext quantifizieren zu können. Ein weiteres Merkmal ist die semantische Vieldeutigkeit, vor allem der Substantive, zumal sie nur 9 mal als Satzsubjekte auftauchen gegenüber 81 mal dem Einsatz von Pronominalsubjekten, zumeist vertreten durch das sehr unbestimmte "das". Dadurch entsteht beim Zuhörer zwar Assoziationsreichtum, gleichermaßen aber auch ein Präzisierungsbedürfnis. Beispiele dafür sind der Gebrauch des Wortes "Verfugung" oder der Satzpassage "eingebildet im Zimmer sitzen". Übliche Ankerbegriffe für Präzisierungen geben nicht genügend Halt oder fehlen ganz, wie etwa ein Appell an geläufige Denkmuster, ein Wechsel zwischen Metaphorik und Konkretion oder gar ein Einsatz metakommunikativer Mitteilungen mit Humor, Selbstironie oder direkter Erläuterung des Gemeinten. Mehrdeutigkeiten entstehen damit sowohl auf der Wortebene wie auf der Satzebene, wobei vor allem die Mehrdeutigkeiten auf Wortebene bisweilen den Charakter eines Wortspieles annehmen könnten, wäre nicht der Gesamttext so diffus. So aber ist der bestimmende Eindruck, daß die Mehrdeutigkeit nicht gezielt zur Expression von Ambivalenz, mehrschichtigen Wahrnehmungen oder sonst unbewußten Konnotationen des Wort- oder Satzfeldes eingesetzt wird, sondern daß eine Präzisierung nicht verfügbar ist und daß die Mehrdeutigkeit eine Art Vagheit des Subjektcharakters der Rede wiederspiegelt. Damit lassen sich auch die eingangs bei Holm-Hadulla und Tress zitierten Phänomene des Intermingling und der Verminderung des Deixis in diesem Text feststellen.

Es wird dadurch die intendierte Aussage des Textes aus der Sprachstruktur selbst kaum oder gar nicht verständlich, eher dann, wenn der Situationskontext als Informationsquelle den notwendigen Standpunkt und Subjektcharakter der Aussage substituiert.

Gibt es eine Gemeinsamkeit der beschriebenen Funktionsabweichungen, und wie kann man sie konzeptualisieren? Mir scheint eine Gemeinsamkeit der beschriebenen Funktionsabweichungen und -eigentümlichkeiten - also Vieldeutigkeit, Mangel an Ich-Gebrauch, Mangel an Substantiven, Mangel an Prädikaten, Gebrauch von durchgängigem Präsens, Iterationen und Reihung statt Konditionalisierung von Satzgliedern, Gebrauch diffuser Pronominalsatzsubjekte - darin zu liegen, daß die Geschlossenheit und Pointiertheit der Aussage im Ich-Du-Kontext gemindert ist. Wichtig ist, daß nicht die Vieldeutigkeit an sich das Abnorme ist, - sie kommt auch in bestimmten Literaturformen vor, sie kann in witzigen ironischen Anspielungen enthalten sein -, sondern das Festgelegtsein auf sie, die mangelnde Verfügbarkeit alternativer und präzisierender Ausdruckmöglichkeiten, und damit das Fehlen eines indirekten metakommunikativen Kenntlichmachens der Vieldeutigkeit als so gemeinter, was allein schon durch ihre Kontrastierung mit präzisen Aussagen möglich wäre, aber auch durch inhaltliche Abhebung; kurz, man müßte irgendwie die Intention spüren. Andererseits kann eine Präzisierung des Bedeutungshalo von Wörtern, Metaphern, ganzen Satz- und Denkfiguren durch den Kontext der ganzen Rede geschehen, - man wehrt sich bekanntlich gegen ein entstellendes Zitat mit dem Hinweis, es sei aus dem Zusammenhang gerissen. Aber auch diese kontextuelle Präzisierung bleibt hier auf halbem Wege stehen.

Für die Konzeptualisierung dieser Störung kommen alte gestaltpsychologische Ansätze in den Sinn, wie sie seinerzeit von CONRAD in die Schizophrenielehre eingeführt worden sind, mit der Beschreibung der epikritischen und protopathischen Durchgliederung der Gestalt im Zuge der Figur-Hintergrund-Differenzierung; jüngst hat KNOLL wieder darauf Bezug genommen.

Mir scheint im vorliegenden Fall aber eine weitere Dimension der Störung essentiell zu sein, nämlich der Mangel an Rückbezüglichkeit vom sprechenden Subjekt zu seinem Gegenüber und wieder zurück auf das sprechende und sinngestaltende Subjekt, sei es durch direkten Austausch, sei es durch Perspektivenwechsel mit imaginierter Übernahme der Position des sozialen Anderen. Die Patientin formuliert selbst dieses Problem unentwegt mit dem Thema der "Verfugung", der "Darstellung", etc., die ganze Rede kreist inhaltlich darum. Die Entschlüsselung des Textes gelingt gerade von diesen rudimentären Ansätzen zu einer Bezogenheit auf das Gegenüber. Wohl ist die Wirkung der Rede durchaus auf den Zuhörer hin entworfen, das untergründige Imponieren-Wollen durch den Jargon, die Rechtfertigungansätze und der Schameinbruch zum Schluß deuten darauf hin; es mangelt aber an der präzisierenden Kontrolle durch den intrapsychisch mithörenden sozialen Anderen oder ein konkretes Eingehen auf den Untersucher mit dem Element der Erläuterung, Verdeutlichung, eben einem dialogisch-dialektischen Prozeß der Feinabstimmung, der Verständigung auf eine gemeinsame Sinngestalt. Die Sprachstruktur legt den Verdacht nahe, daß hinter diesem Mangel an Intersubjektivität ein Mangel an Subjektivität liegt, die eigene Stellungnahme vage bleibt. Ich erinnere an den seltenen Ich-Gebrauch, die zahlreichen unbestimmten Pronominalsatzsubjekte, die prädikatlosen Sätze und den Inhalt der Aussage. Ich habe an anderer Stelle vorgeschlagen (MUNDT 1984), diese Fähigkeit zur Sinnsetzung in der dialektischen Abstimmung mit dem sozialen Anderen als Intentionalität zu bezeichnen unter Bezugnahme auf die Geschichte dieses Begriffes bis zu HUSSERL, wie sie von SPIEGELBERG (1936) gegeben wurde und in jüngster Zeit mit GOSZTONYI (1972) auch wieder in der Psychologie aufgegriffen wurde. Nicht gemeint sind damit Antriebsqualitäten, wie sie mit diesem Begriff bei DÜHRSSEN und RUDOLF in der Tradition der SCHULTZ-HENCKE-Schule angezielt werden. Neuerdings ist in der analytischen Philosophie des Geistes wieder von intentionalen Systemen die Rede, z.B. bei BIERI und TRESS, die den Begriff operational nehmen im Hinblick auf Kommunikationsleistungen und -kompetenz und das Subjekt gewissermaßen als black box betrachten.

Für den schizophrenen Patienten bedeutet eine Störung intentionaler Leistungen mit Entordnungsphänomenen zuallererst eine Beeinträchtigung des Subjektcharakters seines Erlebens, Denkens und Handelns. Dieser Subjektcharakter von Erleben und Handeln scheint untrennbar mit der Fähigkeit zur

Sinnsetzung verbunden zu sein. Gleichzeitig scheint die Entwicklung des Subjektcharakters ebenso unlösbar und ohne ein Vorher oder Nachher mit einer funktionierenden Intersubjektivität verbunden. Der Text der Patientin weist damit aber auch über die kognitivistischen Vulnerabilitätshypothesen der Schizophrenie hinaus, denn die Störung manifestierte sich hier gerade nicht in der straffen Reizreaktionssituation der gezielten Fragen, sondern in der liberaleren, offenen Situation der Selbstexplikation. Gerade die Offenheit der Situation, die vermehrt die intentionalen Leistungen des Subjekts fordert, macht den eigentlichen "Streß" für den Schizophrenen aus.

4. Therapeutische Konsequenzen

Für die Überlegungen zu möglichen therapeutischen Konsequenzen aus diesem Verstehensansatz der Störung stellt sich zunächst die Frage, inwieweit die beschriebene Störung vom sprachlichen kommunikativen Bereich verallgemeinbar auf den gesamten Weltbezug der Patientin ist. Hier gibt es offenbar ganz erhebliche Schwankungen der intentionalen Leistungen. Trotz des Unfalls und einer gewissen Verwahrlosungsneigung hatte sich die Patientin doch über wahrscheinlich sechs Jahre des Krankheitsverlaufs hin stets selbst versorgen können. Man muß also annehmen, daß, je enger und unerbittlicher die Leitschiene der vorgegebenen Sinngestalten ist, umsoweniger die Pathologie der Patientin in Erscheinung tritt, wie etwa der Explorationsmodus der direktiven Fragen zeigt, die keine Sprachstörung bei der Patientin zeitigten oder ihr weitgehend zweckmäßiger Umgang mit den unbelebten Dingen etwa in der Haushaltsführung oder vor der Begutachtung über Jahre auch im Verkehrsverhalten, wo eine Fehlhandlung sich unmittelbar rächen würde. Das geordnete Verhalten langjährig schwerst defekter Anstaltspatienten, z.B. bei Brandkatastrophen, das in älteren Lehrbüchern als luzides Intervall immer wieder erwähnt wird, würde sich so einordnen lassen. Man kann also wohl von der Sprachstörung auf die Existenzstörung des gesamten Weltverhältnisses verallgemeinern; die Stabilität, Präzision und Flexibilität intentionaler Leistungen scheint aber in verschiedenen Lebensbereichen ganz unterschiedlich zu sein. Provozierend für die Störung scheinen vor allem solche Situationen zu sein, die entweder Selbstexplikation oder sonst losgelöst von konkreten und präzisen Führungslinien Sinnkonstituierung erfordern. Je mehr Ambiguität eine Situation erlaubt, je mehr das ausgewogene Zulassen von problematischen oder peinlichen Gefühlen und Tendenzen, etwa in Anspielung, Ironie, Humor gefordert wären, um so gefährdeter erscheinen die intentionalen Leistungen. Andererseits fühlen sich die Patienten gerade von der beherzten Kommunikation, in der ein präpotentes Sinnangebot des Kommunikationspartners gemacht wird, rasch alieniert, wiederum umsomehr, je kontroverser die Intentionen sind und je mehr ambivalent besetzte Erlebnisinhalte und Strebungen des Patienten ins Spiel gebracht werden. Dieser Prozeß ist in der älteren familiendynamischen Literatur mit der Frage, wer hat die stärkere Wirklichkeit in der Familie Schizophrener, thematisiert worden und experimentalpsychologisch durch D. Reiss gut belegt, der nachweisen konnte, daß im Gegensatz zu neurotischen Patienten Schizophrene eigene richtige Lösungsansätze für eine vorgegebene Aufgabe unter dem Einfluß hinzutretender Schlüsselangehöriger zu falschen Lösungen modifizieren.

Für die dyadische therapeutische Beziehung, aber auch für sozialtherapeutische Ansätze gilt es damit einen dem Patienten bekömmlichen Mittelweg zwischen zudringlicher Überfremdung durch Sinnvorgaben und Provokation der Intentionalitätsschwäche durch zuviel Unstrukturiertheit und Ambiguität zu steuern. Der Einsatz der Beziehung zum Patienten als therapeutisches Instrument fordert in diesem Verständnis behutsame Substituierung von Sinnsetzungen an Stellen, an denen der Patient gefordert ist und sie nicht leisten kann, gleichzeitig aber Respektierung von Abschirmtendenzen des Patienten gegenüber Intentionsdruck, etwa durch Rückzugsverhalten aus zu engen und intensiven Beziehungen, wozu auch eine therapeutische Beziehung gehören kann. Klare Orientierung, klares Setting, kurze häufige Kontakte erleichtern dem Patienten das Intendieren, eventuell auch das Umgehen von Ambitendenzen.

Auch präventive Gesichtspunkte können aus diesem Ansatz abgeleitet werden. Beispielsweise überfordert ein zu abstinentes Therapeutenverhalten, wie es gelegentlich in psychoanalytischen Settings vorkommen kann bei gleichzeitiger Stimulierung unbewußter Fantasien und Impulse die Sinnsetzung für die Selbstexplikation maximal; ebenso legt aber umgekehrt die forcierte Konfrontation mit einer präpotenten Wirklichkeit Anderer, in bestimmten Selbsterfahrungsgruppen, die schizophrene Wehrlosigkeit im Kontakt gegenüber Intentionen des sozialen Anderen offen. Beide Therapiesettings sind vielfach aus Auslösekonstellationen für psychotische Schübe studiert worden. In jüngerer Zeit hat Brücher (1988) in einer Studie über die alltagsweltliche Sinnkonstituierung Schizophrener in geschützten Wohnheimen auf die Gefahren falsch verstandener Therapie hingewiesen, bei der ein Patient, der in die Gemeinschaft nicht hineinwächst, nun noch mit zusätzlicher Therapie "beschossen" wird. Die Verwurzelung im durchaus banalen, unverfänglichen, unambiguösen, nicht problematisierten Alltagsleben dürfte sowohl in dyadischen wie gruppentherapeutischen Arrangements die Basis für eine Festigung der intentionalen Leistungen Schizophrener darstellen. Dies könnte auch ein Grund dafür sein, daß Arbeitstherapie mit ihrer Restriktion von Problematisierungen auf instrumentelle Aspekte des Verhaltens unter Ausblendung der Persönlichkeit und dem klar sich aufdrängenden Nützlichkeitsaspekt der Sinnkonstitution so versichernd für schizophrene Patienten wirken kann. Ähnlich wirkt die Einführung eines medizinischen Krankheitsmodells mit Anleitung zu coping -Verhalten.

Die therapeutisch heikelste Problematik bleibt aber sicher die Substitution von Sinnsetzungen, zu der die Patienten bewußt oder unbewußt herausfordern, wenn diese Substitution nicht als unverbindliches alltagsweltliches Milieuangebot, sondern als gezielter Vorschlag mit Aufforderungscharakter an die Patienten gelangt. Vielleicht sollten solche Interventionen überhaupt ganz vermieden werden; wenn sie gewagt werden, stellen sie besondere Anforderungen an die Stetigkeit und emotionale Positivität der therapeutischen Beziehung, an das Gespür für die relevanten und progressionsfähigen Inhalte im Seelenleben und die Fähigkeit des Therapeuten, zusammen mit dem Patienten Ambivalenz und Unabgeschlossenheit der Sinnfindung auszuhalten. Die Positivierung des schizophrenen Selbsterlebens darf, wie BENEDETTI (1983) einmal erläutert hat, dadurch jedenfalls nicht gefährdet werden.[1]

Zusammenfassung: Ein schizophasischer Text wird präsentiert, der im Rahmen einer Anamneseerhebung einen bestimmten biographischen Abschnitt erzählt. Aus dem kommunikativen Zusammenhang läßt sich der emotionale Gehalt des zunächst weitgehend unverständlichen Textes erschließen. Anhand einiger linguistisch präzisierbarer Eigentümlichkeiten des Textes werden die Abwandlung seines Subjektcharakters, seiner Intersubjektivität und damit der in ihm wirkenden Intentionalität erörtert. Die Interpretation der Störung als Ausdruck instabiler Intentionalität weist für die therapeutischen Konsequenzen auf die stets prekäre Balance zwischen notwendiger Stützung von Sinnsetzungen durch den Therapeuten und zu vermeidender Alienation des Patienten durch eine präpotente Wirklichkeit des sozialen Anderen hin.

On the Intentional Structure of a Schizophasic Text

Summary: The paper starts with the presentation of a schizophasic text, in which a patient relates some biographical matters. The emotional contents of the otherwise riddled text can be deciphered in the context of the communicative situation. Certain linguistic features, idiosyncrasies and anolmalies, point to a disturbance of the patient's subjective and intersubjective character and manifest a deformed intentionality. This interpretation of the schizophasic text emphasizes the fact that the patient hovers precautiously between his/her search for a settled and stable sense of reality as offered and supported by the therapy and the protection against the intensive and alienating reality as experienced in intensive social contact.

Literatur

BENEDETTI, G. (1983): Die Positivierung schizophrenen Erlebens im therapeutischen Symbol. Nervenarzt **54**, S. 150-157.

BLANKENBURG, W. (1984): Störungen von Auffassung und Sprache bei Schizophrenen. Nervenarzt **55**, S. 488-495.

BLANKENBURG, W. (1987): Zur Subjektivität des Subjekts aus psychopathologischer Sicht. In: H. NAGL-DOCEKAL und H. VETTER (Hg.): Tod des Subjekts?, S. 164-189. R. Oldenbourg, Wien, München.

BRÜCHER, K. (1988): Therapie und Alltag im Wohnheim - Ausschnitte einer Ethnographie. Fortschr. Neurol. Psychiat. **56**, S. 193-203.

CONSOLI, S.: Erzählungen Schizophrener. In: A. KRAUS, CH. MUNDT (Hg.): Sprache und Schizophrenie. Thieme, Stuttgart, im Druck.

GOSZTONYI, A. (1972): Grundlagen der Erkenntnis. Beck, München.

HOLM-HADULLA, R. (1982): Der "Konkretismus" als Ausdruck schizophrenen Denkens, Sprechens und Verhaltens. Nervenarzt **53**, S. 524-529.

---

1 Ich bin Herrn Dr. WOLFGANG HOFMANN zu Dank für wertvolle Anregungen bei der Interpretation des Textes verpflichtet.

LANG, H. (1973): Die Sprache und das Unbewußte. Suhrkamp, Frankfurt.

LANG, H. (1980): Struktural-analytische Aspekte der Subjektivität. In: KITTLER, F.A. (Hg.): Austreibung des Geistes aus den Geisteswissenschaften. Programme des Poststrukturalismus. Schöningh, Paderborn, S. 188-203.

MUNDT, CH. (1982): Die schizophrene Primärpersönlichkeit im Lichte psychopathologischer und tiefenpsychologischer Ansätze. In: W. JANZARIK (Hg.): Psychopathologische Konzepte der Gegenwart. Enke, Stuttgart, S. 158-166.

MUNDT, CH. (1984): Der Begriff der Intentionalität und die Defizienzlehre von den Schizophrenien. Nervenarzt **55**, S. 582-588.

PETERS, U.H. (1981): Schizophrene Sprachstörungen. In: HUBER, G. (Hg.): Schizophrenie. Stand und Entwicklungstendenzen der Forschung. Schattauer, Stuttgart, New York, S. 11-20.

PETERS, U.H.: Untersuchungen zu den Verwerfungen im Sprach- und Textverhalten Schizophrener. In: A. KRAUS, CH. MUNDT (Hg.): Sprache und Schizophrenie, Thieme, Stuttgart, im Druck.

REISS, D. (1968): Individual thinking and family interaction III. An experimental study of categorization performance in schizophrenics. J. nerv. ment. Dis. **146**, S. 384-403.

SPIEGELBERG, H. (1936): Der Begriff der Intentionalität in der Scholastik, bei Brentano und bei Husserl. Philosophische Hefte **5**, S. 75-91.

TRESS, W., PFAFFENBERGER, U., FROMMER J., (1984): Zur Patholinguistik schizophrener Texte. Eine vergleichende Untersuchung an Schizophrenen, Depressiven, Hirnorganikern und Gesunden. Nervenarzt **55**, S. 488-495.

Dies und nicht das – dies mag das Problem sein: Formal-logische Betrachtungen der schizophrenen Denkstörungen

R. Hess

1. Einleitung

Seit BLEULER 1911 die Assoziationsstörungen Schizophrener als Primärsymptome bezeichnet hat, die eine direkte Folge des hypothetischen organischen Substrats darstellen, sind die Denkstörungen *bzw. kognitive Störungen* ins Zentrum des pathogenetischen Interesses gerückt. KLOSTERKÖTTER (1982) hat die assoziationspsychologische Betrachtung BLEULERS der heutigen lernpsychologischen HUBERS (vgl. z.B. HUBER 1979, S. 400ff; SCHÜTTLER et al. 1981, S. 194f) gegenübergestellt und weitgehende strukturelle Übereinstimmung festgestellt. Die Terminologie ist entsprechend den unterschiedlichen Betrachtungsweisen verschieden und die Hypothesen über das zugrundeliegende organische Substrat haben sich gewandelt. Trotz einer Vielzahl von klinischen Beobachtungen und experimentellen Untersuchungen ist man jedoch dem eigentlichen Ziel, der Kenntnis der morphologischen oder physiologischen Veränderung, die die kognitiven Störungen bedingt, nicht wesentlich näher gekommen.

Was wird heute unter dem Begriff der *Kognition* verstanden? NEISSER (1967) faßte darunter alle Schritte der zentralnervösen Informationsverarbeitung von der Aufnahme über Filterung, Speicherung, Abruf von Speicherinhalten, emotionale Färbung und Bewertung, Verknüpfung von Wahrnehmungs- und Denkinhalten mit- und untereinander (dem eigentlichen Denken), bis hin zur Abgabe von Information durch Bewegung, Mimik und Sprache. Entsprechend der Vielzahl verschiedener Aspekte der Kognition sind eine große Anzahl von klinischen Beobachtungen und experimentellen Untersuchungen durchgeführt worden, die Störungen der kognitiven Funktionen bei Schizophrenen auf den verschiedenen Ebenen der Informationsverarbeitung nachgewiesen haben. Die meines Erachtens beste Zusammenfassung und kritische Bewertung dieser Ergebnisse findet sich bei CHAPMAN und CHAPMAN (1973). Ergänzend dazu seien die Review-Artikel von NUECHTERLEIN und DAWSON (1984) und HOLZMAN (1986) sowie aus dem deutschen Sprachraum COHEN und PLAUM (1980), RUCKSTUHL

(1981), und zum immanenten Problem der Aufmerksamkeitsstörungen die Monographie von HARTWICH (1980) genannt.

2. Die Theorien der schizophrenen Denkstörungen[1]

Tabelle 1 zeigt die verschiedenen Theorien schizophrener Denkstörungen und jeweils ihre wesentlichen Vertreter. Im folgenden Kapitel soll an vier Beispielen dargelegt werden, daß möglicherweise die inhaltlich scheinbar divergierenden Hypothesen formal auf eine gemeinsame Grundstörung der zentralnervösen Informationsverarbeitung zurückgeführt werden können. Um die formale Vorgehensweise zu verdeutlichen, sei zuvor ein Rekurs auf den formalen Ablauf und das Ziel unsrer Bemühungen gestattet.

Tabelle 1: Die Theorien der kognitiven Störungen

1.) Assoziationsstörungen	BLEULER
2.) Excessive yielding to normal biases	CHAPMAN
3.) Loss of abstract thinking	VYGOTSKY, GOLDSTEIN
4.) Errors in syllogistic reasoning	VON DOMARUS, ARIETI
5.) Overinclusion	CAMERON
6.) Regression to an early stage of development (der psychoanalytische Standpunkt)	FREUD, JUNG, ARIETI
7.) Response to emotional problems	JUNG, CAMERON, SULLIVAN, HALEY
8.) Loss of major set	SHAKOW
9.) Defects of attention and information processing	BROEN, CHAPMAN, CROMWELL
10.) Drive theory and schizophrenic conditions	MEDNICK, BROEN, STORMS

Wir beobachten in der Klinik oder im Experiment menschliches Verhalten. Die Grundlage für dieses Verhalten sind neuronale Prozesse, in denen sich Intentionen und Gedanken manifestieren und die schließlich die Äußerungen des Organismus, also das Verhalten steuern. Beobachten wir in einer bestimmten Situation unübliches, von einer Norm abweichendes Verhalten, so stellt sich die Frage, ob dieses Verhalten durch eine besondere, individuelle frühere Erfahrung bedingt ist, die das Individuum sich in dieser Situation so und nicht anders verhalten läßt. Solches Verhalten wäre inhaltlich begründet und würde daher nur in bestimmten, ähnlich erscheinenden Situationen auftreten.

Von dieser inhaltlich zu begründenden Situation ist die zu unterscheiden, in der das beobachtete andersartige Verhalten durch eine organische Fehlfunktion verursacht ist. Hier würde das Fehlverhalten immer dann auftreten, wenn im Handlungsablauf die gestörte Teilfunktion benötigt wird, unabhängig vom jeweiligen Sinnzusammenhang. Wollen wir Erkenntnisse über die Art der gestörten Teilfunktion gewinnen, so hilft daher nicht die inhaltliche Beschreibung, sondern die formale Betrachtung der gestörten Handlungsabläufe.

Zur Veranschaulichung des Gesagten wollen wir den Weg eines Autos betrachten, dessen Lenkung nach links blockiert ist. Ein solches Fahrzeug kann noch alle gewünschten Orte erreichen, es wird nur immer dann, wenn links abbiegen erforderlich wäre, statt dessen drei Mal

1 Wir folgen in unsrer Übersicht der Darstellung von CHAPMAN und CHAPMAN (1973).

rechts abbiegen, um in die gewünschte Richtung zu fahren. Die inhaltliche Beschreibung, wie das Auto gefahren ist, mit Überlegungen warum es diesen Weg gewählt hat (z.B. der Fahrer wollte noch Freunde besuchen, einkaufen etc.) führt im Hinblick auf das Verständnis der Störung nicht weiter. Die formale Betrachtung aber, daß der Wagen unabhängig vom Ziel geradeaus vorwärts und rückwärts gefahren ist sowie vielfach rechts, nie aber links abgebogen ist, läßt den Schluß zu, daß möglicherweise die Lenkung nach links blockiert ist und dies den ungewöhnlichen Weg des Autos erklärt.

Bei der Erforschung endogener Psychosen stehen wir vor einem ähnlichen Problem. Der Begriff *endogen* impliziert eine hypothetische organische Ursache, auf die wir aufgrund der Psychopathologie bzw. des abweichenden Verhaltens zu schließen versuchen. Ähnlich wie im Beispiel des Autos kommt es hierbei nicht auf den inhaltlichen Aspekt des Verhaltens an, da dieser von der je eigenen Erfahrung des Individuums abhängt. Schon BLEULER schrieb, daß jemand, der noch nie von Jesuiten gehört hat, sich auch nicht von ihnen verfolgt fühlen kann (BLEULER 1911, S. 285). Einzig entscheidend für einen sinnvollen Rückschluß auf eine organische Ursache pathologischen Denkens oder Verhaltens ist dessen formaler Ablauf. Im Begriff der formalen Denkstörung, die zumindest mit zu der diagnostischen Beurteilung der Schizophrenie herangezogen wird, ist diese Überlegung schon enthalten, sie scheint jedoch bei der divergierenden und teilweise konkurrierenden Interpretation verschiedener Ergebnisse zu kognitiven Störungen Schizophrener nicht ausreichend beachtet worden zu sein.

3. Eine Fehlfunktion des logischen *exklusiven oder* als gemeinsames Merkmal der kognitiven Störungen Schizophrener?

3.1 BLEULERS Theorie: *Gestörte Assoziationen* und *Ambivalenz*

BLEULER sieht das Wesen der Assoziationsstörungen im Verlust der Zielgerichtetheit des Denkens. Die Gedankengänge sind nicht mehr logisch oder durch nachvollziehbare Erfahrung geordnet, es brechen vielmehr immer wieder unerwartet ungewöhnliche Aspekte in den Verlauf der Assoziationen oder des Gedankens ein. Für den Zuhörer fehlt die übliche Organisation des Gesagten und die gewohnten inneren Beziehungen, sodaß das Gesagte unverständlich wird. Einzelne Assoziationen eines Wortes oder der Teilaspekt eines Sinnzusammenhangs können dabei durchaus nachvollziehbar bleiben.

Als ein konkretes Beispiel führt BLEULER die Benennung eines Elternteils mit "Eltern" statt mit Vater oder Mutter an. Hieran wird deutlich, inwiefern die Assoziationsstörung als mangelnde Exklusion verstanden werden kann. Eltern sind Vater und Mutter, ein einzelner Elternteil offensichtlich entweder Vater oder Mutter, also Vater und nicht Mutter oder umgekehrt. Dieser letzte Schritt in der logischen Begriffsbildung wurde anscheinend nicht durchgeführt oder verlief fehlerhaft, daher die falsche Benennung mit Eltern.

Ein weiteres Beispiel stellt auf die Frage: "Liegt Ihnen etwas schwer auf der Seele?" die Antwort dar: "Ja, Eisen ist schwer". Hier wird die aus dem Sinnzusammenhang ersichtliche übertragene Bedeutung des Wortes "schwer" nicht erfaßt, andere, ebenfalls mögliche Bedeutungen von schwer können nicht ausgeschlossen werden und die Antwort erfolgt nach einer in diesem Zusammenhang falschen, sonst jedoch häufigen Assoziation, nämlich "Eisen ist schwer".

Die Ambivalenz Schizophrener wird von Bleuler als "eine so direkte Folge der schizophrenen Assoziationsstörung" angesehen, "daß ein vollständiges Fehlen unwahrscheinlich wird" (Bleuler 1911, S. 43). Den Begriff der Ambivalenz umschreibt Chapman (1973, S. 108) treffend als "gleichzeitige Erfahrung sich wechselseitig ausschließender Impulse, Wünsche und Ideen". Unter Ambivalenz leiden heißt also, eine der sich widersprechenden Alternativen nicht unterdrücken bzw. ausschließen zu können. Die menschliche Wirklichkeit stellt uns häufig vor solche Ambivalenzsituationen, in denen wir uns für eine Alternative entscheiden müssen, auch wenn weder logisch eine Entscheidung zu treffen ist, noch aufgrund von Erfahrung die Tragweite des Entschlussses zu übersehen ist. Der psychisch gesunde Mensch ist zu dieser Leistung offenbar fähig. Aus der Neurosenlehre ist Ambivalenz als auslösender Faktor für die Komplexbildung in Teilbereichen des Erlebens wohl bekannt. Bei Schizophrenen bleiben Ambivalenzen auf mehreren Ebenen des Erlebens unaufgelöst bestehen, was darauf hindeuten könnte, daß der Mechanismus, eine der Alternativen auszuschließen, auf verschiedenen Ebenen der Informationsverarbeitung gestört ist.

Angeregt durch Bleulers Überlegungen wurden die Assoziationsstörungen Schizophrener mit einer Vielfalt psychologischer und psychophysischer Methoden untersucht und auf deren Ergebnisse aufbauend weitergehende Theorien, wie schon erwähnt, entwickelt, von denen noch einzelne beispielhaft auf ihre Vereinbarkeit mit der hier vorgetragenen Überlegung geprüft werden sollen.

3.2 Camerons *Overinclusion*-Hypothese

Die Formulierung *overinclusion* drückt das gleiche aus wie "*mangelnde Exklusion*", so daß sich begriffliche Erläuterungen erübrigen. Es sollen aber noch die experimentellen Grundlagen skizziert werden, die zu der Formulierung der Hypothese führten.

Cameron gab seinen Patienten die Aufgabe, Gegenstände nach vorgegebenen Merkmalen zu sortieren. Er bemerkte dabei, daß sie häufig unkorrekte Antworten gaben, weil sie ihre Aufmerksamkeit nicht auf die vorgelegten Gegenstände beschränken konnten und andere im Raum befindliche mit in die Aufgabe einbezogen. Selbst nach einem Hinweis, dies nicht zu tun, blieben sie bei ihrem Verhalten. Ein Patient, dessen Äußerung zitiert wird (Cameron 1947) sagt sinngemäß, daß er sich nicht auf die Aufgabe beschränken kann und Dinge aus dem Raum hinzunehmen muß. D.h. eben, daß er sie *nicht* aus seinem Bewußtseinsfeld *ausschließen* kann, daher "Overinclusion".

Payne und Mitarbeiter (1959) führten weitere Untersuchungen durch, um Camerons Hypothese zu überprüfen. Es sei hier nur ihr Test zur Klassifizierung von Gegenständen, der die deutlichsten Ergebnisse lieferte, kurz dargestellt.

Der Test bestand aus 4 Dreiecken, 4 Quadraten und 4 Kreisen, die sich in Gewicht, Dicke, Größe, Material, sowie Farbe und Helligkeit der Farbe unterschieden. So konnten die Gegenstände in 10 verschiedene Gruppierungen sortiert werden. Die Versuchspersonen wurden aufgefordert, die auf dem Tisch liegenden Gegenstände nach irgendeiner Ordnung zu sortieren. War dies geschehen, so wurde nach dem Grund für diese Ordnung gefragt und danach aufgefordert, sie weiter nach so vielen Aspekten wie möglich zu ordnen.

Wie erwartet nahmen Schizophrene mehr Aspekte an den Gegenständen wahr, als zur Lösung der Aufgabe relevant waren, und sortierten so nach abweichenden Prinzipien wie z.B. nach den Schatten, die die Gegenstände warfen, oder nach Kratzern auf der Oberfläche. Insgesamt machten Schizophrene die etwa vierfache Anzahl inkorrekter Antworten im Vergleich zu Kontrollpersonen, wobei Ersterkrankte eine höhere Fehlerzahl aufwiesen als chronisch Schizophrene oder Normalpersonen. Die Ergebnisse wurden als Bestätigung von CAMERONS Overinclusion-Hypothese gewertet (PAYNE 1962).

3.3 *Excessive yielding to normal biases* (CHAPMAN)

Die CHAPMANschen Untersuchungen betrafen das Sprachverhalten von Schizophrenen und befaßten sich mit den ungewöhnlichen, von der Norm abweichenden Antworten auf bestimmte Fragen. Seine Hypothese geht davon aus, daß Begriffe vieldeutig sind und ihre zutreffende Bedeutung aus dem Sinnzusammenhang erschlossen werden muß. Bei Schizophrenen fand er gehäuft Antworten, die im Sinnzusammenhang falsch waren, jedoch durchaus einer möglichen Bedeutung des Wortes entsprachen. Als Erläuterung mag das erwähnte Beispiel von BLEULER dienen, in dem auf die Frage, ob etwas schwer auf der Seele liege, die Antwort: "Ja, Eisen ist schwer" erfolgt.

Die von CHAPMAN tatsächlich gestellten Fragen folgten dem Muster:

Robert says he likes rare meat.
This means:
He likes the kind of meat that is exceedingly uncommon.
He likes meat with bones in it.
He likes partially cooked meat.

In Kontrollversuchen wurde das Wortverständnis der Versuchspersonen geprüft, insbesondere das Verständnis der gefragten Begriffe, also z.B. "rare". Es wurde festgestellt, daß das Spektrum der Wortbedeutungen bei Schizophrenen und Normalpersonen ähnlich war, und auch daß die Verteilung zwischen bevorzugter und nicht bevorzugter Wortbedeutung vergleichbar waren. Die Ergebnisse zeigten, daß Schizophrene vermehrt auf die bevorzugte Wortbedeutung antworteten, auch wenn diese Antwort aus dem Kontext heraus falsch war.

Die theoretischen Erklärungsversuche der CHAPMANschen Befunde sind vielfältig (siehe Tabelle 2) und werden von ihm ausgiebig gewürdigt (CHAPMAN und CHAPMAN 1973, S. 134-135). Sie spiegeln zu einem großen Teil die veschiedenen Hypothesen zur Genese der schizophrenen Denkstörungen wieder und können hier nicht im einzelnen erörtert werden.

Formal betrachtet lautet die Aufgabenstellung der Versuche, aus einer Vielzahl von Reizaspekten oder möglichen Begriffsbedeutungen die aufgrund des Kontextes richtige auszuwählen und dabei von einer nach Erfahrung, Häufigkeit des Gebrauchs etc. bevorzugten abzusehen. Den Schizophrenen gelingt dies nicht, ihre Antworten folgen vielmehr jeweils einer bevorzugten, im Zusammenhang aber unrichtigen Bedeutung. In unserem Sinne formuliert heißt das, daß sie die bevorzugte, aber nach dem Kontext unrichtige Alternative nicht ausschließen können, um die ihnen durchaus bekannte richtige zu nennen.

CHAPMAN selbst schließt, daß das Prinzip der Bevorzugung starker Reize oder Begriffsbedeutungen eine Vielzahl der bei Schizophrenen beschriebenen

Phänomene erklären kann, darunter auch die im nächsten Abschnitt behandelten Irrtümer des logischen Schließens.

Tabelle 2: Theoretische Erklärungsversuche der Befunde von CHAPMAN (nach CHAPMAN und CHAPMAN 1973)

1. Unfähigkeit, auf Hinweise aus dem Kontext zu achten.
2. Unfähigkeit, die Aufmerksamkeit von bevorzugten Bedeutungen bzw. Reizen abzulenken.
3. Verminderte Aufmerksamkeit.
4. Eingeengte Aufmerksamkeit.
5. Erhöhter "drive".
6. Mangelnde Motivation sich zu Verständigen.
7. Rückschritt zu Primärprozeßdenken

3.4 Irrtümer im *logischen Schließen* (VON DOMARUS, ARIETI)

In seiner Arbeit von 1944 vertritt VON DOMARUS die Hypothese, daß Schizophrene nach anderen Gesetzen der Logik argumentieren als Normalpersonen. Er illustriert sie mit folgenden Beispielen:

> Normales Denken folgt den Gesetzen der Logik, wie im Nachweis der Sterblichkeit von Sokrates dargelegt.
>
> Alle Menschen sind sterblich.
> Sokrates ist ein Mensch.
> Daher ist Sokrates sterblich.
>
> Seine Erfahrung mit schizophrenem Denken wird folgendermaßen erklärt:
>
> Manche Indianer sind schnell.
> Hirsche sind schnell.
> Also sind manche Indianer Hirsche.
>
> Dieser Schluß ist natürlich falsch, da alleine aus der gemeinsamen Eigenschaft, schnell zu sein, keine Identität folgt. Nach VON DOMARUS ist diese Eigenart, von einem gemeinsamen Prädikat auf Identität zu schließen, typisch für schizophrenes Denken, das er dann paralogisch nennt.

ARIETI hat VON DOMARUS' Hypothese erweitert und durch einen Erklärungsversuch ergänzt. Die von ihm erwähnten Beispiele legten nahe, daß das falsche Schließen inhaltlich durch die Befriedigung emotionaler Bedürfnisse Schizophrener bestimmt wird (vgl. ARIETI 1962).

Experimentelle Überprüfungen der VON DOMARUSschen Hypothese ergaben, daß 1. auch Normalpersonen zu einem erheblichen Teil zu Schlüssen neigen, die den paralogischen der Schizophrenen ähnlich sind, und 2., daß der wesentliche Unterschied in den bizzarren Inhalten der Schlüsse von Schizophrenen liegt (vgl. CHAPMAN und CHAPMAN 1973, S. 188).

Die Fehler Schizophrener im logischen Schließen schienen zunächst das ideale Beispiel zu sein, an dem sich die Fehlfunktion einer logischen Operation nachweisen lassen sollte. Bei genauerer Betrachtung erwies es sich jedoch als schwierig, ja die Darstellung von VON DOMARUS schien sogar der hier untersuchten Hypothese zu widersprechen. Bei dem Schluß auf Identität aus einem einzigen gemeinsamen Prädikat scheinen ja gerade die anderen, unterscheidenden Merkmale ausgeschlossen worden zu sein.

Eine genauere Betrachtung der Syllogismen zeigt, daß der hierin angewandte Formalismus etwas anderes ist als die formal logischen Operationen. "Der Syllogismus als ganzer ist auf Grund seiner bloßen Form wahr, doch der Schlußsatz für sich ist nur wahr, wenn auch beide Prämissen wahr sind" (MENNE 1981, S. 93). Die Wahrheit der Prämissen hängt wiederum von der Richtigkeit (und Einheitlichkeit unter verschiedenen Menschen) der Konzeptbildung ab, wie sie in einer Wortbedeutung sich ausdrückt. Wenn im oben angeführten Beispiel von einem Konzept, daß "alle Lebewesen, die schnell sind, sind Hirsche" ausgegangen wird, dann ist der Schluß richtig, daß einige Indianer, die schnell sind, Hirsche sind. Da die Konzeptbildung, wie dargestellt, bei Schizophrenen gestört ist, ist es nicht verwunderlich, daß syllogistische Schlüsse, obwohl formal richtig, in ihrer Schlußfolgerung unwahr werden.

In welcher Form die Konzeptbildung bei Schizophrenen verändert ist, wurde in den Kapiteln 2.2 und 2.3 ausgeführt. Wenn sich also die schizophrenen Irrtümer bei Syllogismen auf ungewöhnliche Konzeptbildung zurückführen lassen, die am besten durch CHAPMANS Hypothese beschrieben wird, so trifft auch für die in Syllogismen gemachten Fehler die Erklärungsmöglichkeit durch fehlerhafte Exklusion im Verlauf der Konzeptbildung zu. Es sei betont, daß diese Überlegungen nur eine Möglichkeit und noch keinen Beweis darstellen. Es wäre schon erfreulich, wenn sie zu neuen experimentellen Überprüfungen Anlaß böten.

4. Diskussion

Die dargelegten Überlegungen lassen sich dahingehend zusammenfassen, daß zumindest ein großer Teil der kognitiven Störungen Schizophrener sich formal so beschreiben läßt, daß im Verlauf der Informationsverarbeitung eine notwendige *Exklusion* nicht oder mangelhaft ausgefürt wird. Was hat dies nun zu bedeuten? Ist es nur eine weitere, allgemeinere, vielleicht zu allgemeine Formulierung und daher ohne Vorhersagewert. Dies wurde bereits kritisch zu CAMERONS *Overinclusion*-Hypothese vermerkt. Ein Problem der Untersuchungen zu CAMERONS Hypothese ist, daß jeweils unterschiedliche Aspekte abnormer Kategorisierung als Hinweis für Overinclusion gewertet werden (vgl. CUTTING et al. 1987). Durch die Vielfalt der so gewonnenen inhaltlichen Aussagen wurde der formale Aspekt von CAMERONS Hypothese in den Hintergrund gedrängt. Wie schon in Abschnitt 2 angesprochen ist aber der formale Ablauf der Denkvorgänge entscheidend, wenn wir auf zugrundeliegende neuronale Prozesse rückschließen wollen. Diese neuronalen Prozesse folgen formal einer begrenzten Anzahl von Operationen, so daß eine scheinbar allgemeine Formulierung wie "Overinclusion" oder "mangelnde Exclusion" durchaus auf einen spezifischen neuronalen Prozeß hinweisen kann. Dies sei durch einige Bemerkungen zur neuronalen Informationsverarbeitung erläutert.

Die Sprache unseres Gehirns sind Folgen von Aktionspotentialen. Sinneseindrücke, Gedanken, Emotionen oder Bewegungsabläufe werden in Form von Folgen von Aktionspotentialen kodiert und weiterverarbeitet. Die Verarbeitung erfolgt durch exzitatorische und/oder inhibitorische Verknüpfung von Nervenzellen. Durch diese Verknüpfung können sowohl assoziative als auch logische Verbindungen hergestellt werden. Die assoziativen sind prinzipiell unbegrenzt und individuell, sodaß die Feststellung fehlerhafter Assoziationen nur Konventionen folgend getroffen werden kann. Die Verknüpfung nach logischen Regeln folgt begrenzten Operationen, wobei die drei Grundregeln das "und", "oder" und die Negation sind. Bereits das "exklusive oder" ist eine zusammengesetzte Operation, die jedoch für die Informationsverarbeitung sehr wichtig ist.

In diesem Zusammenhang sei auf die Arbeit von DÖRNER (1974) verwiesen. Er untersuchte in einer Reihe von Experimenten die kognitive Organisation beim Problemlösen und es gelang, "ein vollständiges und exaktes Abbild" davon "beim Lösen von Interpolationsproblemen zu gewinnen". Weiter konnte gezeigt werden, "daß sich menschliche Informationsverarbeitung beim Problemlösen auf die elementaren Prozesse "aktivieren", "hemmen", "verknüpfen" und "entknüpfen" zurückführen läßt". Diese vier elementaren Prozesse können leicht neurophysiologisch im Sinne von Operationen in Netzwerken interpretiert werden (DÖRNER 1974, S. 352 und 353).

Die hier gewählte Formulierung des *exclusiven oder* auf der logischen Ebene von Denkabläufen dürfte DÖRNERS elementaren Prozeß der Entknüpfung entsprechen. Welcher neurophysiologische Mechanismus eine Entknüfpung erzielen könnte, soll nicht weiter diskutiert werden. Es sei nur erwähnt, daß JOHNSON (1985) in einer Betrachtung der Defizite der peripheren Informationsverarbeitung Schizophrener zu dem Schluß kam, daß eine zu geringe neuronale Inhibition dafür verantwortlich sein könnte. In einem Modellentwurf des neuronalen "cocktail-party-Prozessors", der es uns ermöglicht, selbst bei lauter Gesellschaft uns mit einem einzelnen Partner zu unterhalten, fordern VON DER MALSBURG und SCHNEIDER (1986) eine temporäre synaptische Modulation, um eine notwendige Kopplung synchroner Neurone zu erreichen. Eine solche Kopplung synchron feuernder und gleichzeitige Entkopplung asynchroner Neurone dürfte ebenfalls dem hier beschriebenen Exclusions- oder Entkopplungsmechanismus entsprechen. Die neuronalen Vorgänge hierfür sind noch unbekannt, sie stellen aber ein wichtiges Problem der neurophysiologischen- und Netzwerkforschung dar (VON DER MALSBURG und SCHNEIDER 1986). Die formale Analyse der schizophrenen Denkstörungen mit der Formulierung eines defekten Verknüpfungsmechanismus könnte so die Brücke schlagen zur neurophysiologischen Grundlagenwissenschaft und damit zum wechselseitigen Verständnis und zur Lösung des gemeinsamen Problems beitragen.

Zusammenfassung: Durch formal-logische Betrachtung der inhaltlich sehr vielfältigen Denkstörungen Schizophrener wird versucht, einen gemeinsamen formalen Faktor zu finden, der im Ablauf der jeweiligen Informationsverarbeitung zu den beschriebenen Fehlern führt. Mit 4 Beispielen, BLEULERS *Assoziations*hypothese, CAMERONS *Overinclusion*-Hypothese, dem *excessive yielding to* *normal biases* von CHAPMAN und den *Irrtümern des logischen Schließens* nach VON DOMARUS, wird die Vorgehensweise erläutert.

Es stellt sich heraus, daß eine mangelnde Exklusion oder ein fehlerhaftes *exklusives oder* in allen 4 Fällen die Grundlage für die gestörte Verarbeitung der Information in den jeweils gestellten Aufgaben darstellen könnte.

Es wird diskutiert, daß erstens die beschriebene formale Betrachtung einen gemeinsamen Standpunkt für psychologische und psychopathologische Vorgänge einerseits und neurophysiologische andererseits darstellt und so über gemeinsame Terminologie zu besserem wechselseitigen Verständnis führen könnte. Zweitens scheint es zu gelingen, die verschiedenen und sich inhaltlich scheinbar teilweise widersprechenden Hypothesen der schizophrenen Denkstörungen unter dem gemeinsamen formalen Aspekt einer fehlerhaften Exklusion zusammenzufassen. Drittens kann Exklusion funktionell als "Entknüpfung" verstanden werden, die nach DÖRNER eine von nur vier nötigen Feldoperationen ist, auf die die kognitive Organisation beim Problemlösen zurückgeführt werden kann und die leicht neurophysiologisch interpretierbar ist.

So kann die formal-logische Betrachtung der schizophrenen Denkstörungen Anreize zu weiterer Erforschung der neurophysiologischen Grundlagen ergeben.

This and Not That - That May Be the Problem: Formal Logical Considerations of Schizophrenic Thought Disorder

Summary: Schizophrenic thought disorder, which is very variable in its content, will be considered from a formal-logical point of view in order to find a common factor that may explain the mistakes described in the course of information processing. Four examples will be presented to illustrate the course of thought: BLEULER's hypothesis of *broken associative threads*, CAMERONS' *overinclusion* hypothesis, the *excessive yielding to normal biases* from CHAPMAN and VON DOMARUS' *errors in syllogistic reasoning.*

It will be hypothesized, that in all four examples the basis for the disturbed information processing is due to a malfunction of an exclusion or of the *exclusive or* process.

It will be discussed, that firstly the described formal-logical aspect may be a common point of view for psychological and psychopathological processes on the one hand and neurophysiological processes on the other hand, thus leading to common terminology and hopefully better mutual understanding.

Secondly, it appears possible to view the partially contradictory hypotheses of schizophrenic thought disorder under the unifying concept of a malfunctioning exclusion process.

Thirdly, "exclusion" may functionally be understood as "disconnection" or "detachment", which according to DÖRNER is one of only four basic operations necessary to explain the cognitive organization in problem solving, and which is easily interpreted in physiological terms.

The formal-logical consideration of schizophrenic thought disorder may therefore stimulate further research on underlying neurophysiological processes.

Literatur

ARIETI, S. (1962): The Microgeny of Thought and Perception. A Psychiatric Contribution. Arch. Gen. Psych. **6**, S. 454-468.

BLEULER, E. (1911): Dementia praecox oder die Gruppe der Schizophrenien. Deuticke, Leipzig.

CAMERON, N. (1947): The Psychology of Behavior Disorders. Houghton Mifflin, Boston.

CHAPMAN, L.J., CHAPMAN, J.P. (1973): Disordered Thought in Schizophrenia. Prentice-Hall, Inc. Englewood Cliffs, New Jersey.

COHEN, R., PLAUM, E. (1980): Schizophrenie. In: BAUMANN, U. BERBALK, H. SEIDENSTÜCKER, G. (eds.): Klinische Psychologie, S. 260-286, Huber, Bern, Stuttgart, Wien.

CUTTING, J., DAVID, A., MURPHY, D. (1987): The Nature of Overinclusive Thinking in Schizophrenia. Psychopathology **20**, S. 213-219.

DÖRNER. D. (1974): Die kognitive Organisation beim Problemlösen. Versuche zu einer kybernetischen Theorie der elementaren Informationsverarbeitungsprozesse beim Denken. Huber, Bern, Stuttgart, Wien.

DOMARUS, E.v. (1944): The Specific Laws of Logic in Schizophrenia. In: KASANIN, J.S. (ed.): Language and Thought in Schizophrenia. Norton, New York, S. 104-114.

HARTWICH, P. (1980): Schizophrenie und Aufmerksamkeitsstörungen. Zur Psychopathologie der kognitiven Verarbeitung von Aufmerksamkeitsstörungen. Springer, Berlin, Heidelberg, New York.

HOLZMANN, PH.S. (1986): Thought Disorder in Schizophrenia: Editors Introduction. Schizophrenia Bulletin **12**, 342-347.

HUBER, G. (1979): Hauptströme der gegenwärtigen ätiologischen Diskussion der Schizophrenie. In: PETERS, U.H. (ed.): Die Psychologie des 20. Jahrhunderts. Band X. Ergebnisse der Medizin (2), S. 387-410. Kindler, Zürich.

JOHNSON, J.D. (1985): A Mechanism to Inhibit Input Activation and its Dysfunction in Schizophrenia. British Journal of Psychiatry, **146**, S. 429-435.

KLOSTERKÖTTER, J. (1982): Assoziationspsychologische versus lernpsychologische Schizophrenietheorie. Fortschr. Neurol. Psychiat. **50**, S. 165-170.

MALSBURG, CH.V.D., SCHNEIDER, W. (1986): A Neural Cocktail-Party Processor. Biol. Cybern. **54**, S. 29-40.

MENNE, A. (1981): Einführung in die Logik. Francke, München.

NEISSER, U. (1967): Cognitive Psychology. Appleton-Century-Crofts, New York.

NUECHTERLEIN, K.H., DAWSEN, M.E. (1984): Information Processing an Attentional Functioning in the Developmental Course of Schizophrenic Disorders. Schizophrenia Bulletin **10**, S. 160-202.

PAYNE, R.W. (1962): An object classification test as a measure of overinclusive thinking in schizophrenic patients. British Journal of Social and Clinical Psychology 1, S. 213-221.

PAYNE, R.W., MATUSSEK, P. GEORGE, E.I. (1959): An experimental study of schizophrenic thought disorder. Journal of Mental Science **105**, S. 627-652.

RUCKSTUHL, U. (1981): Schizophrenieforschung. Die theoretischen und empirischen Beiträge der experimentellen Psychologie. Beltz, Weinheim.

SCHÜTTLER, R., GROSS, G., HUBER, G. (1981): Reine Defektsyndrome und Basisstadien schizophrener Erkrankungen. Bedeutung für die nosologische und ätiologische Hypothesenbildung. In: HUBER, G. (ed.): Schizophrenie: Stand und Entwicklungstendenzen der Forschung, S. 189-209. Schattauer, Stuttgart, New York.

Part Two

Delusions

Language Disorders in Psychoses and Their Impact on Delusions

B.A. Maher[1]

1. Introduction

Prominent among the various categories of delusion is the belief that some outside agency is controlling the activities and feelings, and especially the language and thought of the patient. Delusions of control occupy a prominent place in the diagnostic catalogs for schizophrenia, and appear to be the most common form of delusion. The experience that affect, impulses or motor activity are being controlled from outside the body was numbered by SCHNEIDER amongst the first-rank symptoms of schizophrenia. BLEULER regarded schizophrenic delusions, including delusions of control, as secondary to the pathologies of affect, autism, ambivalence and associational disturbance - which he regarded as primary. Nonetheless he did perceive delusions as important components of the schizophrenic syndromes as they are manifested clinically. FREUD, of course, regarded the content of all delusions, including delusions of control, as indicative of the motivational conflicts that he believed to be the pathogenesis of psychiatric disorders generally.

The *Diagnostic and Statistical Manual of the American Psychiatric Association*, Third Edition (DSM-III, 1980) lists delusions of control as one of the six kinds of delusion, hallucination, or thought anomaly, that it defines as reliable diagnostic criteria for schizophrenia. DSM-III defines the specific *Delusion of being controlled* in the following terms:

> A delusion in which feelings, impulses, thoughts, or actions are experienced as being not one's own, as being imposed by some external force ... The symptom should be judged present only when the subject experiences his or her will, thoughts, or feelings as operating under some external force. Examples: A man claimed that his words were not his own, but those of his father ... (p. 356).

Delusions of control are commonly considered to be intrinsically bizarre. Bizarre, in turn, is a term applied to delusions that have "content [that] is

---

1 I am indebted to my wife and colleague, Dr. WINIFRED B. MAHER, for a critical reading of this paper, and for her suggestions for improving it. Deficiencies that remain are entirely my own responsibility.

patently absurd and has no possible basis in fact" (p. 188). This judged bizarreness to delusions of control has tended to differentiate them from other kinds of delusion, a distinction that suggests the possibility that they may reflect a different and more malign pathology than is the case with other categories of delusion. Many delusions have reference to events that are experienced by the patient as originating from identifiable outside agencies, and as operating in the way that such agencies do sometimes operate. These may strike us as pathological - because they seem highly improbable in the actual circumstances in which the patient lives - but not completely impossible. Beliefs that one is being spied upon, poisoned, tortured with electricity, and the like, may be false in the case of the patient, but they are beliefs which, under some special circumstances, can be true. People are sometimes actually spied upon, tortured, and so forth. Delusions such as these describe experiences that do actually happen to some people, albeit infrequently, and in that respect correspond to some normal experience. Every experienced clinician has come across cases where improbable, seemingly delusional, beliefs turned out to be valid. Elsewhere, (MAHER 1988a) it has been useful to refer to these cases as examples of the *Martha Mitchell Effect*.[2]

When we turn to delusions of control, the situation appears to be fundamentally different. Here the delusion is about the patient's *own* behavior, and specifically about what is generally regarded as voluntary behavior. The patient alleges, for example, that the words issuing from his or her own mouth are being generated and controlled by someone else. Nothing in normal experience corresponds to this. We do not know of any actual technique whereby such effects could really be achieved. The patient's claim seems *prima facie* impossible. Hence, we find the delusion bizarre, and regard it as more obviously pathological than we do other kinds of delusion.

It is the purpose of the author to propose that delusions of control are susceptible to explanation within a more general theory of delusion formation. For the time being, the proposal is limited to delusions of control of language utterance, but the general premises of the proposal may be extended to include other kinds of experienced control.

2. Elements of a Model of Delusion Formation

Before we discuss a proposed model of delusion formation, it may be helpful to consider some important methodological considerations. Perhaps the most fundamental of these relates to the selection of a standard of comparison against which the cognitive processes of the deluded patient is to be compared. Some investigators have chosen to compare the apparent logic of delusions to the standards of formal logical validity laid down in text-books of logic. A notable example of this is to be seen in the hypothesis of VON DOMARUS (1944). Accor-

2 Martha Mitchell, wife of the then Attorney-General of the United States, alleged that illegal activity was taking place at the highest levels in the White House. This was interpreted by many to be evidence that Mrs. Mitchell was suffering from some psychological disturbance, - until later discoveries about the Watergate affair cast a new light on her statements.

ding to this hypothesis, the pathology of the deluded patient lies in the tendency to make a specific formal logical error, the error of assuming identity of subjects on the basis of identity of predicates. In essence, the performance of the patient is found wanting when compared to an ideal of perfect performance. However, this comparison is uninformative, unless non-deluded patients can be shown to be less vulnerable to this kind of error, i.e. that control subjects actually do think according to the criteria of the text-books of logic. This test of the hypothesis was applied by WILLIAMS (1964) in a well controlled study, from which the clear conclusion could be drawn that this error is common in all kinds of patients as well as in normal subjects; very few people think in a manner consistent with the canons of formal logic. Hence the study of the ways in which the thinking of deluded patients departs from the standards of meaning provided by formal philosophical and linguistic analysis of their statements is likely to be a *cul-de-sac* unless it is informed by empirical studies of the ways in which non-patients actually speak, write and think in everday life.

A similar consideration applies to the content of delusional beliefs. Not only do most people appear to think heuristically (rather than in formal logical terms), they also often accept and promulgate ideas and beliefs that are either *prima facie* implausible, or fly in the face of the available evidence. The list of such beliefs is long, but in it we might include astrology, the Bermuda triangle, spoon-bending by remote mental control, UFOs, reincarnation, the Abominable Snowman, and so forth, amongst many other popular beliefs that seem to meet the criteria for definition as delusions. The heart of the matter is that if an implausible and empirically unsupported belief is shared by a sufficient number of people, it is nò longer defined as a delusion. BUCKNILL, a British psychiatrist writing in 1854, referred to a patient who had been diagnosed as delusional because he believed in Osiris, as follows:

> " ...had there been a few hundreds or even a few scores of persons entertaining the same belief, his [the patient's] ideas on this subject would have been of infinitely less value as a symptom of insanity" (BUCKNILL 1854, cited in SKULTANS 1975, p. 83).

That it has been found necessary to exclude formal religious beliefs from the category definition of delusion is not merely an expedient concession to social pressures. It is, instead, a recognition of the fact that the large majority of the population does not routinely apply criteria of evidence and plausibility before accepting a belief, and hence failure to apply these criteria is not evidence of pathology of thought.

We may now turn to a brief outline of the model of delusion formation that will be applied. It has been developed and described more fully in earlier papers. (MAHER 1970, 1974; MAHER and ROSS 1984; MAHER 1988a, 1988b). It is influenced by the fact that delusions appear in more than 75 different diseases, psychiatric, neurological and general medical. An acceptable model of delusions must accommodate to this; it cannot turn to processes unique to a particular psychiatric disorder as the basis for explanation.

The formal elements of the present model are as follows:

1. The cognitive processes whereby delusions are formed differ in no important respect from those by which non-delusional beliefs are formed. This propo-

sition is consistent with experimental studies of logical thinking in delusional patients; it is also, of course, consistent with the view expressed by JASPERS (1963) that "since thinking is in order in delusion and even used ingeniously to serve it, we can hardly speak of delusion as thought-disturbance" (JASPERS 1963 p. 195).

2. Delusions are best thought of as theories - much like scientific theories - that serve the purpose of providing explanations that give order and meaning to the empirical data of experience.

3. The necessity for a theory arises whenever nature presents us with a puzzle. Puzzles exist whenever a predictable sequence of events fails to occur in its usual and expected fashion, but occurs instead in a new and unexpected way. When there is a discrepancy between what we expect to observe and what we do observe, we experience surprise and tension. Discrepancies are experienced as significant. We notice them, and are brought into a state of alertness that prompts us to search for the explanation of the discrepancy. It does not seem to be necessary that the discrepancy have been consciously identified in concrete detail before the experience of puzzlement begins. It is not uncommon, for example, for us to notice that "something is different" in the appearance of an acquaintance without yet having detected specifically what has caused the change in appearance. We may examine the matter carefully before finally noticing that a hair-style has been changed, a beard shaved off, etc. The feeling that something is different may thus precede the recognition of what it is that has changed.

4. We continue to search for an explanation until one has been found.

5. Explanations, once created, give rise to feelings of relief - sometimes to feelings of euphoria. This happens when the explanation that has been created can accommodate the discrepant observations as well as the prior non-discrepant observations, and explains the basis for the occurrence of the discrepant event.

6. When the explanation (theory) has reached this stage, and relief has been experienced, the observer becomes relatively resistant to evidence counter to the theory. The theorist becomes selectively aware of confirmatory data, and selectively indifferent to negative data. Data that are consistent with the theory are given a primary role in the explanation, and data that are inconsistent are either ignored or "explained away" - usually in terms that make them appear consistent with the theory.

7. Theories are judged to be delusional by others if:

(a) the experiential data upon which they are based are not available to the others, so that the theory seems to run counter to the data that are available to them.

(b) the data are available to others, but they are not discrepant with their expectation and hence no feeling of puzzlement or significance is experienced.

8. Experiences of puzzlement, significance and relief are assumed to have a real locus in the nervous system. This being so, it is possible for pathological endogenous processes to activate these feelings even though no actual observational discrepancy exist in relation to event sequences in the environment.

9. Delusional theories should be expected to develop whenever any one or more of the following conditions exist.

a) The individual has an unrecognized defect of the sensory system. Good examples of this are to be found in studies reporting high proportions of unrecognized sensory impairment in persons diagnosed as paranoid (COOPER at al. 1976).

b) The individual has a defect in the selective inhibition of irrelevant input, (as is often reported in clinical and laboratory studies of schizophrenia). Such defects create the phenomenological experience that stimulus elements that are irrelevant to the current needs of the person have the same impact as elements that are relevant; the effect of this impact is to invest them with an aura of "relevance" or "significance", which must then be explained.

c) The individual experiences the output of expressive behavior - motor or language - for which no prior plan had been developed, or which departs substantially from what had been planned.

d) The locus in the central nervous system that normally mediates the experience of puzzlement or surprize is activated endogenously in the absence of any actual discrepancy between input and expectations. The concept of delusional mood is congruent with this condition.

e) There is a significant interruption in the normal temporal flow of sensory input and output, such that experiences at the end of the hiatus are unpredictable from those that were in being just before the onset of the hiatus. Thus extended temporary unconscious states - as in prolonged anaesthesia - may be followed by conscious experiences that are discontinuous with those that pertained just before the onset of anesthesia. This discontinuity creates a sense of discrepancy - and may produce brief delusional states.

f) Errors of diagnosis in medical conditions, especially where the diagnostician dismisses as "psychological", sets of experiences that have their source in a genuine biological disorder. The classic cases described by SOUTHARD (1912, 1916) are good examples of this process. A particular version of this may arise when the patient has been correctly diagnosed, but has not been adequately prepared for the somatic sensory experiences that a given disease tends to bring with it.

3. The Distinction Between the Origin and the Content of Delusions

While this model relates the origin of delusions to the presence of discrepant phenomenal personal experience by the patient, it does not deal directly with the nature of the content of the delusion. It is of crucial importance that a careful distinction be made between the patient's phenomenological description of the events that create the necessity for the delusion in the first place, (i.e. those that have been itemized in paragraph 9 above), and the specific type of explanation that provides content to the delusion.

Consider the simple case of a person who is developing unrecognized hearing loss. His subjective experiences include the fact that other people's voices appear inaudible. Ignorant of the fact of his hearing loss, he perceives that other people are speaking *sotto voce*, or whispering. This inference will form a beginning component of the delusional sequence, and faces him with the need to explain why other people are whispering. People usually whisper to each other when they are planning or discussing something that they do not wish others present to know; this something might be pleasant, such as a surprize gift, or something unpleasant such as a plan to swindle somebody out of money, etc. Which of these alternatives will seem probable to him, and his hypothesis about the reasons why they are doing this, will depend primarily upon his cultural background, his personal experiences in life, and the relationships that he has had with the people concerned. Thus his final delusion may include, for example, such elements as (a) that members of his family are whispering whenever he is around, (b) that they are doing so because they are plotting to have him placed in an institution, and (c) that they wish to do so because they resent his past history of sexually abusing them. The *selection of content* is determined by the actual past history of the deluded patient, but the *origin* resides in the anomalous experience - in this case the undiagnosed hearing loss. For such a condition the "cure" is not a lengthy analysis of the sexual problems of the patient - the cure is a hearing aid. It is unfortunate that the impact of the psychoanalytic approach to the study of delusions has been to blur the distinction between these separate elements of delusions; in our hypothetical case, for example, the sexual content of the delusion would be regarded as a clue to the origin of the delusion, a confusion of elements that diverts us from the careful analysis of the sequence of cognitive processes that produce the finished delusion.

From the point of view of the present model, the explanatory functions of the delusion should be articulated into two parts. First of these is the "What" question, i.e. that part of the delusion that describes the patient's experience (and thereby provides some clues as to the nature of the anomalous experience itself). This part may be stated in either descriptive or inferential terms. Thus, the patient might say "People's voices sound fainter" (a purely descriptive account of the auditory experience), or he or she might say "People are whispering" - which includes an inferential element, based upon the accumulated probabilities learned from past experience.[3] The second part consists of the "Why" part of the delusion, i.e. the development of a comprehensive explanation as to why the experiences are occurring. Reactions of incredulity and rejection from other people, who deny the validity of the delusion together with the experience upon which it is based, serve to exacerbate the situation. In due course their denials become a part of the problem to be solved, and being consistent with the notion of a conspiracy, serve to validate the delusion.

We may now turn to consider the application of this model of the formation of delusions to anomalies of expressive behavior - specifically those anomalies of language that are often found in schizophrenia.

---

3 Lest the willingness to make an inferential description seem to point towards a pathological personality disposition to make unwarranted inferences, we should consider how necessary it is to make such immediate inferences in normal life if sensory input is to be processed speedily and usefully. When the normal person hears people actually whispering, he or she does not begin by identifying the diminished loudness of their speech, proceeding thence by conscious logical steps to the inference that they are whispering. The experience and the inference are normally simultaneous.

4. Language in Schizophrenia and Its Contribution to Delusions

What patients say and how they say it, play a significant part in the clinical definition of schizophrenia. Were we compelled to diagnose schizophrenia without observation of the patient's language, we would be faced with a very difficult task indeed. Behavioral scientists concerned with the anomalies of language that occur in schizophrenia have followed one of three general strategies in seeking to explain them. One of these, associated particularly with the conceptions of psychoanalysis, assumes that overt disturbances in utterance are more or less faithful reflections of a basic disturbance in thinking; the basic disturbance is ascribed to the disruptive power of unconscious motivational conflicts. It is assumed that the nature of these conflicts may be ascertained by "correct" interpretation of the latent meanings hidden, like the meanings in a cyphered message, behind the manifest defects in the utterances of the patient. Speech disturbances of this kind are regarded, therefore, as fundamentally different in character from those that are found in the various aphasias, these being attributed to neuropathologies having negligible dynamic significance. For the sake of convenience, we may refer to this is the *Cypher Model.*

A second alternative, the *Social Learning Model,* assumes that the defective utterances of the patient are the end-product of poor training in communication - the poor training being due to the ambivalent and contradictory communications given by parents during the childhood of the future patient. Similar effects may arise, it is suggested, when discriminations between what is significant and what is insignificant are not taught clearly and consistently by parents - leading to a need for hypervigilance.

The third major alternative focuses upon the inability of the patient to inhibit the intrusion of internal associations. This is essentially similar to the schizophrenic difficulty in excluding external intrusions, an inability documented many times, as for example in the work of McGhie and Chapman (e.g. McGhie and Chapman 1971). This model, the *Associational Activation Model,* has been described by the present author in detail elsewhere (Maher et al. 1966; Maher 1972, 1983). Time and space permit only a summary account of its essential elements.

5. Associational Activation and Schizophrenic Utterance

Associational activation refers to a process whereby the activation of any element in language is accompanied by the activation of a network of associations related to that element. Activation of the original element occurs whenever the element is read, heard, spoken or written. Activated associations do not ordinarily enter into consciousness and are of brief temporal duration. However, while it is activated, an association will be recognized more rapidly if it occurs in the environment, as has been repeatedly shown in experimental demonstrations of semantic priming.

For most practical purpose, the basic element that primes the activation of the associational network is taken to be the single word, although common phrases or even syllables might on occasion act as elements. Nor is activation confined to language elements; the same process is assumed to exist in relation to sensory icons in pictorial, musical, etc. form. Network models are numerous and complex, with various hypotheses about the structure of the nets, the possible hierarchies of connection within networks, and so forth.[4]

The main tenet of the associational activation model of schizophrenic utterance is that the pathology of schizophrenia involves an inability to inhibit intrusions from either external stimulation or from internal activations. Normal utterance, according to this model is produced through a sequence consisting of, (a) a preverbal plan for the utterance, (b) the expressive production of the actual form of an utterance consistent with that plan, and (c) the continuous self-monitoring of the utterance, with accompanying recognition whenever the manifest utterance departs from the original plan. Throughout the production of the manifest utterance, associations are activated briefly to each uttered element. They fade rapidly (either by a process of decay produced by inhibition, or through their suppression by the activation of networks by succeeding elements). Effective production of coherent utterance requires attentional effort, an effort that is proportional to the predictability of each element in the sequence of the utterance.

In normal utterance, activated associations only enter into the manifest utterance if they are consistent with the original plan. When this is the case they are not identified as discrepant by the monitoring process and are not experienced as "intrusions". Some examples of these normal intrusions are shown in Figure 1 (from Maher 1983).

In schizophrenia the activation of associations is not effectively inhibited. A major consequence of this is that they intrude into language in ways that are sometimes grossly discrepant with the original plan of the utterance. They are particularly liable to intrude at points in an utterance at which the demand on attentional effort suddenly increases (as at the juncture of clauses and sentences), or where two separate associational networks are activated simultaneously - as in utterances that contain words with more than one meaning. Intrusions that enter into utterances may or may not possess some personal significance for the patient. Whatever the personal experience might have been that has led to the formation of specific associations, it is not the experience as such that has created the vulnerability to intrusions. The vulnerability is more likely to be due to basic neuropathology of the inhibitory processes.

Discovery of personal meanings that some intruding associations may have for the patient may tell us something about the past of the patient, but little or nothing about why he or she is vulnerable to the intrusion of associations, personal or otherwise. When such "discovery" is achieved through *post hoc* interpretation and "translation", it is much more a testimony to the creative ingenuity of the interpreter, than a contribution to our understanding of the psychopathology of the patient.

---

4 Useful accounts of network models are to be found in Neely (1977), Anderson (1980), and Shoben (1982), amongst others.

Fig. 1: A model of the assocional influence process on word choice in normal utterance

A. Plan of utterance:[5]

A career in art has problems.

Possible connections:

Associations		Synonyms
Career	Art	Problems
Work	Painting	Difficulties
Employment	Sculpture	Disadvantages
Job	Gallery	Hardships
etc.	Artists	Obstacles
	Draw	*Drawbacks*
	Engrave	Pitfalls

Actual utterance:

A career in art has ***drawbacks.***

B. Plan of utterance:[5]

This book, written by a man awaiting execution in Sing Sing prison, is quite amazing.

Possible connections:

Book	Man	Execution	Prison	Amazing
Volume	Person	Gallows	Pen	Astonishing
Author	Woman	*Electrocution*	Jail	Stimulating
Library	Human	Hanging	Ceil	*Electrifying*
Binding	Male	Death	Convict	Surprising

Actual utterance:

This book, written by a man awaiting execution in Sing Sing prison, is quite ***electrifying.***

C. Plan of utterance:[6]

China is a giant looking cautiously at the world.

Possible connections:

China	Giant	Looking
Orient	Orge	Watching
Emperor	Large	Gazing
Peking	Jack	Peering
Plate	Beanstalk	*Peeking*

Actual utterance:

China is a giant ***peeking*** *cautiously at the world.*

5 Examples noted by the writer through personal observation.
6 Cited by SKINNER, B.G. In EPSTEIN, R. (1980, p. 291).

From the patient's point of view, the monitoring of his or her own utterances produces, when associations have disrupted the utterance, a profound and disturbing awareness of discrepancy between what had been intended to be said and what was actually said. Discrepancies require explanation - as we have already argued in the first part of this paper. The very fact that the discrepant utterance is unrelated to any meanings that the patient might have intended (conscious or unconscious), provides an initial factor that any explanation will have to handle. As the spoken words do not reflect the patient's intentions, clearly they must represent somebody else's! Necessarily, the delusion focuses upon the possibility that some outside agency has managed to take control of the speech of the patient; insofar as associational intrusions enter into the inner speech of waking thought, the patient's experience may be that his or her thought is also being controlled by somebody else.

From this point on the development of a comprehensive delusion will follow a typical course. As the control of language and/or thought requires invisible mediation, delusions of control by radar, hypnotism, extra-sensory perception, magnetism, spirits of the dead, angels or devils and so forth, are likely to be prominent.

Studies conducted by the writer and his colleagues have indicated that

(a) thought-disordered schizophrenics, i.e. patients showing concurrent disturbances of language, are more effective in the recognition of primed associations than are normal controls or schizophrenic patients without language disturbance (Maher et al. 1987; Manschreck et al. 1988), and

(b) these thought-disordered patients are less able to deploy their attention in relation to redundancies in language utterance (Maher, Manschreck and Rucklos 1980; Maher, Manschreck and Molino 1983).

The associational intrusion model assumes the presence of a neural deficit as the basis of this pathology. It appears probable that this deficit fluctuates in a given patient from one time to another, the fluctuations being perhaps related to the varying severity of stress experienced. Possible relations between experienced stress and disturbed utterance may color the patient's search for the agent responsible for the disturbed utterance, individuals or forces seen to be responsible for the stress becoming primary suspects as controllers. The same inference-by-correlation may mislead the psychodynamic clinician into concluding that the content of the disturbed utterance itself contains a coded clue to the emotional core of the stress.

6. Ichstörungen and the Present Model

It will be clear that the present model proposes that the patient's sense of the control of the behavior self by others is hypothesized to be derivative from the experience of discrepancies between the patient's behavior as it actually occurs and the behavior that the patient had intended to produce. The proposition is made here that the patients, in effect, *deduce* that some outside agency is controlling their behavior because the behavior is discrepant with their intentions. In this volume Spitzer (1988) discusses a major alternative possibility, namely that the sense that one is controlling one's own actions is a primary experience. This brings with it the corollary that, if this experience has a specific neural locus, any direct disruption of its functioning could give rise to the experience in a patient that his behavior was not being produced by him, even if the behavior was in fact congruent with his intentions.

As Spitzer points out, there has not yet been much empirical research into the concept of Ichstörungen. A resolution of the difference between these two hypotheses awaits suitable crucial studies. Such work could be of great significance in furthering our understanding of the delusions of control.

Summary: In summary, this paper presents an explanation of the genesis of delusions of control of language and thought. The explanation emphasizes the role of associational intrusions into language, creating the experience of serious discrepancy between intent and action, and with the consequent need to explain the discrepancy. This, in turn, produces explanations that include concepts of invisible agencies controlling the behavior of the patient while operating from a distance. In this respect, delusions of control may be understood as falling within the general model of delusions as cognitively systematic explanations of anomalous experiences.

Sprachstörungen bei Psychotikern und ihre Relevanz für Wahnphänomene

Zusammenfassung: Es wird eine Erklärung der Genese von Beeinflussungswahn bzw. des Gefühls der gemachten Gedanken und des gemachten Sprechens vorgeschlagen: In die Sprachproduktion des Kranken eindringende Assoziationen bewirken bei ihm die Erfahrung einer Diskrepanz zwischen intendierter und tatsächlich ausgeführter Denk- bzw. Sprachhandlung, woraus sich für ihn das Bedürfnis nach einer Erklärung ergibt. Dies wiederum führt zu Erklärungen, die u.a. Gedanken an unsichtbare Mächte, die sein Verhalten von Ferne beeinflussen, enthalten. So gesehen läßt sich der Beeinträchtigungswahn als Spezialfall einer allgemeinen Theorie der Wahngenese interpretieren, die Wahn als systematischen Erklärungsversuch abnormer Erfahrungen auffaßt.

References

Anderson, J.R. (1980): Cognitive psychology and its implications. Freeman, San Francisco.
Cooper, A.F., Curry, A.R. (1976): Pathology of deafness in the paranoid and affective psychoses of later life. Journal of Psychosomatic Research **20**, pp. 97-105.
Domarus, E. von (1944): The specific laws of logic in schizophrenia. In: J. Kasanin (Ed.): Language and thought in schizophrenia. University of California Press, Berkeley.
Epstein, R. (1980): B.F. Skinner's Notebooks. Harvard University Press, Cambridge.
Jaspers K. (1963): General Psychopathology (trans. J. Hoenig and M.W. Hamilton). Manchester University Press, Manchester.

MAHER, B.A. (1970): The psychology of delusions. Paper presented at the Annual Conference of the American Psychological Association, Miami Beach, Florida.

MAHER, B.A. (1972): The language of schizophrenia: A review and interpretation. British Journal of Psychiatry **120**, pp. 4-17.

MAHER, B.A. (1974): Delusional thinking and perceptual disorder. Journal of Individual Psychology **30**, pp. 98-113.

MAHER, B.A. (1983): A tentative theory of schizophrenic utterance. In: B.A. MAHER, W.B. MAHER (eds.): Progress in Experimental Personality Research. Vol. 12. Academic Press, New York.

MAHER, B.A. (1988a): Anomalous experience and delusional thinking: The logic of explanations. In: T.F. OLTMANNS, B.A. MAHER (eds.): Delusional Beliefs, Wiley-Interscience, New York.

MAHER, B.A. (1988b): Delusions as the product of normal cognitions. In: T.F. OLTMANNS, B.A. MAHER (eds.): Delusional Beliefs, Wiley-Interscience, New York.

MAHER, B.A., MCKEAN, K.O., MCLAUGHLIN, B. (1966): Studies in psychotic language. In: P.J. STONE, D.C. DUNPHY, M.S. SMITH, D.M. OGILVIE (eds.): The general inquirer: A computer approach to content analysis. MIT Press, Cambridge, Mass.

MAHER, B.A., MANSCHRECK, T.C., RUCKLOS, M. (1980): Contextual constraint and the recall of verbal material in schizophrenia. British Journal of Psychiatry **137**, pp. 69-73.

MAHER, B.A., MANSCHRECK, T.C., MOLINO, M.A.C. (1983): Redundancy, pause distributions and thought disorder in schizophrenia. Language and Speech **26**, pp. 191-200.

MAHER, B., ROSS, J. (1984): Delusions. In: H.E. ADAMS, P.B. SUTKER (eds.): Comprehensive Handbook of Psychopathology. Plenum, New York.

MAHER, B.A., MANSCHRECK, T.C., HOOVER, T.M., WEISSTEIN, C.C. (1987): Thought disorder and measured features of language production in schizophrenia. In: P. HARVEY, E. WALKER (eds.): Positive and negative symptoms in psychosis: Description, research and future directions. Erlbaum, Hillsdale, N.J.

MANSCHRECK, T.C., MAHER, B.A., MILAVETZ, J J., AMES, D., WEISSTEIN, C.C., SCHNEYER, M.L. (1988): Semantic priming in thought disordered schizophrenics. Schizophrenia Research **1**, pp. 61-66.

MCGHIE, A., CHAPMAN, J. (1971): Disorders of attention and perception in early schizophrenia. British Journal of Medical Psychology **34**, pp. 103-116.

NEELY, J.H. (1977): Semantic priming and retrieval from lexical memory: Roles of inhibitionless spreading activation and limited-capacity attention. Journal of Experimental Psychology: General **106**, pp. 226-254.

SHOBEN, E.J. (1982): Semantic and lexical decisions. In: C.R. PUFF (ed.): Handbook of research methods in human memory and cognition. Academic Press, New York.

SKULTANS, V. (1975): Madness and morals. Routledge, Kegan Paul, London.

SOUTHARD, E.E. (1912): On the somatic sources of somatic delusions. Journal of Abnormal Psychology **7**, pp. 326-339.

SOUTHARD, E.E. (1916): On descriptive analysis of manifest delusions from the subject's point of view. Journal of Abnormal Psychology **11**, pp. 189-202.

SPITZER, M (1988): Ichstörungen: In Search of a Theory. This volume.

WILLIAMS, E.B. (1964): Deductive reasoning in schizophrenia. Journal of Abnormal and Social Psychology **69**, pp. 47-61.

Melancholie und Wahn

J. Glatzel

1. Einleitung

Sowohl in den frühen und mittleren als auch in den späten Verlaufsabschnitten endogener Psychosen darf Wahn in jeder Gestalt zunächst einmal als Hinweis auf eine schizophrene Persönlichkeitsstörung gewertet werden. Bei jenen zyklothym depressiven Psychosen, die gemeinhin als stilrein bezeichnet werden, wird ein Wahnerleben in der strengen Begriffsbestimmung von JASPERS, GRUHLE und KURT SCHNEIDER gemeinhin nicht erwartet. Wahn ist offenbar mit einer endogenen Depression des typischen Manifestationsalters unvereinbar. In deren späten Verlaufsabschnitten allerdings wird er vergleichsweise häufig angetroffen.

Keiner der Autoren, die sich darum bemüht haben, das Essentielle endogener Depression, deren Leitsymptome, auf den Begriff zu bringen, erwähnt den Wahn. Das gilt für SCHNEIDER ebenso wie für WEITBRECHT, JANZARIK oder TELLENBACH.

Unabhängig von der Frage, ob es einer der gegenwärtig oder in der Vergangenheit diskutierten psychopathologischen Ansätze erlaubt, die zweifellos gegebene Eigenart der stilreinen endogenen Depression sprachlich darzustellen, besteht immerhin weitgehend Einigkeit über eines der zentralen, vielleicht das zentrale Thema depressiven Erlebenswandels. Ich meine die Gewißheit, in Schuld geraten zu sein. Dabei mögen eigenes Handeln bzw. Unterlassen Quellen der Schuld sein oder das Dasein, das Existieren als Mensch schlechthin. Das Besondere dieser Schuldgewißheit des endogenen Depressiven liegt augenscheinlich darin, daß er keine Instanz zu nennen vermag, deren Normen oder Regeln er schuldhaft verletzte. Angesichts der existentiellen Bedrängnis depressiver Schuldgewißheit, die den Umgang mit den anderen ebenso wie das Verhältnis des Kranken zu sich selbst bestimmt, ist es eigentlich erstaunlich, daß sie während des typischen Manifestationsalters niemals zu wahnhafter oder halluzinatorischer Verselbständigung gelangt. Die Externalisierung, d.h. die Wendung des Zeigers der Schuld auf die Außenwelt, wie es SCHEID einmal formuliert hat, begegnet erst im höheren Lebensalter.

Die Tatsache, daß die Schuldgewißheit der stilreinen, idealtypischen endogenen Depression nicht als Wahn erlebt wird, hängt, so glaube ich, mit der besonderen Kommunikationsstörung zusammen, die offenbar von anderer Art ist als die des Schizophrenen. In einer KURT SCHNEIDER gewidmeten Festschrift hat KRANZ (1962) vor Jahren Gedanken zur Rolle des Autismus in den endogenen Psychosen vorgetragen. Hinweisend auf das von SCHNEIDER beschriebene "Gefühl der Gefühllosigkeit" und auf die Arbeit SCHULTES (1961) über das "Nicht-traurig-sein-Können im Kern melancholischen Erlebens" bezeichnete er die zyklothyme Depression als die eigentlich autistische Psychose. Dieser depressive Autismus erschließt sich besonders einer Betrachtung, die die von TELLENBACH (1976) und anderen betonte Räumlichkeit der stets gerichteten Gefühle und Stimmungen bedenkt. In diesem Sinne steht die Depression als eine zentripetal gerichtete Gestimmtheit der zentrifugalen normalseelischen Trauer gegenüber. Es sind nicht Umwelt und Mitwelt, die erdrücken, lähmen, die als übermächtig erfahren werden in der Weise, daß Rückzug und Passivität als die allein angemessenen Haltungen und notwendigen Einstellungen erlebt werden. Um- und mitmenschliche Welt werden vielmehr unerreichbar und unzugänglich, weil die Unfähigkeit zum sozialen Kontakt, die Unfähigkeit, ein Interaktionsbündnis mit anderen einzugehen, als eine primäre Kommunikationsbehinderung erlitten werden. Man vermag mit anderen zu trauern, kann mit der eigenen Trauer den Partner gleichsam anstecken und bei ihm ein Gefühl induzieren, das dem eigenen zumindest ähnlich ist. Die psychotische Depressivität aber ist nicht übertragbar; zwei Depressive vermögen nicht miteinander über das gemeinsame Thema der Schwermut zu kommunizieren. Während Trauer stets auf ein Außen bezogen und insofern beziehungsstiftend ist - man denke an die "Trauergemeinde" -, bleibt die Depression stets auf das Selbst des Schwermütigen verwiesen. Sie führt in Vereinzelung und schließlich Isolierung. Der Traurige vermag seine Verfassung sprachlich darzustellen, dem Depressiven bleibt nur die mittelbare Kundgabe. Der Depressive erlebt sich als Zentrum einer schwermütigen Welt, zu der die anderen keinen Zugang haben und aus der er selber auf dem Weg zu den anderen nicht heraustreten kann.

2. Der Depressive als nicht wahnfähig

Der radikale oder konsequente Autismus des Melancholischen - auch in der manischen Verfassung läßt sich im übrigen der Autismus als ein bestimmendes Element aufzeigen (GLATZEL 1982) - läßt eine Wahnbildung nicht zu, denn Wahn ist - auch - ein kommunikatives, d.h. ein interaktionales Phänomen (GLATZEL 1978, 1981).

Der Vergleich des Wahns mit der Glaubensgewißheit verdeutlicht diesen Sachverhalt. Ein Glaubensinhalt wird bisweilen mit der gleichen befremdlichen Gewißheit vertreten wie ein Wahn. Geglaubtes und Gewähntes können gleichermaßen von hoher subjektiver Evidenz sein. Anders als der Wähnende aber bemüht sich der Gläubige - ebenso wie der fanatisierte Erfinder - darum, den anderen im Gespräch zu überzeugen, ihn für sich zu gewinnen. Er geht in der Beziehung auf ihn zu, ist bestrebt, ihm den Blick für Zusammenhänge zu schärfen, die, wie er meint, den anderen veranlassen müssen, seine Überzeugung zu teilen. Gerade das Fehlen eines entsprechenden Verhaltens aber, das Ausbleiben jedes Überzeugungsversuches kennzeichnet eine Beziehung, die Veranlassung gibt, von wahnhafter Einstellung, von Wahn zu sprechen. Im Umgang mit dem Wähnenden bemerkt nur der Partner, daß der Kranke von einem Situationsverständnis ausgeht, das sich allein diesem erschlossen hat und zu dem der Partner keinen Zugang findet. Der Wähnende unterstellt als selbstverständlich eine Übereinstimmung hinsichtlich der Situationsdefinition, die ihn von der Notwendigkeit entbindet, den Partner von seiner Sicht der Dinge zu überzeugen. Deswegen entsteht beim Partner der Eindruck einer Pseudointimität zwischen ihm und dem Wähnenden, das heißt eines scheinbaren Konsens, wo doch tatsächlich Befremden und Verständnislosigkeit die Beziehung bestimmen.

Aber auch der Wahn, der der Interaktion mit dem Wähnenden den Charakter der Pseudointimität gibt, hat es mit einem Gegenüber zu tun, mit einem dinglichen oder einem menschlichen, einem realen oder einem fiktiven. Das gilt für den Wahneinfall ebenso wie für die Wahrnehmung, für das initiale Trema ebenso wie für die ausformulierte Wahnfabel. Das Wahnhafte liegt in der Art des Umgangs mit diesem Gegenüber, d.h. in der Beziehung, in der sich der Wähnende diesem gegenüber erlebt. Diese Beziehung aber wird vorgegeben durch die subjektive, dem konsentierten Situationsverständnis widersprechende Situationsdefinition, die ihn Elemente bzw. Aspekte als bestimmend erleben läßt, die für den anderen von allenfalls marginaler Bedeutung sind. *Deswegen ist der Depressive, der Welt und Umwelt nicht als ein Gegenüber, sondern als Emanation der eigenen eingefrorenen Befindlichkeit erlebt, nicht wahnfähig. Der Wahn bedarf des Bezuges zu einer realen oder fiktiven Umwelt, um sich im deutenden Umgang mit ihr zu verwirklichen.* Dem im Zentrum seiner schwermütigen Welt eingeschlossenen Depressiven ist wahnhaftes Erleben nicht möglich.

Die depressive Verfassung des höheren Lebensalters, die hier in Anlehnung an einen früheren Sprachgebrauch als Melancholie bezeichnet werden soll, ist offenbar von anderer Art - vermutlich als Ausdruck einer altersabhängigen Modifikation der personalen Struktur.

Der melancholische Wahn alter Menschen imponiert als monoton, was die Themenauswahl angeht; die das jeweilige Wahnthema illustrierenden Wahnfabeln sind demgegenüber nicht selten ungewöhnlich farbig. In einer Arbeit aus dem Jahre 1914 hat Ernst Kretschmer unter dem Begriff *Affektwahn* jene Bilder beschrieben, die bei Dreyfus und Kraepelin als depressiver Wahnsinn begegnen. Er nennt die inhaltliche Ausgestaltung des Wahnerlebens der von ihm untersuchten alten Melancholiker barock und phantastisch. Die Haltung des Gesunden diesen Kranken gegenüber sei durch eine eigentümliche Distanz und Unberührtheit gekennzeichnet, die unbeschadet der bisweilen monströsen wahnhaften Schreckensgemälden stets erhalten blieben.

Wahnerleben dieser Art findet man sicherlich nicht allein bei Melancholien des höheren Lebensalters - auf die bemerkenswerte Tatsache, daß der Wahn hirnorganisch Kranker erscheinungsbildlich nicht selten demjenigen alter Melancholiker ähnelt, hat übriges ebenfalls Kretschmer schon vor Jahren hingewiesen -, er ist jedoch für die späten Verlaufsabschnitte psychotischer Depressionen recht charakteristisch. Wirklichkeit, d.h. die Welt des Depressiven als ein dem erlebenden Ich entgegenstehendes Gegenüber wird im melancholischen Wahn in einer durchaus anderen Weise erfahren als in den frühen Phasen der Erkrankung. Mit der Entwicklung eines melancholischen Wahns wandelt sich die Beziehung des Depressiven zu seiner Wirklichkeit, zu der ihm gegenüberstehenden dinglichen ebenso wie zur humanen.

3. Angetroffene und vergegenwärtigte Wirklichkeit

Zu fragen ist, wie die Wirklichkeit in den frühen, d.h. typischen Verlaufsabschnitten der psychotischen Depression erlebt wird, wenn die depressive Verstimmung als gleichsam frei flottierende Schuldgewißheit in Erscheinung tritt, und wie in den späten Jahren des melancholischen Wahns.

Angesichts der Schwierigkeiten, die gerade auch Psychologen mit dem Wirklichkeitsbegriff haben, scheint ein solcher Ansatz problematisch. Ihn dennoch zu wählen zwingt zur Entscheidung für einen der denkbaren Begriffe.

Einen Rahmen gibt LEWIN (1963) vor, der die Anerkennung der Wirklichkeit einer Gegebenheit davon abhängig machen will, daß diese Gegebenheit spezifische Eigenschaften und Invarianten zeigt. LEWIN verlangt, Wirklichkeit und Realität auseinanderzuhalten. Im Unterschied zur Wirklichkeit umfasse die Realität auch das Mögliche.

Weiterführend und im gegebenen Zusammenhang bedeutsam sind die Überlegungen METZGERS (1968) zu diesem Thema. Er unterscheidet verschiedene Wirklichkeiten in Abhängigkeit von der Weise, in der sie von uns erfahren werden. Als Wirklichkeit ersten Sinnes bezeichnet er die physikalische, d.h. die allgemein erlebnisjenseitige Wirklichkeit. Sie kann außer Betracht bleiben, wenn es um die Erörterung psychotischer Wirklichkeitserfahrung geht, sei sie wahnhaft oder verzerrt durch einen hohen Affektdruck. Die Wirklichkeit zweiten Sinnes umfaßt nach METZGER das Erlebbare, und zwar das angetroffene ebenso wie das vergegenwärtige. "Innerhalb des Erlebbaren, d.h. innerhalb der Wirklichkeit im zweiten Sinne, wird unterschieden zwischen den Dingen, Wesen, Ereignissen, Taten selbst und deren Vergegenwärtigungen, also zwischen von uns Angetroffenem, Vorgefundenem leibhaftig uns Begegnendem, uns selbst also in diesem Sinne Gleichrangigem einerseits - und von uns bloß Gedachtem, Vorgestelltem, Vermutetem, Geahntem, Beabsichtigtem andererseits. Die Vergegenwärtigungen nun haben tatsächlich häufig ... den vielberufenen Charakter der "Intentionalität" ..., sie werden dann als "hinweisend auf" dasjenige Wirkliche oder Mögliche, das sie vorstellen oder bedeuten, unmittelbar erlebt ..." (METZGER 1968, S. 18).

In der nicht-wahnhaften Schuldgewißheit stilreiner endogener Depressionen wird Wirklichkeit erfahren als Wirklichkeit im zweiten Sinne, sie wird wahrgenommen von den Kranken als vergegenwärtigte Wirklichkeit. Da im Vergegenwärtigen etwas Vorgestelltes, eine Bedeutung unmittelbar erlebt wird - das meint dessen Intentionalität - kommt auch der Schuldgewißheit Hinweischarakter zu. Sie verweist auf die Ich-Indentität des Depressiven, d.h. der Depressive identifiziert sich in der Schuldgewißheit dem eigenen Ich gegenüber als ein Schuldiger. Er vergegenwärtigt sich das eigene Schuldigsein und findet die Bestätigung dieser Selbsteinschätzung allein in seinem Wissen. Das Schuldigsein wird zum Bestandteil der Ich-Identität, nicht selten überhaupt zu deren entscheidendem Bestimmungsstück. Zu dieser Identifikation gelangt der

Depressive allein im Umgang mit sich selbst, ein wie auch immer geartetes Außen oder Gegenüber gerät ihm weder bestätigend noch entlastend in den Blick. Der Depressive, so ließe sich verkürzt sagen, hat nicht Schuld auf sich geladen durch irgendein Tun oder Unterlassen, er ist ein Schuldiger ab ovo.

Von der Erlebnisqualität her ist diese Gewißheit von einem im Wahn erlangtem Wissen durchaus abzugrenzen. Auch vom Wahneifall im Sinne KURT SCHNEIDERS unterscheidet sie sich. Die wahnhafte Überzeugung etwa, der wiedergeborene Christus zu sein, bedeutet keine Selbstidentifikation, die der Wähnende allein aus Eigenem vornehmen könnte. Christus sein kann ich nur in Relation zu jener historischen Figur.

Solange also die zentrale Thematik der psychotischen Depression als vergegenwärtigte Wirklichkeit im zweiten Sinne erlebt wird, ist kein Wahn bzw. kann Wahn nicht möglich sein. Deswegen ist der radikale Autismus des Depressiven mit Wahnerleben nicht vereinbar.

In höheren Lebensalter aber werden Schuld und Verschulden anders erfahren. An die Stelle der ebenso vagen wie umfassenden Schuldgewißheit treten konkrete Themen, die bisweilen zu bewegten und bewegenden Fabeln ausformuliert werden. Schuldgewißheit und melancholischer Wahn stehen in einem Verhältnis zueinander, das demjenigen zwischen Angst und Furcht durchaus vergleichbar ist. Die im melancholischen Wahn erlebte Wirklichkeit ist nicht Wirklichkeit als Vergegenwärtigung, sie ist angetroffene Wirklichkeit, im Verhältnis zu der sich der Kranke nicht selbst identifiziert, sondern durch die ihm eine Identität zugeschrieben wird. Das gilt nicht nur für jene gelegentlich grotesken Wahnfiguren im KRETSCHMERschen Sinne, sondern auch für die SCHNEIDERschen Urängste. Die Themen Sünde, Krankheit und Armut definieren eine Beziehung des Betroffenen zu seinem Gegenüber, sei es ein Gott, sei es der eigene Leib, sei es die soziale Gemeinschaft. Und sie können sich deswegen als Wahn konkretisieren, weil sie nicht als vergegenwärtigte, sondern als angetroffene Wirklichkeit erfahren werden. Als angetroffene Wirklichkeit bedeuten sie ein Gegenüber, zu dem der Kranke in eine Beziehung treten kann. Dem Wahn als angetroffener Wirklichkeit fehlt gegenüber der Schuldgewißheit als vergegenwärtigter Wirklichkeit das Moment der Intentionalität, er verweist nicht auf einen stabilen und insoweit vom Betroffenen als kennzeichnend gewußten Aspekt der Ich-Identität sondern wird erlebt als Zuschreibung, und zwar unbeschadet der Tatsache, daß diese Zuschreibung vom Kranken als begründet und insoweit berechtigt beurteilt werden mag. Zuschreibungen implizieren Verhaltenserwartungen, sie erlauben ein Stellungnehmen oder fordern ein solches geradezu heraus. Vor allem aber nötigen sie zur Prüfung, wieweit sie vereinbar sind bzw. übereinstimmen mit anderen Verhaltenserwartungen, die sich aus anderen Zuschreibungen herleiten. Anders ausgedrückt: Die gewähnte Wirklichkeit muß in Relation gesetzt werden zu anderen angetroffenen Wirklichkeiten, die im Wahn verwirklichte Rollenfigur gerät damit notwendig in ein Verhältnis zu anderen Rollenfiguren.

Es war PLESSNER, der den Rollenbegriff um eine anthropologische Dimension erweitert hat. In seiner philosophischen Anthropologie hat er den Gedanken vom Doppelgängertum des Menschen entwickelt und damit, wie DREITZEL es formulierte, die Idee der Rollenhaftigkeit des Verhaltens zur "anthropologischen

Gestalt radikalisiert" (1980, S. 51). Alles, was der Mensch ist, ist er auf dem Umweg über andere. In diesem Sinne heißt es bei PLESSNER. "Am anderen wird der Mensch seiner habhaft. Diesen anderen trifft er auf dem Umweg über die Rolle, genau wie der andere ihn. Immer vermittelt das Rollenspiel als Gelenk den zwischenmenschlichen Kontakt, soweit er sozial relevant ist und dem Austausch von Leistungen dient" (PLESSNER 1966, S. 20). Die Reduktion auf das invariante Selbst, wie sie in der von dinglicher und humaner Umwelt gleichermaßen unabhängigen Selbstidentifikation geschieht, beraubt den Betroffenen der Möglickeit zu sozial relevanten Kontakten. Erst in der Verwirklichung einer Rolle, die an die wirksame Gegenwart eines angetroffenen Gegenüber gebunden ist, wird eine soziale Identität gewonnen und damit die Voraussetzung einer dynamischen Kommunikation.

Der radikale Autismus des Depressiven in den frühen Erkrankungsphasen meint demnach Reduktion auf das invariante Selbst, insoweit also Rollenlosigkeit. Die mit dieser verbundene Orientierungslosigkeit bezüglich der aktuellen Verhaltenserwartungen und damit auch der Situationsdefinition zwingt in den Autismus. Erst wenn die Schuldgewißheit als vergegenwärtigte Wirklichkeit zum Wahn wird als angetroffene Wirklichkeit, erst dann ist soziales Handeln als Rollenhandeln wieder möglich. Der depressive Autismus wird im melancholischen Wahn durchbrochen zugungsten einer allerdings verkürzten und thematisch festgelegten Kommunikation. Die so ermöglichte Kommunikation schafft einen Zugang zu Um- und Mitwelt und läßt diese insoweit relevant werden, als dem Kranken durch sie eine soziale Identität vermittelt wird.

Zusammenfassung: Wahn gleich welcher formalen Struktur und welchen Inhalts gehört nicht zu den differentialtypologisch verbindlichen Leitsymptomen endogener Depressionen des typischen Manifestationsalters. Demgegenüber bestimmt die wahnhafte Aufdeckung der Urängste im SCHNEIDERschen Sinne die Melancholie des höheren Lebensalters. Die von METZGER vorgeschlagene Unterscheidung zwischen vergegenwärtigter und angetroffener Wirklichkeit aufgreifend, wird gezeigt, daß die Entwicklung eines melancholischen Wahns ein Aufbrechen des depressiven Autismus bedeutet. Im Wahn gelingt dem Melancholiker der erste Schritt zurück in eine dynamische Kommunikation mit der dinglichen und humanen Umwelt, die im Autismus der endogenen Depression des frühen und mittleren Lebensalters unmöglich geworden war.
Die Vergegenwärtigung der depressiven Schuldgewißheit im melancholischen Wahn ist zu verstehen als eine den Betroffenen entlastende Syndromprogression ähnlich der, von der Angst zur Furcht, vom Trema zum Wahn.

Melancholia and Delusion

Summary: Delusions of any structure and content do not belong to the necessary symptoms for the diagnosis of a major depression at the typical age of onset. Depression in old age - which here is called melancholia - is characterized, however, by certain delusions which Schneider interpreted as "revealed primary anxieties of man". METZGERS distinction between reality as objectively given and as subjectively represented is adopted and it is shown that the development of delusions in depressed patients correlates with a weakenig of these patients' autism. In developing delusions the elder patient - in contrast to the young and middle aged patient who is hindered by his autism - is able to reestablish dynamic communications with the objective world. This progression of the syndrome is comparable to the progression from (free floating) anxiety to fear (of a certain object or situation) or to the progression from delusional mood to delusions, both of which processes may be accompanied by a sense of relief.

Literatur

DREITZEL, H.P. (1980): Die gesellschaftlichen Leiden und das Leiden an der Gesellschaft. Enke, Stuttgart.

DREYFUSS, G. (1907): Die Melancholie. Fischer, Jena.

GLATZEL, J. (1978): Allgemeine Psychopathologie. Enke, Stuttgart.

GLATZEL, J. (1981): Spezielle Psychopathologie. Enke, Stuttgart.

GLATZEL, J. (1982): Über den manischen Autismus. Schweiz. Arch. Neurol. Psychat. **130**, S. 69-72.

JANZARIK, W. (1988): Strukturdynamische Grundlagen der Psychatrie. Enke, Stuttgart.

KRAEPELIN, E. (1899): Die klinische Stellung der Melancholie. Mschr. Psychiat. Neurol. **6**, S. 325-339.

KRANZ, H. (1962): Der Begriff des Autismus und die endogenen Psychosen. In: Kranz, H. (Hg.): Psychopathologie heute, S. 61-71, Thieme, Stuttgart.

KRETSCHMER, E. (1914): Wahnbildung im manisch-depressiven Symptomenkomplex. Allg. Z. Psychat. **71**, S. 397-412.

LEWIN, L. (1969): Grunzüge der topologischen Psychologie. Huber, Bern.

METZGER, W. (1968): Psychologie. Steinkopff, Darmstadt.

PLESSNER, H. (1966): Diesseits der Utopie. Diederichs, Düsseldorf, Köln.

SCHNEIDER, K. (1950): Die Aufdeckung des Daseins durch die zyklothyme Depression. Nervenarzt **21**, S. 193-197.

SCHULTE, W. (1961): Nicht-traurig-sein-Können im Kern melancholischen Erlebens. Nervenarzt **32**, S. 314-321.

TELLENBACH, H. (1976): Melancholie. Springer, Berlin, Heidelberg, New York.

WEITBRECHT, H.J, GLATZEL, J. (1979): Psychiatrie im Grundriß. Springer, Berlin, Heidelberg, New York.

Karl Jaspers, Mental States, and Delusional Beliefs: A Redefinition and Its Implications

M. Spitzer

1. KARL JASPERS and the Three Criteria of Delusions

No other subject within the field of psychiatry is so central and simultaneously so little understood as delusional beliefs, and a history of psychiatry is always a history of changing ideas about delusions as well. Although clinicians daily diagnose delusions opinion is unanimous in the literature that no-one can specify what a delusion really is. As HUBER (1981, p. 172) puts it, "there exists no satisfactory general definition of delusion".

In view of this situation KARL JASPERS' three criteria of delusional beliefs - (1) subjective certainty [subjektive Gewißheit], (2) incorrigibility [Unkorrigierbarkeit] and (3) impossibility of content [Unmöglichkeit des Inhalts] - have been referred to again and again up to now. However, JASPERS himself has pointed out that the criteria mentioned above are only correct at first glance and do *not define* a delusion[1] so that they do not help to solve the seemingly simple problem 'what is a delusional belief?'.

To avoid misunderstanings of our argument we would like to stress that our present subject is not a new "theory of delusions" in the sense of a theory of the *genesis* of delusions. Those theories describe delusions as a result of a disorder of other psychological, neuropsychological, or neurobiological functions: thus delusions have been related to disorders of perception (ZIMBARDO et al. 1981, MAHER and ROSS 1984, MAHER 1988), of formal thinking, attentional or language processes (BERZE 1903, MAGARO 1980, MAHER, this volume), of affectivity (HAGEN 1870, BLEULER 1906, WEINSCHENK 1965, OEPEN 1988, OEPEN et al., this volume), of motivation (WINTERS and NEALE 1983), of sexual orientation and resulting dynamics of drives (FREUD 1911) or of the endocrine system (RINIERIS et al. 1985). All these theories, however, presuppose that the term "delusion" has already been defined. (To try to define it by these theories is to beg the question.) Nevertheless, very frequently the problem is not investigated but a presupposed solution is rather taken for granted.

1 "... some clinicians have proposed that the term *delusional* should be applied only to those beliefs that are truly incredible or completely impossible (e.g. Jaspers)" (OLTMANNS 1988, p. 3). This statement about JASPERS is simply not true as can be seen in JASPERS' discussion on delusions of jealousy or delusions of religious content (see below).

In the following we want to show that delusional beliefs are epistemologically identical with certain statements a person makes about him- or herself, and that this concept of identity is implied in JASPERS' first two criteria of delusions. Hereby we reach a deeper knowledge of these criteria. Moreover, it would seem that, by adopting an epstemological approach to the problem of delusion, we find ourselves in a position to give a general definition of delusional beliefs, which does more justice to clinical practice than the definitions existing so far.

JASPERS gives a very broad characterization in so far as he defines delusions in general as (a) *judgements* or *statements* and (b) as a *special form of significance.*

Ad a) Delusions always manifest themselves in judgements or statements, "the delusion is imparted to the statement. Delusions can only arise from peoples' thought and judgement. This is why delusional beliefs are called the pathologically false statements" (JASPERS 1973, p. 80).

Ad b) JASPERS clearly states that each experience of a delusion is an experience of significance. Thus delusions are to be interpreted as a type or special form of significance. "All primary delusions are experiences of significance..." (JASPERS 1973, p. 86).

KURT SCHNEIDER and HANS WALTER GRUHLE are probably the most famous European authors who tried to improve on these specifications by giving, in addition to JASPERS' characterizations the well known definitions of the "binary delusional perception" [zweigliedrige Wahnwahrnehmung] (SCHNEIDER) and the "setting of a relation without an occasion" [Beziehungssetzung ohne Anlaß] (GRUHLE), yet without giving new characterizations of delusions. So it is no surprise that the problematic nature of defining delusion in general has not been solved by the authors mentioned above.

OLTMANNS recently has tried to avoid the problem of clearly defining delusional beliefs by providing specific diagnostic criteria. OLTMANNS (1988, p. 5) speaks of "defining characteristics, with none being considered to be either necessary or sufficient" and obviously has in mind the same approach to a symptom, namely delusions, that is followed in current American psychiatry (and especially represented by the DSM-III) with regard to mental disorders in the meaning of nosological entities. The consequence that there are criteria of criteria is not without problems: (a) If there are criteria of criteria (see SPITZER and DEGKWITZ 1986, SPITZER 1987), there could be (and ought to be, if one looks at OLTMANNS' criteria) criteria of criteria of criteria. Thus matters get at least very complicated. (b) If the criteria (e.g. the occurence of specific delusions) of a disease (e.g. schizophrenia) are defined by criteria themselves, how can this approach reasonably be called 'descriptive' as it often is? (c) Furthermore, if some psychiatrists already feel uneasy about the criterial approach to diagnostics because it simply adds up symptoms without giving them a weighed interpretation, how will they feel about not only adding up symptoms to a disease but also features to a symptom? - So this approach does not seem to meet what psychiatrists either want to do or actually do when they make diagnoses. The question still remains: is it possible to tell what a delusion is without merely introducing criteria for a delusion?

As there are patients who do have only one symptom - a delusion - and who are otherwise not outside the range of normality, it is clear that any definition of delusions should *not* refer to other pathological phenomena: delusions should not be explained in terms of abnormal perception, abnormal emotion or abnormal behavior even if a theory of their *causal development* or behavioral *treatment* cannot avoid mentioning these concepts. A definition must be free of them if it wants to meet the clinical pratice in which there certainly are patients who are, psychopathologically speaking, not disturbed with regard to perception, emotion or behavior.

From clinical practise it is obvious, that the notion of *falseness* does *not* delineate delusions from normal statements. Obviously, false statements give *first hints* to a clinician when he talks to a patient and false statements may sometimes be regarded as the clue to the diagnosis of delusions. While this being the fact, there are also cases of delusions of which it cannot be told whether they are true or false for practical or fundamental reasons (see our discussion of religious delusions below). For that reason HEISE (1988, p. 269) concludes that "... practising psychiatrists cannot logically be using falsity as a criterion of thought disorder."

That clinicians always have been in search of a definition of delusions which has *not* to refer to the content of them, is quite obvious: there is no list of contents or of normal contents with the help of which the clinician could decide whether a specific content p represents a delusion or not. The often mentioned "general accepted believes within a certain culture" only point to whether a specific content is believed by others or not but they do not apply to the question of truth. The answers to these questions give first hints and are of course not useless for the diagnosis. Nevertheless, they are not useful for the definition of a delusion.

2. Judgements on Mental States

JASPERS repeatedly emphasized that a delusion is always a (form of) judgement. Generally speaking judgements can be made on various objects, events, topics, or subjects, and they have a different validity in the respective fields. If somebody talks about things he knows well, he is *more sure* than when he makes statements about facts he does not know so well. By the same token *correcting* him in a dispute will be more or less easy depending on his knowledge of the subject in question. However, are there statements of which a person is "absolutely certain" that no possible arguments can correct him? - If such statements exist, they will show *formal*[2] similarities to delusions, because delusional beliefs are uttered with certainty and incorrigibility according to JASPERS' criteria.

If someone speaks about "objective" facts he basically can be right or wrong. However, if a person makes statements about himself it can be the case that any kind of error or deception is excluded, namely, if he talks about himself in a certain manner.

If somebody makes a statement about himself this statement can either refer to an "inner" or an "outer aspect" of the topic. Examples for inner aspects would be "I'm feeling pain", "I'm feeling good" or "I'm thinking at the moment". Examples for a person's statement regarding the other aspect would be "I am 180 cm tall" or "my weight is 70 kg". If a person speaks about an outer aspect of himself, such statements are epistemologically nothing special. Another person can state as well as I can that I weigh 70 kg or that I am 180 cm tall (see SPITZER 1985, 1986). Yet just the opposite is the case with statements characterizing the inner aspect of a person: a person is certain and cannot be corrected concerning statements regarding his inner aspect. Following common philosophical terminology we shall refer to this inner aspect of a person as the *mental states* of that

2 It can be questioned whether the epistemological similarities should be called "formal". As psychopathologists are used to differentiate between content and form of delusions and as the certainty and incorrigibility of delusions are normally regarded as characterizing their *form*, it seems to be justified to speak of a formal similarity.

person. A person cannot be wrong by saying he has a toothache, or by saying he is thinking or feeling this or that. On the other hand, if someone makes statements about other things ("objects") there is always the possibility that he is wrong or mistaken and that he can be corrected in a dialogue. In accordance with this, someone cannot make statements about objects with full certainty. It is, however, not sensible[3] to doubt the statements a person makes concerning his mental states (there are good grounds for regarding questions like "are you sure you are feeling pain?" or "are you sure you are thinking?" as absurd). It should be mentioned that this is not a "speculative" attempt to define the "nature of the self", but a simple argument concerning the epistemological status of a class of statements.

To summarize what we have been discussing so far: There exists a class of statements of which a person is certain and incorrigible by others. However, this puts JASPERS' first two criteria of delusions in a new context: these criteria are met by all statements a person makes about him- or herself, more exactly, about his/her inner aspect. Thus we have a class of statements - besides delusion-statements - which also meet JASPERS' first and second criterion of delusion, however without passing for delusion in clinical or other linguistic usage: statements of a person about her/his mental states.

Before expanding the idea we insert a methodical reflexion to get a somewhat broader view of the matter we have reached with the present state of disscusion. Most current definitions of delusions start with a very general determination ("form of judgements") and try to specify delusions by special features (to mention only a few: falseness with regard to the contents, reference of content to the deluded person and emotional alterations). This situation has changed in the course of the argument presented so far: the interpretation of the first two Jasperian criteria of delusions in the light of general epistemological considerations has shown that these criteria define a certain class of judgements against all other judgements. With the help of this differentiation within the very general field of judgements we have not yet come to a definition of delusions. We can, however, proceed in a new way and try to give a further specification which will aim at distinguishing delusions from statements about mental states.

3. Formal Self-Reference and Delusional Beliefs

Each person is subjectively certain and not to be corrected when speaking about her/his own mental states. The patient with delusions differs from the sane person in so far as he speaks with subjective certainty and incorrigible about facts which do *not* lie within the scope of his mental states: things, events, other persons. Thus the clinician meets in the patient with delusions a person who extends his epistemological "claim to absoluteness" in an inadmissible way to intersubjectively accessible facts, i.e. to facts which are communicable, and with

3 The possibility of lying at first seems to contradict with that point. However, as an analysis of the presuppositions of lying could show, it only can happen because of the epistemic assymmetrical relation two person have to the mental states of one of them.

regard to which there is no asymmetric epistemological relation between two persons.

Thus we can define delusional beliefs as follows: delusions are statements which are uttered formally like statements about a mental state, whose contents, however, are not mental states but rather intersubjectively accessible ("objective") facts. In what follows we will examine the consequences, advantages, apparent drawbacks, and criticisms of this definition.

To begin, the person-referential feature [der "Ich-Bezug] of delusions, which is often regarded as accidental, gains a totally new meaning in light of this new definition: it is no certain characteristics of the *content* of delusions but the *form* of delusions which results in such a very close relation between "I" and "delusion". When we speak of "I" we do not mean the concrete, single mentally disturbed person, but an epistemological point of view shared by each person qua being a person. From this viewpoint one can make statements about a certain subject which formally show the same characteristics as delusion-statements. Thus we can speak of an epistemological-formal analogy between the statement "I'm thinking" of a sane person and the statement "somebody is pursuing me" of an insane. *The person-referential feature of delusions thus turns out to be an epistemological analogy regarding the general form of statements.*

It should be stressed again that the main point of the proposed definition is a formal one: delusions are analoguous formally, i.e. regarding their epistemological claim, to a person's statements about himself (inner aspect). The difference to the sane person lies in the range of application. This definition leads to a new view of some theoretical and clinical-practical problems.

4. The Achievements and Problems of the Proposed Definition

4.1 Advantages Over the Third Jasperian Criterion of Delusions

In many cases of delusions the third criterion of JASPERS - the impossibility of the content - does not hold. JASPERS himself mentions the example of the patient with a delusion of jealousy who continues to be classified as having the disorder delusion of jealousy by the clinician even if the partner has in fact become untrue. In our proposed definition the problem does not arise that the clinical situation (one would like to continue speaking of a delusion) contradicts the third criterion of JASPERS (impossibility of the content). In other words, the clinical situation is not adaquately represented by the term delusion when defined inter alia by the third criterion of JASPERS.

However, if we understand delusions as statements about a topic which does not lie within the scope of a person's mental states and which is nevertheless uttered with certainty and in an incorrectable way, then clinical practice is represented adequately: the clinician can speak of delusions irrespective of the correctness or falseness of the patient's statements. His criteria are the first two criteria of JASPERS coupled with the fact that the uttered content is not a mental state of the person expressing this content.

4.2 Degrees of Certainty and the Problem of Sameness

Psychiatrists agree upon the empirical fact that delusions are stated in various degrees of certainty. With regard to a proposal of STRAUSS (1969) OLTMANNS, for instance, proposes a continuous measuring line of certainty on which a delusion should be placed when being properly described. Clinically it is well-known that in the course of neuroleptic treatment a delusion does not disappear all of a sudden but rather will be less likely to have consequences for the every day life in the first step (while being stated with "absolute" conviction) and secondly will still be stated but with a diminished degree of certainty. Thus, at least for these cases our definition seems to be wrong because it does not match - as it is intended to - the clinical use of the concept of delusion. However, most of the definitions or characterizations in the textbooks will lead into the same kind of trouble. A short look at the possible options will tell us why it could be wise to extend our definition to include statements which had been held by the patient with certainty and in an incorrectable way but are not so anymore.

These possible options are:

(a) One could avoid speaking of delusions and reserve the term to statements which are held with absolute conviction. Clinicians generally feel uncomfortable with this approach because the degree of certainty is just one out of a number of dimensions of their description.[4] Thus, clinicians would have to switch terms in all cases, where there is a change in degree of certainty (which actually can happen more than once), even if other descriptive dimensions are unchanged. This creates a somehow artificial situation that clinicians will not be likely to accept.

(b) One could still speak of delusions, despite the fact that the respective statements are not held with absolute certainty and in an incorrectable way. The problem is, that if one allows a delusion to be characterized by "stated with some degree of conviction, from probability to absolute certainty", the definition of delusions which rests on the epistemological degree of certainty, will collapse. However, this need not be so.

Clinicians refer to a delusion as the same as another delusion, if both are stated by the same patient and do have the same content. Thus, a patient does not have a new delusion every day but is considered to have the same delusion, if the content is the same. Even if the degree of conviction changes, the delusion will be called the same by clinicians, if the content is the same. This clinical use of sameness referring to delusions can be employed to avoid the difficulties with delusions being stated without absolute conviction: a statement p that is held by a patient without absolute conviction may be called a delusion *if and only if this statement p has been held with absolute conviction before*. We propose, that one should speak of "delusions in remission" to indicate the diminished degree of conviction.

4 Other such dimensions are degree of systematisation, degree of relevance for severeal parts of every day life, degree of being accompanied by hallucinations etc. (cf. OLTMANNS 1988, BERNER 1975).

4.3 Delusions with Religious Content

Among others, it was KURT SCHNEIDER who stressed repeatedly that it is impossible to distinguish between religious ideas and delusions with religious contents. A difference between a "religious idea of the non-psychotic life" and a "delusion" was considered "incomprehensible at all events" (SCHNEIDER 1949, p. 30). In another context SCHNEIDER remarks, "principally there cannot be made any psychological distinction between a delusion and a belief whose only criterion is the felt certainty" (SCHNEIDER 1928, p. 50). It seems to be impossible to answer the question of how religious experiences or contents should be distinguished from delusions with religious content. In both cases the statements that are made are held with great personal conviction. Thus JASPERS' first two criteria are also quite applicable to religious contents and therefore to many forms of religion.

Subjective certainty and incorrigibility *may* but need not be characteristics of religious beliefs, as the examples of many religious people show who "wrestle" with their conviction. However, as for many people religion fulfils these criteria, the possibility of doubt (which may be presentis at times or permanently) as a diagnostic means, is inapplicable. We are careful not to go into the question whether religious contents are to be regarded as a description of mental states or not because this is - as a question about the ontological status of god or religious experience respectively - a subject of theology and is answered differently in various religious communities. The seemingly easy "solution" to the question about the existence of delusions with religious contents in the sense that each form of religiousness may be a form of a delusion (FREUD probably is the most famous representative of this thesis) is justified neither regarding JASPERS' criteria nor with regard to clinical practice. JASPERS third criterion for delusions is not applicable in the case of religious contents because the question about the possibility or impossibility of a content is to be understood as an empirical question. Thus JASPERS' third criterion is *only applicable to empirical facts*. It is well known clinically that in diagnosing delusions of religious content, members of the respective religious community (sect, mystic group et.) are most likely to notice changes in the patient's thoughts and are the first to know whether he or she is mentally disturbed or not.[5]

Frequently a kind of statistic standard is applied to answer the question how to differentiate between delusion with religious content and religionsness, as for example in the DSM-III-R (p. 193), "beliefs or experiences of members of religions or other cultural groups may be difficult to distiguish from delusions or hallucinations. If such experiences are shared and accepted by a subcultural group they should not be considered evidence of psychosis". There are, however, many objections to the criterion of intersubjectivity which amounts to saying that a delusion is an *individual's* belief and a religious belief is a *collective* phenomenon. First, according to this definition the founders of religions must needs be classified as having a delusional disorder according to this criterion. Secondly, not each religion contains the idea of mission, i.e. the aspect of communication, as LENZ (1973, p. 376) has pointed out. Thirdly, the criterion of intersubjectivity is not applicable to those cases where a delusion is adopted by others.[6] In the fourth place the criterion of of intersubjectivity is not applicable to all cases of induced delusions which by no means concern always just two persons. *Clinically*, religious delusion has been and always is stated *indirectly*.

5 For some striking examples see MURPHY 1967.
6 For a very impressive case also see MURPHY 1967.

Indirect signs for delusions with religious contents are the presence of other symptoms of a mental disorder, inconsistencies between uttered content and ways of acting (both criteria of symptomatology) as well as a time-course criterion, which sees a criterion of pathology in the development of the person, in the reduction to stiffness or torpidity of his/her thought, feeling or acting.

The attempt to come to general statements about religions delusion involves the danger of dogmatic "solutions" (inapplicable for clinical purposes), which may either lie in the "theologisation" of psychopathological facts (see KAHN 1929, p. 438) or in the "psychopathologisation" of theological facts (see FREUD 1927). The question, whether to speak of religions delusion or true religiousness can only be decided in each specific case, as HEIMANN (1961, p. 490) has already pointed out.

Our proposed definition of delusions admittedly meets the clinical use of "delusion with religious contents" just as little as other definitions. We therefore must extend the characterization of delusions: statements about religious contents are also to be characterized as delusions if adequate indirect hints are present.

4.4 Analytical Statements

Besides judgements about his or her own mental states other statements are to be found of which a person can claim to be subjectively certain and incorrigible: analytical judgements, i.e. sentences like "all singles are not married". Everybody knows that this sentence is correct without an empirical verification but that is only because everybody knows the meaning of the term "single" and the term "not married".

Why could this class of statements completely be overlooked in the discussion so far? The reason is, that clinically nobody feels motivated to distinguish between true analytical statements and delusions, because the question whether a true analytical statement could be a delusion does not arise. Nevertheless we must add to our definition of delusions the triviality, that the class of analytical statements has to be excluded from the class of delusions as defined according to our definition.

This is not the end of the discussion yet, because what remains to be classified are *false* analytical statements uttered by patients, i.e. statements like the following: "singles are married". In fact the clinician often has to deal with false analytical statements. It is not difficult to classify them into the psychopathological systematic representation if one looks at the principles of analyticism, which are logical relations and semantic rules. However, inasmuch as a patient violates logical and/or semantic rules we do not speak of a *contentual* thought-disorder (i.e a delusion) but of a *formal* thought disorder. Therefore the psychopathological characterization of false analytical statements does not create difficulties for our definition.

4.5 Other Judgements Which We Are Certain About and a Speculative Extension: Mismatching Epistemic and Psychological Certainty

There are many judgements which are not analytical and not about mental states, which we would regard as certain: for me it is hard to doubt that I am Manfred Spitzer, am married, work as a psychiatrist, have two children etc. All these statements, though empirical, belong to a set of things I do not know how to doubt reasonably. However, as LUDWIG WITTGENSTEIN already has pointed out, this kind of certainty does not refer to a certain *single* statement. The point here is, rather, that to doubt one of these statements always means to take a variety of other ones for sure.[7] Thus, with regard to a certain statement p of the kind mentioned above, there is not the same certainty as with regard to mental states.

One could further argue[8] that all the statements we are able to report could be ranked by their epistemic certainty, at least in principle: on one end of the ranking we would find cogito-certain statements and on the other end we would find statements of empirical facts. In between, opinions, scientific theories, metaphysical claims, religious beliefs and so on had their place. Then we could evaluate a certain person's psychological ranking of examples of the above mentioned statements with regard to their certainty. Normally, we would achieve corresponding rankings with regard to epistemic and psychological certainty. In the case of delusions, there would be a mismatch of epistemic and psychological certainty-ranking, i.e. the psychological ranking of certain statements would be more on the certain-end than we would expect looking at the ranking of epistemic certainties.

What about a mismatch in the other direction? Is there any clinical correlate, i.e. other patients, who claim utterances which would be epistemically ranked as certain, with less psychological certainty? - Perhaps hebephrenic schizophrenics could be in a very broad sense described that way. What often has been called a "läppische Einstellung" might be described as a mismatch of psychological and epistemic certainty-ranking in the way that the patients will not regard anything as certain.

4.6 Problems of Delusions with a Content Referring to the Deluded Person and Their Solution

Delusions with a content referring to the delusional person do not seem to be compatible with our definition because they do not seem - at least in part - to be concerned with statements about "objective" facts which are stated in the manner of statements about mental states. A closer look at this counter-argument is rewarding, because it reveals further advantages of our definition.

No difficulties arise if the content refers to intersubjective aspects of the person (the outfit, name, height, weight etc.). If, however, the mental states of a person are concerned, our definition is not applicable, i.e. it excludes the phenomena from beeing delusions by definition.

Let us take a closer look at the detailed clinical facts which are relevant here. No problem arises in nearly all frequent themes of delusions because the topic already indicates that it is a question of an intersubjectively accessible fact, as for

7 For details of the argument see WITTGENSTEIN, *On Certainty*.

8 This argument has been proposed by Prof. H.-N. CASTAÑEDA during a discussion at the conference. He has also made some very valuable comments on the whole article and I would like to express my special thanks to him.

example the delusions of jealousy, persecution, love, poverty or the paranoia querulans.

Two large fields merely lead to the assumption that there are possibly statements about ones own mental states which are clinically referred to as delusions (and as such leading to contradictions between clinical practice and its theory) - the field of delusions of reference and the field of the "affective" delusions of grandeur and of belittlement.

4.6.1 Delusions of Reference

Let us start discussing the problem with a view to delusions of reference. When we come to the conceptual classification of the delusions of reference, the third Jasperian criterion of delusions leads to confusion. If the experience of a patient who says for example that the chime of the church-tower clock is immediately connected with his thoughts, is to be characterized as a delusion, it must be understood - in accordance with JASPERS and most of the psychiatric literature - as an incorrigible, subjectively certain, yet *false* statement with regard to its contents (the church tower clock or its chimes respectively). Thus the delusion of reference is understood as a statement about *something else*: either the clock (an object), the chime (an event) or the relationship of clock or chime to the insane person (conceptualized as something which can be referred to by other persons as well).

This understanding, however, of a delusion of reference does not seem to represent the phenomenon adequately. The term "delusion of reference " should rather be understood as *characterization of a patient's certain immediate way of experience*. The experience "that the chime of the church-tower clock is immediately connected with me" is thus not interpreted as s statement about an object, event or a relation (i.e. about "objective", viz., intersubjective facts) but as a statement about the *patient's own immediate experience*. It is his own immediate experience which is disturbed, irrespective of special contents but with regard to the relation of the experiencing person to the experienced contents. According to this interpretation the patient's reported experiences of reference are not to be understood as a "delusion" but as reports of disordered immediate experience, which correctly have to be characterized as "Self-disorders"[9] in psychopathology.

This does not mean to deny that a delusion can develop from experiences of reference. In this case the patient's immediate experience of reference would be interpreted by him or her, and such logical conclusions drawn by the patient about causes or backgrounds of his way of experience would rightly be called delusions. This could be one possible way in which systematized delusions could develop as secondary, i.e. as a result of a disordered immediate experience of the self.

We can therefore meet the objection that delusions of reference are a matter of statements about mental states, which are clinically referred to as delu-

9 There exists no English Translation of the German term "Ichstörung", which seems to most appropriate. "Depersonalization" does not meet the scope of "Ichstörungen" and "Ego-disorders" probably leads to a mix-up with psychoanalytic theory (see also my contribution on Ichstörungen, this volume).

sion (which would contradict our definition) as follows: A patient's reported experiences of reference can be interpreted either as *false* statements about the "*objective*" *world* (according to the third criterion of delusion[10]) or as *correct* statements about his *immediate experience*. Thus the terminus "delusion of reference" is part of a tradition which can be traced back to JASPERS. The experiences that are meant by this term, however, could just as well be subsumed under the term "immediate experience of reference" and be regarded as a "self-disorder". This is, in our opinion, a better interpretation of the clinical facts.

There are two quite heterogeneous considerations fostering this interpretation: primarily the patient is taken seriously. His reports of immediate experiences of reference are taken for what they really are. The patient is not thought - as in what we may call the Jasperian interpretation of his or her statements - to make a false statement about objective things. He is rather thought to try to express adequately his way of immediate experience. Our second consideration takes into account the frequency of the experiences discussed here: "delusions of reference" are the most frequent "type" of delusions with an incidence in schizophrenic psychoses of about 70%, independent - as far as we know - of temporal and cultural factors. Thus it is obvious that the matter is not a thought disorder with regard to its contents (which is regarded as contingent and may vary optionally depending on the patient's life-story or cultural realities) but a way of experiencing which is immediately connected with the schizophrenic disorder.[11] Consequently we consider what has so far been called "delusion of reference " as much too important to remain in the status of a merely disorder of contents.

4.6.2 "Delusions" of Grandeur and Belittlement

The alterations in thinking reported by patients with affective psychoses have to be interpreted in the same way as above. The patients for example report that they found it hard to think, that they did not get any further in everyday situations, that they were inhibited or were extremely fast thinkers, could comprehend connexions in no time and had generally speaking an extreme perceptive faculty. In so far as these statements refer to the patient's own thoughts and not to the patient as a whole person, they should *not* be understood as s *false* description of reality but as a *correct* description of the patient's own immediate experience. Therefore such statements are not cases of delusions but descriptions of formal thought disturbance which occur in depressed or manic patients. Utterances are only to be characterized as delusions when they refer to the person as a whole ("I am the greatest", "I am not worth anything at all"), i.e. when they also comprise the outer aspect of the person.

This again suggests the question whether delusions in affective psychoses might be understood as conclusions resulting from the patient's formal thought disorders experienced in these

10 Of course, this criterion does not *define* a delusion, as we argued above. But nevertheless, that a statement is false is often the first hint in clinical settings that it might be delusive. In addition one could say that at least according to the clinical practice of today delusions are regarded as false.

11 It should be mentioned that we feel strongly in accordance with E. BLEULER, who also saw the "Ichstörung" [disorder of the Self] as the most basic symptom of schizophrenia.

psychoses. We consider such an origin of delusions as possible, but we want to stress again that this is in no way the only possible genesis of delusion (for a detailed discussion see SPITZER 1988).

What we wanted to show was that statements about one's own experience or thinking are not capable of being called a "delusion" according to our definition. This, however, is not a drawback but an advantage, and we have put foreward arguments for our opinion.

4.6.3 Contentual Relations to the Person

In older and as well more recent psychiatric literature the reference of delusions to the deluded person ["Ich-Bezug"] is treated again and again. As a rule, this means that the delusional content is somehow connected with the deluded person: It is the disturbed person who is persecuted, who tends to megalomania, who is jealous etc. By the same token the personal reference ["Ich-Bezug"] of delusions is indeed mentioned in literature, it is, however, considered to be accidental, i.e. it is not thought to be a part of the nature or definition of delusions. This does not mean the structural analogy of delusions to statements of a person about his or her mental states. Rather it is a matter of references with regard to the contents of delusions to the deluded person.

The presence of such references in all cases of delusions was discussed controversially in the past. E. BLEULER accepts it, whereas SATTES denies it. Although a final empirical affirmation is still to be made, we agree with the opinion which is most frequently found in literature that in many (all?) delusions there are contentual relations to the deluded person. The problem whether there is a connexion between the contentual relations and the formal analogy of delusion to statements about mental states represents a field of general and clinical-psychopathological research that has not yet been investigated.

5. Concluding Remarks

Delusions are statements which are formally uttered like statements about a mental state, whose contents, however, do not refer to mental states but to intersubjectively accessible ("objective") facts.

As far as the clinical practice is concerned, our definition of delusion immediately leads to the following conclusion: the diagnosis of delusions is not a matter of an empirical validation or falsification of patients' statements but an exact registration of the way how a person claims certain statements. Statements of the immediately experienced reference of an object or event towards oneself should not be interpreted as false statements about reality but as correct statements about one's own experiences, i.e. as self-disturbances. Statements of depressive or manic patients about their mental states should also be interpreted as true statements about their thinking and experiencing and not as delusions. Analytical judgements are no delusive judgements (the exclusion of correct analytical judgements is trivial; false analytical judgements belong into the field of formal thought disorders). Delusions with religious content can only be stated indirectly.

Furthermore our discussion of the clinical phenomena leads to a number of hypotheses that might stimulate empirical-psychopathological research in the future: the conditions of the genesis and the development of delusions have indeed been studied empirically. However, many questions remain undecided partly because it is not clear under which conceptual assumptions the data were obtained. Thus the questions concerning the connexion between delusion and affect, between delusion and formal thought-disturbances as well as between delusion and disturbances of perception have not been solved definitely to the present day. Pathological alterations of affectivity, formal thinking, perception or motivation again and again are made responsible for the genesis of delusions and are discussed as "basic disturbances" [Grundstörungen]. However, as long as the question still remains unsolved what has to be characterized as delusion at all these approaches remain vague and their results contradictory. Especially since neurobiological and neuropsychological methods have become more and more refined by now, it seems important to take into account the consequences of our definition, and to try to assign biological and neuropsychological correlates to the now possible differentiations.

Only when the question "what is a delusion" is solved, the questions asking for the "how" of the diagnosis and the "why" of the origin can be answered sensibly and effectively.

Summary: Proceeding from Jaspers' criteria for delusional beliefs and founded on general considerations regarding the epistemological degree of certainty of judgements a new definition of delusions is proposed: delusional beliefs are uttered formally like assertions about mental states. Their contents, however, are not mental states but intersubjectively accessible ("objective") facts. As it is shown, this definition implies (a) that the clinical diagnosis of delusions has nothing to do with an empirical validation or falsification of patients' statements but with the exact registration of the manner how a person makes certain statements. (b) Delusions of reference (i.e. the immediate experience of a relationship of facts or events towards oneself) should not be interpreted as false statements about reality but as statements about one's own experience (i.e. as Ichstörungen [disturbances of the self]). (c) Statements of depressive or manic patients about their mental states should also be interpreted as valid assertions about their thinking and experiencing and not as delusions (i.e. false statements about "objective" reality). (d) Analytical judgements have to be excluded (for the exclusion of correct analytical judgements is trivial; false analytical judgements are to be classified as formal thougt-disorders). (e) Religious delusions do not fall within the scope of the definition and can only be diagnosed indirectly.

KARL JASPERS, mentale Zustände und Wahn: Eine neue Definition und ihre Implikationen

Zusammenfassung: Es wird eine neue Definition von Wahn vorgeschlagen, die von den JASPERSschen Wahnkriterien abgeleitet ist und systematisch auf allgemeine Überlegungen zum erkenntnistheoretischen Gewißheitsgrad von Urteilen gründet: Beim Wahn handelt es sich um Aussagen, die formal wie Aussagen über einen mentalen Zustand geäußert werden, bei deren Inhalten es sich jedoch nicht um mentale Zustände, sondern um intersubjektiv zugängliche ("objektive") Sachverhalte handelt. Aus dieser Definition ergibt sich unmittelbar, (a) daß es klinisch bei der Diagnose von Wahn nicht um eine empirische Validierung oder Falsifizierung von Patientenaussagen geht, sondern um die genaue Erfassung der Art, wie eine Person bestimmte Aussagen vertritt. (b) Erlebnisse der Eigenbeziehung sollten nicht als falsche Aussagen über die Realität, sondern als richtige Aussagen über das eigene Erleben, d.h. als Ichstörung interpretiert werden. (c) Aussagen depressiver oder manischer Patienten über ihre mentalen Zustände sollten ebenfalls als wahre Aussagen über ihr Denken und Erleben und nicht als Wahn aufgefaßt werden. (d) Analytische Urteile sind keine Wahnurteile (der Ausschluß richtiger analytischer Urteile ist trivial; falsche analytische Urteile sind als formale Denkstörungen zu klassifizieren). (e) Religiöser Wahn läßt sich mit der vorgeschlagenen Definition nicht als Wahn abgrenzen und kann nur indirekt festgestellt werden.

References

AMERICAN PSYCHIATRIC ASSOCIATION (1987): Diagnostic and statistical manual of mental disorders (3rd ed., Revised) (DSM-III-R). American Psychiatric Association, Washington, DC.

BERNER, P. (1975): Zum heutigen Stand der Wahnforschung [On the current state of research in the field of delusions]. Psychiatria Clin. **8**, pp. 1-13.

BERZE, J. (1903): Das Primärsymptom der Paranoia. Marhold, Halle.

BLEULER, E. (1906): Affektivität, Suggestibilität und Paranoia. Marhold, Halle.

BLEULER, E. (1911): Dementia praecox. Deuticke, Leipzig, Wien.

FREUD, S. (1911/1978): Über einen autobiographisch beschriebenen Fall von Dementia Paranoides. Werke VIII, pp. 239-320, S. Fischer, Frankfurt.

FREUD, S. (1927/1976): Die Zukunft einer Illusion. Werke XIV, pp. 323-380, S. Fischer, Frankfurt.

GRUHLE, H.W. (1951): Über den Wahn. Nervenarzt **22**, pp. 125-126.

HAGEN, F.W. (1870): Studien auf dem Gebiete der ärztlichen Seelenheilkunde. Besold, Erlangen.

HEIMANN, H. (1961): Religion und Psychiatrie. In: GRUHLE, H.W., JUNG, R., MAYER-GROSS, W., MÜLLER, M. (eds.): Psychiatrie der Gegenwart, Bd. III, pp. 471-493. Springer, Berlin.

HEISE, D.R. (1988): Delusions and the construction of reality. In: OLTMANNS, T.S., MAHER, B.A. (eds.): Delusional beliefs, pp. 259 - 272. Wiley, New York, Chichester, Brisbane, Toronto, Singapore.

HUBER, G. (1981): Psychiatrie. Systematischer Lehrtext für Studenten und Ärzte. Schattauer Verlag. Stuttgart, New York.

JASPERS, K. (1973): Allgemeine Psychopathologie. Springer, Berlin.

KAHN, E. (1929): Über Wahnbildung. Archiv f. Psychiatrie **88**, pp. 435-454.

LENZ, H. (1973): Glaube und Wahn. Fortschr. Neurol. Psychiat. **41**, pp. 341-359.

MAGARO, P.A. (1980): Cognition in schizophrenia and paranoia. Lawrence Erlbaum, Hillsdale, New Jersey.

MAHER, B.A. (1974): Delusional thinking and perceptual disorder. Journal of Individual Psychology **30**, pp. 98-113.

MAHER, B.A. (1988): Anomalous experience and delusional thinking: The logic of explanations. In: OLTMANNS, T.S., MAHER, B.A. (eds.): Delusional beliefs, pp. 15 - 33. Wiley, New York, Chichester, Brisbane, Toronto, Singapore.

MAHER, B.A., ROSS, J.S. (1984): Delusions. In: ADAM H.E., SUTKER P.B. (eds): Comprehensive Handbook of Psychopathology, pp. 383-409. Plenum Press, New York.

MURPHY, H.B.M. (1967): Cultural aspects of delusion. Studium Generale **20**, pp. 684-692.

OEPEN, G., FÜNFGELD, M., HÖLL, T., ZIMMERMANN, P., LANDIS, T., REGART, M. (1988): Schizophrenia - an emotional hypersensitivity of the right cerebral hemisphere. Internat. J. of Psychophysiol. **5**, pp. 261-264.

OLTMANNS, T.S. (1988): Approaches to the definition and study of delusions. In: OLTMANNS, T.S., MAHER, B.A. (eds.): Delusional beliefs, pp. 3 - 11. Wiley, New York, Chichester, Brisbane, Toronto, Singapore.

RINIERIS, P., MARKIANOS, M., HATZIMANOLIS, J., STEFANIS, C. (1985): A psychoendocrine study in male paranoid schizophrenics with delusional ideas of homosexual content. Acta psychiatr. scand. **72**, pp. 309-314.

SATTES, H. (1948): Über Wahnbildung ohne Ichbeziehung. Archiv f. Psychiatrie **181**, pp. 110-135.

SCHNEIDER, K. (1928): Zur Einführung in die Religionspsychopathologie. Mohr, Tübingen.

SCHNEIDER, K. (1949): Zum Begriff des Wahns. Fortschr. Neurol. Psychiatr. **17**, pp. 26-31.

SPITZER, M. (1985): Allgemeine Subjektivität und Psychopathologie. Haag und Herchen, Frankfurt a.M.

SPITZER, M. (1986): Erfahrung - Aspekte einer Begriffsklärung. Nervenarzt **57**, pp. 342-348.

SPITZER, M. (1987): Symptom and criterion in medicine and psychiatry. In: WEINGARTNER, P., SCHURZ, G. (eds.): Logic, Philosophy of Science and Epistemology (Proceedings of the 11th international Wittgenstein-Symposium), pp. 183-185.

SPITZER, M. (1988): Untersuchungen zum Wahnproblem. Ein Beitrag zur allgemeinen und klinischen Psychopathologie. In print (see also for further references).

SPITZER, M., Degkwitz, R. (1986): Zur Diagnose des DSM-III. Nervenarzt **57**, pp. 698-704.

STRAUSS, J.S. (1969): Hallucinations and Delusions as Points on Continua Function. Arch. Gen. Psychiat. **21**, pp. 581-586.

WEINSCHENK, C. (1965): Üer die Wirksamkeit der pathologischen Affektivität bei der Wahnentstehung der endogenen Psychose. Schweizer Archiv f. Neurol. Neurochirurg. u. Psychiat. **95**, pp. 91-119.

WINTERS, K.C. , NEALE, J.M. (1983): Delusions and delusional thinking in psychotics: a review of the literature. Clinical Psychology Review **3**, pp. 227-253.

WITTGENSTEIN, L. (1979): Über Gewißheit. Suhrkamp, Frankfurt.

ZIMBARDO, P.G., ANDERSEN, S.M., KABAT, L.G. (1981): Induced hearing deficit generates experimental paranoia. Science **212**, pp. 1529-1531.

Part Three

The Experiencing I and Its Disturbances (Ichstörungen)

Bewußtsein und Selbstbewußtsein

F. A. Uehlein

1. Einleitung

Die Menschen, mit denen wir leben, die Dinge um uns, für und gegen uns, und die Welt, in der wir zusammen da sind, erlebend, denkend und handelnd, sind uns ganz selbstverständlich. Wir kennen uns hier ziemlich aus, und im Horizont dieser selbstverständlichen Bekanntschaft, in dieser Welt unseres Handelns und unserer Erfahrung begegnet uns Neues, Befremdliches und Gefährliches, wie Vertrautes und Gewohntes. Wir *beginnen* stets im natürlichen Erfahrungsbewußtsein, wenn wir uns besinnen, wenn wir fragen, beschreiben und begründen. Unser Bewußtsein ist immer schon erfüllt, lebensweltliches Bewußtsein mit dem Reichtum seiner Erfahrung, auch wenn wir seinen Anfängen nachgehen und seine Genese fassen wollen, oder phänomenologisch beschreiben, was sich uns gibt und in transzendentaler Besinnung aufdecken, welche subjektive Leistungen diesen Gegebenheiten entsprechen (HUSSERL), wenn wir die apriorischen Strukturen der Erfahrung und des Handelns entdecken (KANT), die Geschichte des Selbstbewußtseyns (re)construieren (SCHELLING) oder das nicht reduzierbare und unabdingbare autonomous self of ideas (TH. NAGEL, D. PARFIT) erforschen.

Ich trete im folgenden hinter diesen *Beginn* zurück. Ich behandle das Thema "Bewußtsein und Selbstbewußtsein" nicht vom natürlichen Erfahrungsbewußtsein aus. Nicht vom Mitleben und seinen Handlungszusammenhängen in der gemeinsamen Welt, nicht von der Lebenswelt, ihrer Selbstverständlichkeit und ihrem Erfahrungsreichtum gehe ich aus.

Bei meinem Thema "Bewußtsein und Selbstbewußtsein" interessiert insbesondere, wie dies alles *bewußt* werden kann, so daß es uns selbstverständlich, bekannt und neu, gefährlich und gewöhnlich ist, daß wir von ihm erzählen können als unseren Geschichten, daß wir es aber auch in bestimmter Allgemeinheit benennen, in seinen Strukturen beschreiben und bewußt zum Beginn philosophischer, psychologischer und soziologischer Überlegungen nehmen können.

Somit beginne ich mit dem Denken und schließe mit einer Bemerkung zum Ich als unableitbarem ursprünglichen Selbstbewußtsein.[1]

2. Exposition des Themas

Wird überhaupt gedacht, dann wird etwas gedacht, etwas Bestimmtes gedacht, wird etwas in Gedanken bestimmt.

So in Gedanken bestimmt, ist es bewußt. Gedanken sind Gedanken von etwas. Gedanken sind aber nicht nur Gedanken von etwas, sie sind auch Gedanken eines Ich. Ein Ich erzeugt sich Gedanken - es denkt -, sonst gibt es keine Gedanken und kein Gedachtes-Bewußtes.

Bewußtsein meint also, daß ein Ich sich Gedanken von etwas erzeugt. Bewußtsein ist ein Sein, das sich Gedanken von etwas erzeugen kann. So bin ich ein Bewußtsein und habe das Bewußtsein von etwas, das ich mir in meinen Gedanken bestimmt habe.

Was aber meinen in diesen Sätzen "ich" und "sich"? "Ich" meint ein Seiendes, das gerade eben jenen Gedanken erzeugen kann, nach dem es genannt ist - oder besser, mit dem es sich selber nennt: Ich.

Dieser Sachverhalt hängt nicht an dem Wort "ich", sondern an der Erzeugung einer bestimmten semantischen Struktur. Es muß daher auch nicht ein einheitliches Wort geben, das dieses natürliche Ichbewußtsein bezeichnet, durchaus kann "ich" in verschiedenen intersubjektiven Kontexten in verschiedenen Wörtern, Morphemen oder verschiedener syntaktischer Fügung zum Ausdruck gebracht werden.

Ferner: der Wortlaut *ich*, die verschiedenen Morpheme und Syntagma werden gelernt. Aber die Erzeugung der semantischen Struktur, die sich im richtigen und kreativen Gebrauch (CHOMSKY) dieser Sprachelemente äußert, ist nicht erlernbar. Das natürliche Ichbewußtsein bzw. die Erzeugung dieser semantischen Struktur ist die Voraussetzung des Lernens. Entwicklungspsychologisch gesprochen: das Kind erzeugt aus sich jene Struktur, jenes natürliche Ichbewußtsein und kann daher lernen, jene Sprachelemente richtig und kreativ zu gebrauchen.

Was *ist* das Kind aber, wenn es diese Struktur erzeugen und "dieses vielsagende Wort ICH sagen kann"? Es wird nicht nur natürliches Ich sein und sich in seinen vielen lebensweltlichen Verhältnissen wissen, sondern auch "vernünftige Seele, die ein Bewußtsein dessen hat, was sie ist".[2] "Ich" kann Vielfaches bedeuten, zum einen das natürliche Ichbewußtsein einer Person in ihrem je anderen Erleben (das Ich der in intentio recta gesprochenen Sätze), zum anderen gerade aber auch jenes Moment ihres Seins, aufgrund dessen sie sich alles dies zu Bewußtsein bringt, in Gedanken faßt (unter ihnen auch jenes natürliche Ichbewußtsein) und diese Gedanken als die ihren hat. Die Frage, was eine Person *sei*, die sich als natürliches Ich weiß und sich anderer Personen und

1 Zum ganzen Gedankengang vgl. besonders WOLFGANG CRAMERS *Grundlegung einer Theorie des Geistes*, 1975, und den programmatischen Aufsatz *Vom transzendentalen zum absoluten Idealismus*, 1960.

2 LEIBNIZ, *Discour de Métaphysique* (1958), S. 86: "Mais l'ame intelligente connoissant ce qu'elle est, et pouvant dire ce MOY, qui dit beaucoup".

Gegenstände und Sachverhalte bewußt ist, wird den Gedanken auf das Ich als ursprüngliches Selbstbewußtsein hinführen. Der Gedanke "ich" treibt über seine Bedeutung hinaus, die er in intentio recta gesprochenen Sätzen hat: er geht auf das, was ich (schon) bin, wenn ich (es) denke.

Gedanken sind Gedanken von etwas. Der Gedanke "ich" ist der Gedanke vom eigenen Sein, das Bewußtsein ist, sich Gedanken erzeugt und in diesem Gedanken "ich" sich selber bestimmt. Ich erzeuge mir das Bewußtsein von mir selbst: ich bin selbstbewußtes Sein.

Der Gedanke "ich" beinhaltet - bis jetzt - folgende Bestimmungen: Ein Sein, das Denken ist und somit Gedanken erzeugt, Gedanken von etwas; *sich* diese Gedanken erzeugt und also Bewußtsein ist; und all diese Bestimmungen selber *ist*, indem es sie selber *vollzieht*: denkendes selbstbewußtes Sein.

Die beiden Begriffe meines Themas - Bewußtsein und Selbstbewußtsein - sind also verflochten.

Gedanken sind Gedanken von etwas.
Gedanken gibt es aber nur, wenn ein Bewußtsein sich Gedanken erzeugt.
Gedanken sind *seine* Gedanken.
Ein Bewußtsein ist somit auch Selbstbewußtsein, damit es sich Gedanken erzeugen kann.[3]

Ich gehe im folgenden dieser Verflechtung nach und fasse Bewußtsein von etwas oder Gegenstandsbewußtsein einerseits und Selbstbewußtsein andererseits als Punkt und Kontrapunkt. Gegenstandsbewußtsein und Selbstbewußtsein, Punkt und Kontrapunkt, sind weder auseinander ableitbar oder eines auf das andere reduzierbar, noch sind sie eines ohne das andere.[4] Ich möchte also - in Konturen - zeigen, wie sie sich gegenseitig bedingen und wie nur so uns 1. das Bewußtsein voneinander, Ich und Ich, und von Gegenständen der uns gemeinsamen Welt und ihrer Sachverhalte und damit 2. das bestimmte Ichbewußtsein einer jeden konkreten Person in ihrer Geschichte entstehen kann.

3. Bewußtsein

Nur in Gedanken gefaßt ist etwas für uns da, so daß wir sagen könnten, es sei und sei von dieser Art, Qualität und Relation. Auch das noch so Objektive, das angeblich von außen Gegebene, ja das schlechthin Vorgegebene sind für uns nur objektiv, draußen, gegeben, gar vorgegeben, wenn wir sie in unserem Denken dergestalt bestimmt haben. Denn "in" das Bewußtsein kommt nichts hinein und

---

3 Zur Selbstzuschreibung und dem Gedanken der Meinigkeit vgl. KONRAD CRAMER (1987). Ein Spektrum der gegenwärtigen Diskussion gibt der Sammelband *Theorie der Subjektivität*, hrsg. von CRAMER, FULDA, HORSTMANN, und POTHAST.
Die im folgenden Argumentationsgang auftauchenden Momente von Subjektivität, wie Meinigkeit, Vereinzelung, Intersubjektivität, Leibhaftigkeit, Selbstunterscheidung, Gegenstandsbezug und Einheit (Identität) könnten auch für Psychopathologie von Bedeutung sein. Vgl. hierzu M. SPITZER (1985): *Allgemeine Subjektivität und Psychopathologie*.

4 Damit ist nicht bestritten, daß es Wesen geben kann, die erleben und vorstellen, ohne daß sie sich dessen auch bewußt sind. Sie haben Vorstellungen von etwas, also in gewisser Weise auch "Bewußtsein". Ohne Selbstbewußtsein zu sein, so daß sie sich auch noch bewußt sein könnten, etwas vorzustellen, etwas *als* Vorstellung zu haben und daß diese Vorstellungen *ihre* sind, wird ihr "vorstellendes Bewußtsein" nicht zum Bewußtsein von Gegenständen und Sachverhalten.

wird Erlebtes, Wahrgenommenes und Bewußtes, was das Bewußtsein sich nicht selbst erzeugt hat, also auch jenes erlebte und begriffene Sein, das nicht erst durch diese Erzeugung *existiert*, wohl aber erst durch diese Erzeugung empfundenes Anderes und gewußtes Sein ist.

Von äußeren Gegenständen beispielsweise wissen wir erst und können wir erst reden, wenn wir sie für uns bestimmt haben. Keineswegs richten wir uns einfach auf sie hin und hinaus, bevor wir sie uns zu Bewußtsein und Begriff gebracht haben. Erst dann, wenn wir sie dergestalt für uns erzeugt haben, können wir wissen und sagen: sie sind und sind reales Seiendes ganz unabhängig von unserem Erleben und Begreifen. Das Ich muß sich also losreißen können von seinen Erlebnissen und Gedanken und sich unterscheiden von dem, was es erlebt hat und sich bewußt macht, damit das Erlebte-Bewußte ihm zum Gegenstand wird. Wir werden sehen, wie diese Unterscheidung gelingt und Bewußtsein von Gegenständen entsteht, da ein Bewußtsein auch Selbstbewußtsein ist.

Ein wichtiges Moment unseres Selbstseins haben wir noch nicht zur Sprache gebracht: unsere Individualität. Ein Bewußtsein und Selbstbewußtsein ist eines, nur eines, ein Ich ist ein *einzelnes Ich*.

3.1 Vereinzelung

Im natürlichen Lebensvollzug ist es uns klar, daß wir nicht die Erlebnisse eines Anderen selbst erleben, noch seine Gedanken denken können, mögen wir auch Gleiches, ja das Selbe erleben und denken und uns darüber verständigen.[5] Einsicht in dieses Bekannte, in unser Einzelsein, unsere Individualität, können wir gewinnen, wenn wir unser Bewußtsein bedenken - als denkendes selbstbewußtes Sein können wir dies.

Bewußtsein, so sahen wir, ist ein Sein, das sich Gedanken erzeugt. Ich denke dies und dies und jenes. Freilich integriere ich die wechselnden vielen: es sind meine Gedanken. Nur von meiner *Einheit* aus und der Dimension ihrer *Vereinigung* zum einen Bewußtseinsleben kann ich sie auch als *viele* abfolgende identifizieren. Aber auch so bleibt klar: meine Erzeugung von Gedanken, mein Bewußtseinsleben ist zeitlich-endlich, nur dieses eine. Ich bin ein Ich, ein Bewußtsein und Selbstbewußtsein, nicht einzig oder Ich schlechthin, sondern ein einzelnes. Somit habe ich im Bewußtsein, ein einzelnes Ich zu sein, unmittelbar das Bewußtsein möglicher anderer Iche gleich mir. Anders gesagt: Subjektivität ist - weit davon entfernt solipsistisch verschlossen zu sein - von Grund auf intersubjektiv, da sich das Ich als vereinzeltes, als einen Fall von Subjektivität weiß.

Wie aber kann ein Ich einzelnes und gerade als solches eines unter anderen und mit anderen sein? Wie können sie vereinzelt jedes für sich und doch zusammen da und für einander Ich und anderes Ich sein? -

5 Der Vollzug eines Gedankens ist je meiner, aber zum Inhalt eines Gedankens, zum Gedachten, gehört es überhaupt nicht, mein zu sein.

3.2 Leib

Wir müssen das Bewußtsein von uns selbst, von unserem Selbstsein, jetzt ergänzen; das Bewußtsein der eigenen Vereinzelung treibt uns dazu.

Das einzelne Ich muß durch eine Ordnung bestimmt sein, in der es mit gleichen Einzelnen zusammen sein kann, eine Ordnung, in der sie füreinander sein können. Die Ordnung, in der Einzelnes, Vieles auseinander dasein und koexistieren kann, ist das Raum-zeitlich-Sein.

Es läßt sich zeigen, daß eine weniger reiche Ordnung nicht ausreichte. Als bloß Räumliches wären Einzelne wohl auseinander geordnet, aber in vermittlungsloser Gleichgültigkeit. Sie wären prozeßlos in sich und wirkungslos aufeinander. Ihre Relation wäre eine rein geometrische, kein Wirkungszusammenhang; sie wären damit *von sich her beziehungslos zu einander*. Ihre Relation, in der sie als räumlich Geordnete stünden, könnte höchstens für einen Betrachter sein, der sie von außen anblickte. Der wäre dann aber selber ein zeit-räumliches Wesen und "erzwänge" auch für das, was er anblickt, eine Zeitlichkeit, nämlich Dauer, zumindest für die Zeitspanne, während der er anblickt. Der Gedanke zerfällt. Als bloß Räumliches kann Einzelnes nicht bestehen.

Als bloß Zeitliches wären Einzelne wohl prozeßhaft, aber im baren Auseinander bloßer Sukzession. Sie beständen nie zusammen und wären, dergestalt wirkungslos, nie für einander.

Sollen Einzelne bestehen, und als Einzelne bestehen, also zusammen bestehen, zusammenwirken und füreinander sein, dann müssen sie (mindestens) raum-zeitlich sein.[6]

So ist jedes Einzelne als solches räumlich-zeitlich (auch ganz abgesehen davon, ob es auch Bewußtsein und Selbstbewußtsein ist). Was zugleich und für einander sein kann, ist da im körperlichen Wirkungszusammenhang. So ist ein vereinzeltes Ich auch ein körperhaftes Wesen; es hat einen Leib. Der Leib ist somit nicht erste kontingent in der Erfahrung gegeben, er gehört vielmehr zur Struktur vereinzelten Bewußtseins. Als Einzelnes ist das Ich leibhaftig. So kann es Ich für Ich sein. Sein Leibkörper steht aber auch noch in Wirkungszusammenhang mit anderen Raum-zeitlichen, im dynamischen Zusammenhang der Natur. Es ist selber auch naturhaft da und lebt naturhaft mit. (Das leibhafte Ich unter möglichen Anderen, die füreinander sein können, nennen wir Person.)

3.3 Erleben

Nur in Gedanken gefaßt - so sagten wir - ist etwas für uns da, so daß wir sagen könnten, es sei, sei dieses Eine da und sei von dieser Art, Qualität und Relation. Aber von dieser inhaltlichen Bestimmtheit der Gedanken war bisher noch nicht die Rede. Die Frage, wie ein Bewußtsein sich bestimmte Inhalte zu erzeugen

6 Vgl. LEIBNIZ (1966 I), S. 134f., 151 und (1966 II) 401 und MONIKA OSTERHELD-KOEPKE (1984) S. 79-87.
Angemerkt sei, daß die zeitliche Struktur des Erlebens und Denkens nicht als eine solche bare Sukzession einzelner Erlebnisse und Gedanken gefaßt werden kann. Die Integration des Gewesenen (z.B. des gehabten Gedankens) und das Aussein auf Neues (neue Gedanken, Weiterdenken) *im* Jetzt bestimmen die Zeitlichkeit des Subjekts.
Geht man von einzelnen Erlebnisgeschehnissen und Gedankenvorkommen (mental events) aus, die sich dann nach immanenten Gleichheitsrelationen verknüpfen sollen (*concatenation*; vgl. den Beitrag von CASTAÑEDA in diesem Band), so wäre zu fragen, in welcher Ordnung sie allererst bestehen und zusammenbestehen, damit sie sich verknüpfen können. *Mental events* sind kaum als frei flottierende Entitäten zu fassen. Erst von der *Einheit* des denkenden, selbstbewußten Seins (Ich) her und aus der Dimension ihrer *Vereinigung* (Integration und Aussein auf Neues) zum einen Bewußtseinsleben sind sie als *einzelne, viele*, abfolgende zu identifizieren.

vermag, kann jetzt beantwortet werden, nachdem seine Vereinzelung, anderes Einzelnes und das Raum-zeitlich-Sein als die Ordnung, in der sie füreinander sein können, thematisch geworden sind. Als Einzelnes ist das Ich leibhaftig, ist es Person. In ihrem Leibkörper steht die Person im Wirkungszusammenhang mit anderem Raumzeitlichem. Sie ist selber auch naturhaft da und lebt naturhaft mit. Sie ist determiniert. Von ihrer Determiniertheit her kann klar werden, wie sie sich bestimmte Inhalte erzeugt, die sie dann - als Bewußtsein und Selbstbewußtsein - in Gedanken faßt. Das Vermögen solche Inhalte zu erzeugen nennen wir *Erleben.*

Hätte das Ich nur einen Körper, stünde es nur im Wirkungszusammenhang mit anderem Raum-zeitlichen, wäre es nur naturhaft da, dann könnte es "Körper", "Wirkungszusammenhang", "Natur" und "Mitleben" nicht wissen, geschweige denn als die Bestimmungen seiner selbst (seines *bewußtlosen Selbstseins*) wissen. Das Ich ist nicht nur Bewußtsein und Selbstbewußtsein sondern auch Erleben. Als solches erzeugt es sich Erlebnisse, sonst gibt es keine Erlebnisse und nichts Erlebtes. Es erzeugt sich seine Erlebnisse als Vereinzeltes, also in Bezug auf sein leibhaftes Dasein mit anderen Einzelnen, in Bezug auf sein Determiniertsein. *Es erlebt sein Mitleben.*[7] Empfinden, Fühlen, Sich-befinden, in Zuständen sein und Wahrnehmen sind die Weisen des Erlebens.[8] Hier ist das einzelne Ich und anderes Einzelnes, Naturhaftes und Gemachtes (von seinem Ursprung aus dem menschlichen Handeln einmal abgesehen), Ich und Ding, Ich und Natur, Ich und Welt (als Inbegriff des objektiven Seins gefaßt) vermittelt. So wenig das Ich solipsistisch verschlossen, sondern von Grund auf intersubjektiv ist, so wenig ist es eine weltlose, bloße Formalität zum Erleben und Denken, die sich zu nichts Seiendem in Beziehung brächte. Mitlebend ist es da: Einzelnes mit Einzelnem; erlebend erzeugt es sich die Anschauung und Vorstellung von dem, mit dem es da ist. Es ist ihm gegeben. Im Erleben (Empfinden, Fühlen) ist das Ich unmittelbar und ungeschieden mitlebend bei dem Erlebten, jenem Empfundenen, Gefühlten, das ihm - kann es sich sein Erleben nur unterscheiden und in Gedanken fassen - zu seinem Anderen, anderen Personen und den Gegenständen der gemeinsamen Welt wird.

4. Methodische Überlegung

Aus unserer Vereinzelung, dem je einzelnen Selbst-bewußt-sein, tritt uns das andere einzelne Selbst und die natürliche Welt zusammen hervor. Zudem wird das bisher nur anklingende Moment, unser Erleben, bewußt. Wir können diese Momente unseres Seins - Leiblichkeit, Mitleben und Erleben - dem Bewußtsein

7 Die Differenzierung des Körpers zum Leib bleibt hier unausgeführt. Sie wäre vom Erleben her durchzuführen. Einzelnes ist raum-zeitlich. Es ist Körperliches bestimmter Qualität im dynamischen Wirkungszusammenhang der Natur. Gemäß seiner Art ist Einzelnes als Körper bestimmt. Der Körper eines Erlebenden ist auch Organismus und Sensorium: Leib. Somit hat der Leib des Erlebenden, grob gesprochen, folgende Seiten. Er ist Sensorium, Organismus und chemisch-physikalisches Naturding.

8 Alfred North Whitehead hat die Weisen des Erlebens und bewußtlosen und der sozusagen vorprädikativen Erfahrung reich differenziert. Wäre Erleben thematisch, dann müßte seine kosmologische Theorie mit der transzendental-ontologischen konfrontiert werden.
In Betracht zu ziehen wären ferner die Ergebnisse der Erforschung des "ratiomorphen Apparates", der subliminalen Wahrnehmung und Bildung einer vorrationalen Lebenswelt.

nicht subsumieren. In das Ich kommt eine Differenz, die wir im Bewußtsein, Einzelne zu sein, schon angesprochen haben, die aber gerade nicht auf Bewußtsein zu reduzieren ist. Und doch gehören diese Momente zusammen. Mitleben und Erleben werden nur gewußt, wenn ein selbstbewußtes Sein sie in Gedanken faßt. Was es da aber faßt, sind gerade die Momente seines eigenen unbewußten Daseins und Mitlebens, seines noch unbewußten Erlebens und seiner begrifflosen 'Erfahrung'. Das Ich weiß hier um Momente seines Selbstseins, die im Bewußtsein nicht aufgehen. Das Bewußtsein des Einzelnen ist Bewußtsein der Differenz von Bewußtsein, Erleben und Mitleben.

Ich fasse zusammen. Die Person ist ein einzelnes Bewußtsein und Selbstbewußtsein; Erleben und Denken, Ursprung ihrer Erlebnisse und Gedanken; leibhaft da. Sie lebt mit und erlebt ihr Mitleben, ihre wechselnden Zustände, und jenes Mannigfaltige, Wechselnde, mit dem sie lebt; und sie faßt sich und anderes in Bestimmungen. Vereinzeltes Selbst-bewußt-sein macht sich Einzelnes in seinen Bestimmungen bewußt.

5. Selbstbewußtsein und Gegenstandsbewußtsein

Diesem letzten Punkt müssen wir nun nachgehen, um den Zusammenhang von Selbstbewußtsein und Gegenstandsbewußtsein zu klären.

Solange die individuelle Person in ihrem Mitleben und Erleben versenkt ist - nur Auge, nur Ohr - gehen ihr die Erlebnisse, die sie erzeugt, als wechselnde Zustände dahin. Sie kann in solchem Erleben sich nicht von ihren Erlebnissen unterscheiden, noch weniger ein Erlebtes/Anderes aus der Unmittelbarkeit ihres Erlebens abheben. In ihrem anderen Moment ist die Person aber ein Sein, das Denken ist, Gedanken erzeugt, Gedanken von etwas, sich diese Gedanken erzeugt und also Bewußtsein ist; und all diese Bestimmungen selber ist, indem sie sie selber vollzieht: denkendes selbstbewußtes Sein. Sie *hat* sich ursprünglich und unableitbar: Ich. Sie hat sich *in* ihren wechselnden Zuständen. Jene sind *ihre* wechselnden, vergehenden Zustände. So kann sie sich selber in ihren wechselnden Zuständen unterscheiden und sich losreißen von dem, was sie mitlebend erlebt.

In der Selbstunterscheidung unterscheidet sich die Person ihre Zustände inhaltlich, gegenständlich. Sie ist in je anderen Zuständen, fühlt anders, da sie mit je anderem mitlebt, anderes erlebt, das sie affiziert und modifiziert. Sie unterscheidet sich in ihrem Erlebnis das Erlebte als das andere Einzelne gleich ihr, als andere Person, oder als erlebten, ihr gegebenen Gegenstand.

Im Empfinden und Begreifen der Empfindung bestimmt die erfahrende Person fortschreitend jenes Andere, gemäß der Art und Weise, wie sie modifiziert empfindet; erzeugt sie mit Bezug auf ihr Modifiziertsein selbsttätig den Begriff jenes Anderen und unterscheidet es als selbständiges anderes Sein, das ist und so bestimmt ist, ob sie es denkt oder nicht.[9] Sie selber *wird* in diesen Akten der Selbstunterscheidung aus dem bestimmten Erleben zur konkreten

9 Die Vereinzelung bestimmt gegenständliches Begreifen kategorial. Als vereinzelte erlebt und begreift und unterscheidet die Person anderes unter dem "Vorurteil" des *anderen Ich* und Gegenstände und Sachverhalte im Horizont der *gemeinsamen Welt*.

Person in ihrer Geschichte. S.T. COLERIDGE hat in diesem Zusammenhang notiert (Notebook, 1813-1815): "Wir ziehen uns selber weg von unserer eigenen Erzeugung, reißen uns los von unserer Selbstversenkung im Erleben, und uns so selber verwirklichend, unterscheiden wir uns von unserer Selbstverwirklichung."[10] Andere Personen, die Gegenstände der gemeinsamen Welt und die je bestimmte Selbstverwirklichung der Person kommen in einem Beziehungsgeflecht zusammen hervor.

Bewußtsein und Selbstbewußtsein sind nicht ohne einander, sind aber auch nicht auseinander ableitbar. Ihr Verhältnis ist assymetrisch. Ohne Selbstbewußtsein zu sein, käme die Person nie zum "Bewußtsein dessen, was sie ist"[11], noch zum natürlichen Ichbewußtsein, zu anderen Personen, Gegenständen und zur Welt, die zusammen in einem Beziehungsgeflecht hervorkommen. Sie bliebe in der Zuständlichkeit und vorprädikativen Erfahrung des Erlebens. Ohne Selbstbewußtsein zu sein, käme die Person nie zu Bewußtsein. Sie wäre ein (nur) erlebendes Wesen.

Versucht man dagegen Selbstbewußtsein unter Absehung von Bewußtsein zu fassen, so erscheint es als die bloße Dynamis zum Denken, die, so für sich, nicht ist. Dieser Dynamis wollen wir im abschließenden Punkte nachgehen.

6. Ursprüngliches Selbstbewußtsein

Im Attribut "ursprünglich" steckt die These, daß diese Dynamis aus nichts ableitbar sei, auf nichts anderes reduzierbar, noch von anderem her begründet.[12]

Im Gedanken "Ich", jetzt als Ausdruck des ursprünglichen Selbstbewußtseins gefaßt, liegt keine Subjekt-Objekt Beziehung vor wie im Bewußtsein von etwas, im natürlichen Ichbewußtsein oder gegenständlicher Erkenntnis. Das Beziehende selber, das Bestimmende aller Bestimmung von Gegenständen (welcher Art auch) bringt sich im Begriff "Ich" zum Ausdruck. "Ich" ist nicht der Begriff von etwas, das im Erleben gegeben werden könnte und somit von diesem Gegebensein abhinge, es ist vielmehr der Selbstbegriff des Beziehenden, Bestimmenden, auf das hin es allererst Gegebenes gibt. Es ist der Selbstbegriff des Ursprungs, von dem her die Momente des eigenen Selbstseins bewußt werden

---

10 " - we abstract form our own product - the Spirit snatches itself loose from its own self-immersion, and self-actualizing distinguishes itself from its Self-realization - But this is absolutely impossible otherwise than by a free Act - ".
Die Begrenzung des Gedankenganges, die das Thema auferlegt, wird hier empfindlich spürbar. *Self-realization* und *free Act* bedürften weitergehender Ausführungen, um einigermaßen ihren vollen Sinn zu erhalten. So konnte nicht gezeigt werden, wie ein vereinzeltes (zeitlich-endliches) Bewußtsein auch ein Sprachwesen ist, noch wie sich die Person schon als erlebende, leibhafte zu äußerem Tun bestimmt, noch wie sie als selbstbewußte, denkende in ihren Determinationen selbstbestimmt handeln kann.

11 Siehe Anm. 2.

12 Trotz und gerade wegen ihres andersartigen, metaphysischen Gedankenganges ist PLOTINS Enneade V 3 höchst aufschlußreich für das anstehende Problem. Vgl. ferner HENRICH (1982a) und meinen Versuch, die Philosophie S.T. COLERIDGES auszulegen (UEHLEIN 1982).
Zum Gedanken einer nicht mehr transzendentalen und erst recht nicht empirischen Begründung, vielmehr einer Begründung des Ich im Absoluten vgl. die genannte Enneade, ferner *Realisierung des Bildes* in BEIERWALTES (1985), *Fichtes Ich* in HENRICH (1982a) und UEHLEIN (1982, S. 30ff. und das Kapitel *Endliches und Absolutes Ich*). Es handelt sich um den metaphysichen Begründungsgang, daß das Ich von einem ihm transzendenten, absolut-denkenden Sein her *ist*.

können. Beides ineins gefaßt: es ist der Selbstbegriff des einfach *einen Ursprungs*, von dem her *vieles Bewußtes* sein kann - die Momente des eigenen vereinzelten Daseins und die Strukturen des Erlebens und Denkens und das andere (von welcher Art auch) -, das er zum bestimmten, erfüllten Bewußtsein vereinigt.

Auch der Versuch, das ursprüngliche Selbstbewußtsein in einem Reflexionsakt entstehen zu lassen, scheitert. Die Person müßte sich schon haben; ich muß schon ein Ich sein, um auf mich zurückkommen zu können. Der Reflexionsakt hebt schon bei dem an, was er als Resultat erzielen soll. Wer begönne den Akt, wer erzeugte diesen Reflexionsgedanken, wenn erst an seinem Ende Ich sein soll?

Reflexionsakte kann die Person dagegen *in* ihren bewußten Erlebnissen und bestimmten Gedanken vollziehen, da sie der Ursprung ihrer Gedanken ist. In jedem ihrer Gedanken kann sie mit apodiktischer Gewißheit auf sich zurückkommen, weil sie selbstbewußtes Sein ist. "Ich denke mich" bezeichnet somit den Reflexionsakt und gibt den allgemeinen Titel für den Prozeß der Selbstbestimmung. Akt und Prozeß aber sind Vollzüge eines (schon) selbstbewußten Seins.

Eine konzise Fassung dieser Struktur, die Vollzug ist, nicht außer oder ohne diesen Vollzug, und die aus nichts anderem ableitbar, vielmehr Grund dafür, daß anderes für uns ist, bietet EPIKTETS Satz (I. 1.4) "He dynamis kai hauten theorusa kai talla panta." Das ursprüngliche Selbstbewußtsein ist das einfache eine Sehen, das seiner selbst inne ist und alles andere sieht.

Daher kann die Person sich selber unterscheiden (A) und anderes sich unterscheiden (B). Als Unterscheidung der einfach einen Dynamis bleibt das Unterschiedene geeint (A) und bezogen (B).

(A) Die Person "kann ein Bewußtsein dessen haben, was sie ist". (Wir haben dieses eigene Sein in den Momenten Bewußtsein und Selbstbewußtsein, Vereinzelung, Leib, Erleben und Mitleben zu fassen gesucht.) Sie bestimmt sich ferner - erlebend und denkend, bewußt und unbewußt - und hat sich je und je als natürliches Ich in ihrer Geschichte. Natürliches Ich aber ist sie (B) in der Beziehung, im Leben mit Personen und Dingen im Horizont der Welt.

Zwei Vorschläge, Selbstbewußtsein abzuleiten, möchte ich noch skizzieren. Das Ich entstünde aus dem Prozeß der Sozialisation. LACANS Spiegelmodell können wir so lesen (vgl. LACAN 1966, 1986). Das Kind, das sich selber sieht, stehe als Metapher für den umfassenden Prozeß, durch den es Ich wird. Indem es sich in anderen Personen gespiegelt sieht, erkennt oder mißkennt es sich und komme so zu seiner Identität, werde Ich.

Richtig ist, daß ein konkretes Ichbewußtsein sich nur im Leben mit anderen Personen und in der gemeinsamen gegenständlichen Welt herausbildet. Dazu muß das Kind aber schon ursprünglich ein Ich sein. Es kann dies nicht *an Anderen lernen*, muß vielmehr diese Struktur aus sich entfalten, um sich andere Personen aus dem Mitleben *unterscheiden* zu können, an denen es sich spiegelnd erkennt oder mißkennt.

Andere Theorien (seit HUME insbesondere[13]) fassen das Ich als Bündel seiner Erlebnisse und Gedanken und als Komplexion von Bewußtseinsvorkommnissen. Das Ich entstünde als die veränderliche Vereinigungseinheit vieler einzelner

13 Vgl. hierzu UEHLEIN 1982, S. 2-5; 9-22.

impressions und ideas oder sei die Komplexion (complexion, concatenation) vieler einzelner Bewußseinsvorkommnisse und ihrer einzelnen Ichgestalten.

Richtig ist, daß die Dynamis, das einfach eine Sehen zur bestimmten Sicht, Selbst-Bewußtsein zum bestimmten Ichbewußtsein *sich vollzieht* im vielfältigen Erfahrungs- und Bewußtseinsleben. Wiederum aber liegt keine Ableitung vor, denn bewußte Erlebnisse[14] und Gedanken gibt es nur vom Ich her, das jene erzeugt, sich unterscheidet und integriert zum erfüllten Bewußtsein. Erst von seiner ursprünglichen *Einheit* und der Dimension ihrer *Vereinigung* her sind jene als einzelne identifizierbar und Bündel und Komplexionen bestimmter Gestaltung.

Zusammenfassung: Bewußtsein und Selbstbewußtsein sind nicht ohne einander, sind aber auch nicht auseinander ableitbar. Ihr Verhältnis ist assymetrisch. Ohne Selbstbewußtsein zu sein, käme die Person nie zum Bewußtsein dessen, was sie ist, noch zum natürlichen Ichbewußtsein, zu anderen Personen, Gegenständen und zur Welt, die zusammen in einem Beziehungsgeflecht hervorkommen. Sie bliebe in der Zuständlichkeit und vorprädikativen Erfahrung des Erlebens. Ohne Selbstbewußtsein zu sein, käme die Person nie zu Bewußtsein. Sie wäre ein (nur) erlebendes Wesen. Versucht man dagegen Selbstbewußtsein unter Absehung von Bewußtsein zu fassen, so erscheint es als das Vermögen zum Denken und der Einheitspunkt vielfältigen Bewußtseins, die, so für sich, nicht sind. Das ursprüngliche Selbstbewußtsein ist der *einfach eine Ursprung*, von dem her *vieles Bewußtes sein kann*, seien es die Momente des eigenen vereinzelten Daseins und die Strukturen der Erlebens und Denkens, oder sei es das viele Andere (von welcher Art auch), das es erfaßt und zum bestimmten, erfüllten Bewußtsein vereinigt.

Consciousness and Self-Consciousness

Summary: Consciousness and selfconsciousness do neither exist apart from each other nor can they be derived one from the other. Their relation is asymmetrical. A person needs must be selfconscious in order to become conscious of what he/she is, on the one hand, and to become aware of his/her own natural self, of other persons, things and of the world which emerge together in one net of correlations on the other hand. Otherwise an individual person would remain in the shifting states and unjudged, ungraspable feelings of experiencing life. Without being selfconscious a person would never be conscious. Taken apart from consciousness, however, selfconsciousness appears as the mere power of

14 Wie weit ein Erleben, das nicht - kantisch gesprochen - vom "Ich denke" begleitet werden kann, das *eine 'Subjekt'* seiner Erlebnisse ist, bleibe hier unerörtert. Der monadologische Grundzug der vorstehenden Überlegungen spricht für eine solche Lösung. Auch unbewußte Erlebnisse sind, sofern sie *Erlebnisse* sind, keine irgendwie vorhandenen, frei schwebenden Ereignisse, sondern Ereignisse, die in einem Erleben vorkommen und Zustände, in denen sich ein Erlebender befindet. Erlebnisse sind von einem Erlebenden erzeugt, sie sind seine Erlebnisse. Zu berücksichtigen wäre bei dieser Erörterung die spezifische monadologische Theorie WHITEHEADS. Für ihn ist jedes wirklich Seiende (actual entity) eine Monade und in seinem physischen und mentalen Pol Erleben und Erzeugen von Erlebnissen (prehensions, feelings). Alles dauernde Erleben und Bewußtsein und Selbstbewußtsein bilde sich dann aus den Komplexionen und Vergesellschaftungen solcher actual entities. In diesem Punkte bestehen Ähnlichkeiten zu HECTOR-NERI CASTAÑEDAS Theorie des Selbst und der Ichgestaltungen (vgl. seinen Beitrag in diesem Band und CASTAÑEDA 1987, insbesondere S. 135-140).

thinking and the unifying pole of the manifold consciousness, which, thus splendidly isolated, does not exist. "Original Selfconsciousness" - as this structural moment of a person will be called in the paper - is the *one* and *single origin of thought* in virtue of which there can be *many thoughts* and thought contents; the specific moments of a person, the structure of experiencing life and of thinking, and the many things, the other (of what kind soever) which it grasps and *unifies* into one concrete and rich consciousness.

Literatur

BEIERWALTES, W. (1985): Denken des Einen. Klostermann, Frankfurt a.M.

CASTAÑEDA, H.-N. (1987): The Self and the I-Guises, Empirical and Transcendental. In: CRAMER, K. et al. (Hg.), S. 105-140, Suhrkamp, Frankfurt a.M.

CHOMSKY, N. (1966): Cartesian Linguistics. Harper and Row, New York and London.

COLERIDGE, S.T. (1973): The Notebooks, vol. 3, (1808-1819), ed. by KATHLEEN COBURN. Routledge and Kegan Paul, London.

CRAMER, K. (1987): Über KANTS Satz: Das: Ich denke, muß alle meine Vorstellungen begleiten können. In: CRAMER, K. et al. (Hg.): Theorie der Subjektivität, S. 167-202, Frankfurt a.M.

CRAMER, K., FULDA, H.F., HORSTMANN, R.-P., POTHAST, U. (Hg.; 1987): Theorie der Subjektivität. Suhrkamp, Frankfurt a.M.

CRAMER, W. (1960): Vom transzendentalen zum absoluten Idealismus. Kant-Studien **52**, S. 3-32.

CRAMER, W. (1975): Grundlegung einer Theorie des Geistes, Klostermann, Frankfurt a.M.

EPIKTET (1925): The Discourses as reported by Arrian, the Manual, and the Fragments. With an English Translation by W.A. OLDFATHER. Loeb, London, Cambridge (Mass.).

HENRICH, D. (1976): Identität und Objektivität. Eine Untersuchung über Kants transzendentale Deduktion. Carl Winter, Universitätsverlag, Heidelberg.

HENRICH, D. (1982a): Selbstverhältnisse, Reclam, Stuttgart.

HENRICH, D. (1982b): Selbstbewußtsein und spekulatives Denken. In: Fluchtlinien. Philosophische Essays. Suhrkamp, Frankfurt a.M.

HUME, D. (1739/40; 1886): A Treatise of Human Nature. Edited with Preliminary Dissertations and Notes, by T.H. GREEN and T.H. GROSE. Longmans, London.

HUSSERL, E. (1963): Cartesianische Meditationen und Pariser Vorträge, herausgegeben und eingeleitet von S. STRASSER. Husserliana, Bd. I. Nijhoff, Haag.

LACAN, J. (1966; 1986): Schriften I. Ausgewählt und herausgegeben von N. HAAS, Quadriga, Weinheim und Berlin.

LEIBNIZ, G.W. (1966): Hauptschriften zur Grundlegung der Philosophie. Meiner, Hamburg.

LEIBNIZ, G.W. (1958): Discours de Métaphysique. Meiner, Hamburg.

NAGEL, Th. (1986): The View from Nowhere. Oxford University Press, Oxford.

PARFIT, D. (1984): Reasons and Persons. Oxford University Press, Oxford.

OSTERHELD-KOEPKE, M. (1984): Der Ursprung der Mathematik aus der Monadologie. Haag und Herchen, Frankfurt a.M.

PLOTINS Schriften (1960), übersetzt von R. HARDER, Neubearbeitung mit griechischem Lesetext und Anmerkungen fortgeführt von R. BEUTLER und W. THEILER, Bd. V, Meiner, Hamburg.

SCHELLING, F.W.J. (1800; 1975): System des transzendentalen Idealismus. In: Schriften von 1799-1801. Nachdruck der Ausgabe 1858ff, Wissenschaftl. Buchgesellschaft, Darmstadt.

SPITZER, M. (1985): Allgemeine Subjektivität und Psychopathologie. Haag und Herchen, Frankfurt a.M.

UEHLEIN, F.A. (1982): Die Manifestation des Selbstbewußtseins im konkreten 'Ich bin'. Meiner, Hamburg.

WHITEHEAD, A.N. (1929/1978): Process and Reality. (Corrected edition, edited by GRIFFIN, D.R., SHERBURNE, D.W.) The Free Press, London.

Ichstörungen bei Modellpsychosen

L. Hermle, G. Oepen, M. Spitzer, A. Harrington

1. Einleitung

Unter Ich-Störungen wird in der Psychopathologie eine Reihe von Symptomen verstanden, für die es schwerfällt, einen gemeinsamen Nenner anzugeben und die mit unterschiedlichen Begriffen belegt wurden. Man spricht vom "Ausgeliefertsein der Patienten an willentlich unbeeinflußbare Erlebnisse", um die "Einschränkung der Selbstverfügbarkeit", die "Störung der Meinhaftigkeit des Erlebens" (SCHNEIDER 1980), den Verlust der "Ich-Umwelt-Balance" (AVENARIUS 1976), der "Ichgrenzen" (PETERS 1984), des "Ich-Bewußtseins" (JASPERS 1973), des "Ich-Erlebens" (SCHNEIDER 1980) sowie des "Körper-Erlebens" (HUBER 1957) zu beschreiben. "Bestimmte Handlungen und Zustände werden als von außen, von einer ichfremden Instanz gelenkt, gemacht oder beeinflußt erlebt" (PETERS 1984, S. 263).

Man spricht weiterhin von "Depersonalisation" oder "Derealisation", wobei manche Autoren diese Begriffe offenbar für Erlebnisweisen verwenden, bei denen die Umwelt als fremd, unwirklich, traumhaft und unvertraut erlebt wird, die Erlebnisveränderungen jedoch nicht auf Außeneinflüsse oder Fremdbestimmtheit zurückgeführt werden, d.h. es sich nicht um Erlebnisse des sog. "Gemachten" (SCHNEIDER 1980) handelt.

Gelegentlich wird auch von "Erlebnissen der Passivität" (BERINGER 1927, MULLEN 1986) gesprochen, worunter letztlich die Erstrangsymptome im Sinne KURT SCHNEIDERS gemeint sind, d.h. Beschreibungen von Erlebnisweisen, daß die eigenen psychischen Vorgänge und Zustände als von außen und von anderen gelenkt, gemacht und beeinflußt erscheinen. Weiterhin findet sich in der Literatur eine Reihe von Hinweisen darauf, daß ein gestörtes Zeiterleben mit Ichstörungen in Zusammenhang steht (FISCHER 1929, MELGES et al. 1970).

Gleiche oder zumindest sehr ähnliche Erlebnisweisen können bei Temporallappenepilepsie auftreten, werden in der Neurologie jedoch interessanterweise *nicht* als Ichstörungen, sondern als Störungen der Wahrnehmung und/oder des Bewußtseins beschrieben bzw. konzeptualisiert (vgl. die Beiträge von OEPEN et al. sowie HARRINGTON et al. in diesem Band). Dies verdeutlicht die Abhängigkeit der "Beschreibung" solcher Erlebnisse von dem jeweils - mehr oder weniger explizit bzw. reflektiert - angenommenen Interpretationsrahmen (vgl. den Beitrag von SPITZER zu Ichstörungen in diesem Band).

Im folgenden soll sowohl die Heterogenität der mit "Ich-Störung" bezeichneten Erlebnisse (Heterogenität der "Daten") als auch die Heterogenität der zur

Bezeichnung derartiger Erlebnisse verwendeten Begriffe und Erklärungsversuche dargestellt werden (Heterogenität der "Konzepte").[1] Wir beziehen uns dabei vor allem auf Beobachtungen bei experimentell erzeugten Meskalinintoxikationen. Zudem stand uns bisher unveröffentlichtes Material aus den dreißiger Jahren zur Verfügung, das damals im Rahmen der Forschungen an der Freiburger Universitätsklinik unter KURT BERINGER erhoben worden war, jedoch bisher noch nicht zur Auswertung gelangte.[2]

Ich-Störungen gelten als nosologisch unspezifisch und werden bei Schizophrenie (insbesondere zu Beginn), bei affektiven Erkrankungen (vor allem bei endogener Depression), bei Neurosen, Persönlichkeitsstörungen, im Drogenrausch wie auch bei Gesunden (meist unter extremer affektiver Anspannung) beschrieben. Bei der Heterogenität der Daten wie auch der verwendeten Begriffe erscheint allerdings Vorsicht geboten im Hinblick auf die nosologische Spezifität, könnte sich doch die häufig behauptete nosologische Unspezifität als ein Charakteristikum der Konzepte und nicht der Daten erweisen. KURT SCHNEIDER beispielsweise war von der Unterscheidbarkeit schizophrener Ichstörungen von Ichstörungen anderer Genese überzeugt (vgl. SCHNEIDER 1980, S. 122). Das Material von BERINGER erscheint auch vor diesem Hintergrund von besonderem Interesse, waren doch klinisch erfahrene Ärzte an den Experimenten beteiligt, deren Belastung mit festgefügten Erwartungen noch nicht dem entsprach, was heute in Anbetracht der langen Tradition experimentell-psychopathologischer Forschung angenommen werden kann.

2. Methodik

Die Auswertung der oben genannten Protokolle aus den Forschungen unter BERINGER (im folgenden zitiert als "BERINGER-Materialien") erfolgte nach inhaltsanalytischen Gesichtspunkten. Es wurde versucht, jeweils besonders eindrückliche Beispiele aus dem Bereich der Modellpsychose den verschiedenen, vor allem aus der Literatur zu schizophrenen Psychosen bekannten Begriffen zuzuordnen.

Eigene Untersuchungen zum Meskalinrausch wurden im Zeitraum Oktober 1987 bis März 1988 in der Freiburger Klinik durchgeführt (vgl. OEPEN et al. 1988).

Probanden: Unsere eigenen Meskalin-Selbstversuche wurden mit 12 männlichen Probanden (im Folgenden als "Vp" zitiert) im Alter zwischen 27 und 47 Jahren durchgeführt. Alle Vpn wurden über die Wirkungen und Nebenwirkungen des Meskalins informiert und nahmen nach schriftlicher Erteilung ihres Einverständnisses an der Studie teil. Die notwendige Genehmigung seitens des BGA wurde gewährt, die Zustimmung der Ethikkommission lag ebenfalls vor.

Jeder Proband erhielt morgens um 8.30 Uhr nüchtern 500 mg Meskalinsulfat, entsprechend einer durchschnittlichen Dosierung von ca. 7 mg pro kg Körpergewicht. Die lückenlose Überwachung und der experimentelle Ablauf umfaßte einen Zeitraum von 12 Stunden, entsprechend der ca. 10stündigen Dauer der Intoxikation.

1 Vgl. hierzu auch die Beiträge von BLANKENBURG, HARRINGTON et al. sowie SPITZER in diesem Band.

2 Für die Überlassung des umfangreichen (in Form von Typoskripten und Handschriften) vorliegenden Materials möchten wir uns bei Herrn Prof. em. R. DEGKWITZ bedanken.

Pharmakologie: Die Verabreichung von 0,4 - 1,5 g Meskalinsulfat per os erzeugt beim Menschen einen bis zu 10 Stunden andauernden Rausch. Meskalin (chem. 3.4.5.-Trimethoxy-ß-phenyl-ethylamin) ist ein weißer, kristalliner Stoff, der innerhalb von 24 Stunden zu 83 %, innerhalb von 48 Stunden zu 92 % ausgeschieden wird. Seine Halbwertzeit beträgt 6 Stunden (Charalampous et al. 1966).

Die Struktur von Meskalin und die neurobiochemischen Wirkungen ähneln den Strukturen der Catecholamine (Noradrenalin, Dopamin) und dem Amphetamin. Diese Beobachtungen sowie die rasche Antagonisierung von Meskalin- und Amphetamineffekten durch Neuroleptika bei Mensch und Tier sprechen für eine Beziehung der Meskalin-induzierten Veränderungen zum schizophrenen Syndrom (Kety 1972, Aghajanian 1982).

Der *Intoxikationsablauf* ist initial durch eine vegetative Phase mit Schwindel, Brechreiz und Bewegungsunruhe geprägt. Der Rauschverlauf ist bei vorhandener Vigilanz typischerweise durch Wahrnehmungsveränderungen (optisch, akustisch, Körpersphäre) geprägt. Der Berauschte schildert den Eindruck der Entfremdung (Depersonalisation, Derealisation), Störung des Zeitgefühls, Konzentrations- und Aufmerksamkeitsstörungen. Störungen des Denkens und der Sprache sind weitere typische psychopathologische Auffälligkeiten.

3. Ergebnisse

Bei 10 unserer 12 Vpn traten im Laufe der Intoxikation variabel ausgeprägte psychopathologische Veränderungen auf. Anhand der Selbstschilderungen und des semistandardisierten Interviews haben wir die Veränderungen des Ich-Erlebens näher analysiert. Parallel hierzu stellen wir Auszüge aus den alten Rausch-Protokollen vor. Wir betrachten dabei die Sachverhalte jeweils unter einem bestimmten Gesichtspunkt.

Passivitätserlebnisse können im Zusammenhang mit *formalen Denkstörungen*, aber auch mit Körperbewegungen vorkommen. Das "nicht-mehr-so-gut-Können" von Denken und Sprechen hat zunächst nur leichtes passives Gepräge.

> "Zugleich merke ich, daß mir die Sprache nicht mehr so zur Verfügung steht wie sonst, ich drücke mich ungeschickt aus, finde manche Worte nicht, stottere. Es fällt mir nicht ganz leicht, mich auf bestimmte Dinge zu konzentrieren" (Beringer-Materialien).

Mit zunehmender Wirkung des Meskalins trat bei den meisten Vpn eine mehr oder weniger ausgeprägte formale Denkstörung auf, die unterschiedlich erlebt wurde. In diesem Rahmen kann z.B. ein eigentümliches "Außerhalbstehen" erlebt werden, als würden die eigenen Gedanken als fremd erscheinen, da man sie sich für den Augenblick gar nicht zutraut. Die Äußerungen können wie geäußerte Erlebnisse der Depersonalisation oder der Spaltung klingen.

> "Es scheint, als ob eine zweite Instanz denkt und redet, während das eigentliche Ich gar nicht in der Lage ist, einen kompletten Gedanken zu entwerfen: Am Ende des Satzes weiß ich nicht mehr, wie er begonnen hat, merke jedoch an der eigenen Zufriedenheit und der Reaktion der Umgebung, daß es so schlimm gar nicht gewirkt haben kann, wie ich es empfinde" (Vp 1; 37 Jahre).

Die Passivität kann auch als *Ausgeliefert-sein* erlebt werden und hat dann mitunter eine starke *affektive* Komponente.

> "Etwa um diese Zeit kommt es auch zu unangenehmen Erlebnissen. Vom Flur her höre ich die Stimmen des Klinikpersonals, die Geräusche der Essenwagen und des Aufzugs, welche als unartikuliertes Gerufe, Hydraulikgeräusche, NS-Medizin, Schlachthaus etc. assoziiert wird, dem ich nicht entrinnen kann" Vp. 7; 31 Jahre).

Das Erleben der Passivität kann sich auch auf *Körperbewegungen* beziehen:

"Meine Bewegungen erscheinen mir künstlich, fremd, automatenhaft, wobei ich mich wundere, daß ich noch sicher gehen kann" (Vp 2; 37 Jahre). An anderer Stelle berichtet dieselbe Vp: "der Mund ... bewegt sich ohne mein Zutun."

Die Selbstschilderungen verdeutlichen, daß all das, was man mit "geordneter Ich-Aktivität" bezeichnen könnte, mehr oder weniger nicht mehr vorhanden ist. Der Berauschte ist seinem Denken, seinen Affekten und seinen Bewegungen eher passiv ausgeliefert, als daß er sie aktiv vollzöge. BERINGER sprach hier von einem Passivitätssyndrom mit Entfremdung des Ichs und Zurücktreten der Außenweltwahrnehmung: "Das Ich als Persönlichkeit mit all seinen Strebungen, Wünschen, mit seiner Verbundenheit mit der Welt, tritt immer mehr zurück, hat schließlich keinen Platz mehr. ...desgleichen treten in solchen Zuständen stärkster Passivität keine Denk- oder Willensakte mehr auf" (BERINGER 1927, S. 73).

Dieses Erleben der Passivität kann sich bis zum völligen *Verlust der Meinhaftigkeit* steigern.

"Dabei war mir unangenehm, daß ich mich und vor allem auch meinen Mund sprechen sah, als ob nichts wäre, während die Sätze, die daraus quollen und die ich hörte, mir fremd waren und nicht von mir zu stammen schienen" (Vp 10; 32 Jahre).

Die Störung der Meinhaftigkeit kann sich nicht nur in Passivität ausdrücken, sondern auch in "Gedankenausbreiten".

"Ich hatte gewußt, was der Golem dachte, andererseits wußten alle, was in mir vorging" (BERINGER-Materialien).

Was wir soeben unter die Begriffe "Passivität" und "Verlust der Meinhaftigkeit" faßten, ließe sich auch als "*Depersonalisation*" fassen. Dieses Erlebnis, daß das eigene Denken und daß eigene Bewegungen eher passiv erscheinen, kann auch den *Affekt* betreffen.

"... es gelingt mir nicht, versuchsweise beim bewußten Gedanken an nahestehende Personen irgendwie emotional zu reagieren, alle scheinen mir sehr weit weg zu stehen, auf die Frage nach der Suizidalität im Untersuchungsbogen wird mir klar, daß ich mich, falls ich zu diesem Zeitpunkt auf dem Münsterturm stünde, vermutlich ohne innere Regung hinunterstürzen würde" (Vp 7; 31 Jahre).

Auch Störungen der *Abgrenzung "Ich-Anderes"* kommen vor. Ein Proband BERINGERS berichtet, wie die gesehenen Bewegungen in der Umgebung plötzlich auf ihn übergehen.

"Dieses Gefühl des Hineingezogenseins in eine wallende, fließende Bewegung ist etwas Neues, mit allem von mir bisher Erlebten in keiner Weise Vergleichbares und nicht näher Beschreibbares. Ich kann nur sagen, daß es mit einer sehr starken Alteration des Persönlichkeitsgefühls einherging, so daß ich auf dem Höhepunkt dieser Erlebnisse geradezu das Gefühl des Untergangs meiner Persönlichkeit hatte, am ehesten vergleichbar etwa noch mit dem sexuellen Orgasmus, jedoch nur im Sinne des Ausströmens des Ich, ohne genitale Erregung oder Lustempfindung (wie überhaupt spezifisch sexuelle Empfindungen, Gedanken oder Bilder im ganzen Rausch völlig fehlen). Dieses Gefühl des Versinkens meines Ich ist durchaus bedrohlich, Angst erregend, so daß ich eine Zeitlang fürchte, ich könnte in eine Psychose hineingeraten" (BERINGER-Materialien).

Formale Denkstörung, gestörte Meinhaftigkeit und Störung der Abgrenzung "Ich-Anderes" sind in den folgenden drei Berichten kaum zu trennen.

"Ich selber hätte, so erklärte das Sprachzentrum, die Ich-Umweltbeziehungen abgebrochen, und ich war erstaunt, daß ein Vorgang von so außerordentlicher Bedeutung mit einem kurzen Satz ausgedrückt werden konnte; das war fremdartig" (BERINGER-Materialien).

"Dem Grammophon war ich preisgegeben. ... Aufdringlich hörte ich das Kratzen der Nadel, die Klänge waren ungeordnete Geräusche, und vor allem lief die Platte bald schneller, bald langsamer, wie mir schien. Damals allerdings war ich unfähig, den Gesamteindruck zu analysieren, ich war in einem Gestrüpp von Geräuschen verfangen" (BERINGER-Materialien).

"Die Veränderung des Denkens beschrieb ich mit den Worten einer Abhandlung über schizophrene Denkstörungen, und ich war glücklich, daß die Worte so sinnvoll sich aneinander reihten. Über diese Fähigkeit verfügte ich also noch. Das heißt, eigentlich war nicht ich der Redende, sondern das Sprachzentrum, das blau-graue Ding in der dauernd gesehenen Scheibe war es, welches meine Denkstörung beschrieb ... Indessen mir wurde nicht geglaubt. Wie von ganz weit her vernahm, wie einer der Ärzte bestritt, was das Sprachzentrum erzählt hätte, ich könne unmöglich, meinte er, wohlgeformte Sätze sprechen und dabei denkgestört sein. Es war kränkend und ärgerlich, doch schlimmer als das, ich vermochte mich nicht zu wehren, ich stand hilflos da und hoffte vergeblich auf Hilfe vom Sprachzentrum. Aber diesem fiel nichts ein in der noch nie erlebten Situation" (BERINGER-Materialien).

Die Ichstörungen im Meskalinrausch werden nicht selten von Störungen des Körpererlebens begleitet (Zusammenhänge im Sinne einer ein- oder wechselseitigen Verstärkung oder Bedingung werden im Beitrag von HARRINGTON et al. am Beispiel des Gesichtererlebens diskutiert).

"An der linken Seite zog eine sonderbare Empfindung entlang, die Seite war wie taub, und später war ein völlig unbekanntes und unbeschreibbares Gefühl dort. Es war etwa so, als streiche ein Lufthauch entlang und ich war erinnert an das, was Galen als Aura beschreibt. Danach hatte ich an der linken Seite die Empfindung körperlicher Begrenzung verloren, jenes Seltsame war eher ein Hauch in mir oder ich war dort ein Hauch, der langsam und ohne Grenze in die Umgebung überging. Diese Sensation hielt stundenlang an" (BERINGER-Materialien).

Der *eigene Körper* wird als verändert erlebt, als zunehmend ausdruckslos, maskenhaft starr, er zerfällt schließlich in isolierte Teilobjekte.

"Beim Betrachten meines nackten Unterarms sehe ich mit Erstaunen, daß dieser spinnenförmig lang ausgezogen ist und um 180 Grad in sich torquiert ist. Finger und Daumen sind unproportional groß aufgetrieben. Es fällt mir ein, daß Dali einen solchen Arm in einem seiner Bilder dargestellt haben muß. Meine ganze Aufmerksamkeit ist auf diese klobig aufgetriebene Hand gerichtet, die mir fremd und als nicht zu meinem Körper gehörend erscheint" (Vp 2, 37 Jahre).

Insbesondere spielen sich auch Veränderungen im Bereich der *Wahrnehmung von Gesichtern* ab (siehe hierzu auch den Beitrag von HARRINGTON et al. in diesem Band).

"Ein- oder zweimal setzte sich der Verfallprozeß bis zum völligen Fehlen des Gesichtes fort, und ich sah mich im Spiegel ohne Kopf, was ich in diesem Augenblick keineswegs beängstigend, sondern lediglich interessant fand, gelang es mir doch, mit einem Augenzwinkern meinen Kopf wieder im Spiegel zu sehen" (Vp 4, 30 Jahre).

10 von 12 Vpn berichten über *Störungen des Zeiterlebens*, wobei das Zeitempfinden teils verlangsamt, teils beschleunigt oder auch ganz aufgehoben war. Wie Vp 7 schildert, ist die Aufhebung des Zeitgefühls für Vergangenheit und Zukunft möglich.

"Die anfängliche Überempfindlichkeit gegenüber äußeren Reizen weicht einer zunehmenden Unempfindlichkeit, Selbstzufriedenheit, Wohligkeit und starken Verlangsamung des Zeitgefühls.... Das Bewußtsein von der unaufhaltsamen, verstreichenden Zeit, vom Leben als unweigerlich zum Tode führendes Insuffizienzgefühl - all diese Eckpfeiler des Lebens - sind zu meiner größten Überraschung wie abgeschüttelt, und ich bin ohne Wunsch und ohne Bedürfnis."

Wie hier im Beispiel deutlich wird, kann das aufgehobene Zeitgefühl zu ekstatischen Glückserlebnissen führen.

Auch das Bewußtsein vom Umfang der vergangenen Zeit ist häufig gestört; Überschätzungen, ebenso wie Unterschätzungen sind möglich: "Ich weiß nicht, ob ich erst Sekunden, Stunden, Tage oder Jahre im Meskalinrausch bin..." (Vp 2). Zwei Stunden nach der Meskalineinnahme berichtet Vp 7: "Seit ich das eingenommen habe, kommt es mir vor, als seien viele, viele Stunden vergangen, wie wenn es jetzt spätabends wäre".

Auch die Probanden BERINGERS berichteten nicht selten über entsprechende Erlebnisse.

"Wie lange diese Höhe des Rausches gedauert hat, vermag ich nicht zu sagen. Ich habe das Gefühl für den Ablauf der Zeit ziemlich stark verloren..." (BERINGER-Materialien).

"Die Zeit war endlich einmal ausgeschaltet, und es war sehr schön, nur die Gegenwart zu erleben, ohne jeden Gedanken an die Zukunft oder an die Vergangenheit" (BERINGER-Materialien).

"Eine Zeitlang - ich weiß es nicht genau, denn meine Zeit stand still, mochte es so gewesen sein, das seltsame Gefühl klang wieder ab..." (BERINGER-Materialien).

Nachdem ein weiterer Proband BERINGERS zunächst die Bewußtseinsklarheit und Orientiertheit in der Selbstschilderung hervorgehoben hatte, hält er fest: "Vergangenheit und Zukunft werden belanglos, das eigene Erleben vollzieht sich auf dem Höhepunkt der Vergiftung in einer seltsamen Bezugslosigkeit zu unserem früheren Dasein, wie auch zu unserer eigenen Zukunft. Der Vergiftete weiß, daß er dieser oder jener ist, mit dieser Vergangenheit oder jener Zukunftsabsicht. Aber die beiden Kategorien haben zum Erleben im Rausch keinerlei Bezug mehr, sie schmelzen gleichsam weg, sie bilden nicht mehr den sonst üblichen Hintergrund, auf dem sich ja alles und unser aktuelles Leben abspielt, der sonst stets mitgegeben ist" (BERINGER-Materialien).

Die Erlebnisse eines gestörten Zeiterlebens sind damit untereinander bemerkenswert ähnlich.

4. Diskussion

Wie die Zitate zeigen, handelte es sich bei den Versuchspersonen zum Teil um psychiatrisch erfahrene Ärzte, die ihr Erleben teilweise bereits in einer psychopathologisch adäquaten Begrifflichkeit zu beschreiben versuchten. War dies in anderen psychopathologischen Dimensionen (Denken oder Wahrnehmung) relativ einfach (vgl. HERMLE et al. 1988), so gelang dies bei den Ich-Störungen nur schwierig. Dies hat sicherlich nicht zuletzt den Grund, daß in der psychiatrischen Literatur unterschiedliche Konzepte zu Ich-Störungen bestehen und unterschiedliche Hypothesen über deren "eigentliches Wesen" oder über deren Ursache vorliegen. Im folgenden sollen die Konzeptualisierungsversuche von Ich-Störungen schlaglichtartig angeführt werden, um nicht nur die Variabilität der Phänomene, sondern auch die Variabilität der psychiatrischerseits erfolgten Reflexionen zu diesen Phänomenen zu verdeutlichen.

Affekt

Die letzte obengenannte Selbstschilderung macht den Zusammenhang zwischen Ich-Störungen und Affekt sehr deutlich. Es wundert daher nicht, daß Ich-Störungen mit Veränderungen der Affektivität in Beziehung gebracht wurden, wie beispielsweise von BECKER (1949, S. 430), der von einer "Verhinderung der erlebnismäßigen Verwirklichung der Affekte" bzw. von einer "Störung der emotionalen Ich-Besetzung" (BECKER 1949, S. 428) spricht. Auch unsere Versuchspersonen konnten lachen oder weinen, ohne Freude oder Trauer zu empfinden. Es schien ihnen, als ob sie neben sich stünden und distanziert die eigenen Gefühle beobachteten. BECKER spricht hier auch von einer "Entfremdung in sich selbst" bzw. von "affektiver Anästhesie". Man spricht in solchen Fällen auch von "dissoziiertem Affekt".

Passivität, Antriebsmangel, Autistischer Rückzug

Nicht selten tritt im Meskalinrausch eine Antriebshemmung deutlich zutage. Damit kann eine Hinwendung auf das eigene (psychotisch veränderte) Erleben einhergehen sowie ein Rückzug der Außenwahrnehmung.

Bereits 1927 sprach BERINGER vom "Passivitätssyndrom" in der Modellpsychose. Die Versuchsperson erlebt sich als inaktiv, zurückgezogen, rein rezipierend und unfähig zur Kontrolle von Denken, Erleben und Verhalten. BERINGER sah einen engen Zusammenhang zwischen dem inaktiven Zustand bzw. dem "Passivitätssyndrom" im Rausch und der Entfremdung des Ich-Bewußtseins in der schizophrenen Psychose.

Zeit

Über ein vollkommen aufgehobenes Zeiterleben bei schizophrenen Psychosen berichtet bereits 1929 SIEGFRIED FISCHER. Ihm fiel auf, daß bei Schizophrenen die Zeit weder langsamer, noch schneller abläuft (dies ist der Fall nach den Schilderungen mancher Patienten mit affektiven Psychosen), sondern gleichsam fragmentiert erscheint oder ganz fehlt. Entsprechendes wurde auch in der Modellpsychose berichtet: Die Zeit erscheint entweder verkürzt, gedehnt oder aber ganz aufgehoben. Insbesondere Schilderungen wie "Ich weiß nicht, eine Sekunde, ein Tag oder ein Jahr" machen deutlich, daß auch Berichte über die scheinbare Dehnung von Zeit eher als Berichte über die aufgehobene Zeit interpretiert werden müssen.

Das gestörte Zeiterleben kann, wenn sie auf eine halluzinogenbedingte euphorische Grundstimmung trifft, zu ekstatischen Glückserlebnissen führen (BECKER 1949, S. 436). Umgekehrt können bei drogenbedingten ängstlich-depressiven Verstimmungen Gefühle von Angst und Unheimlichkeit durch den Eindruck verstärkt werden, daß die Zeit nicht mehr fortschreitet. HEIMANN (1961) beschreibt Störungen des Zeiterlebens bei der Psilocybin-induzierten Psychose im Zusammenhang mit zunehmender Ich-Nähe der übrigen Drogenwirkungen, und MELGES et al. (1970) fanden einen deutlichen Zusammenhang zwischen gestörtem Zeiterleben und Ichstörungen während einer Marihuana-Intoxikation bei acht Probanden.

Kontrolle, Meinhaftigkeit
Nicht nur von Vp 1 wurde berichtet, daß Bewegungen subjektiv als automatenhaft, unharmonisch, schwerelos etc. empfunden wurden, bzw. daß sich die eigenen Bewegungen der bewußten Kontrolle entziehen. Äußere und innere Wahrnehmungen schienen irgendwie nicht mehr steuerbar zu sein. Passagenweise kann dazu das Gefühl des körperlich Aus-sich-heraus-Tretens bestehen oder auch das Gefühl, daß das Ausdrucksverhalten nicht mit dem Auszudrückenden übereinstimmt, daß z. B. der Gesichtsausdruck oder andere Bewegungen dem Willen entzogen sind (Paramimik oder Parakinesen, vgl. Vp 2).

Neben (motorischen) Ausdrucksphänomenen sind auch (sensible) Erlebnisqualitäten des Körperlichen betroffen. Interessant hierbei ist die von der Versuchsperson aus BERINGERS Meskalinexperimenten geschilderte Begrenzung der "unbeschreibbaren Empfindung" auf die *linke* Körperhälfte, was oft auch bei sensorischen Erlebnissen im Rahmen von *dreamy mental states* und *Hysterie* beschrieben wurde (vgl. HARRINGTON 1987; dort auch weiter Literatur) und für eine besondere Rolle der rechten Hemisphäre bei der Entstehung und Ausgestaltung solcher Erlebnisweisen spricht (vgl. OEPEN et al. 1987, 1988, HERMLE et al. 1988, sowie OEPEN et al., in diesem Band).

Eng mit dem Begriff der Kontrolle verbunden ist der Begriff der Meinhaftigkeit: Er wird angewandt in privativem Sinn, d.h. im Sinne des Fehlens der Meinhaftigkeit. Das Denken wird nicht mehr als eigenes, die Wahrnehmung nicht mehr als eigene, der Wille nicht mehr als eigener und die Bewegungen nicht mehr als eigene erlebt. Damit einhergehen kann das Gefühl, daß das Denken nicht nur nicht von mir, sondern von jemand anderem initiiert wird, d.h. Erlebnisse der Fremdbestimmung. Bis heute unklar und auch anhand unserer Untersuchung nicht entscheidbar ist die Frage, ob sich die Erlebnisse der gestörten Meinhaftigkeit bei Schizophrenen von denen bei drogeninduzierter Psychose qualitativ unterscheiden, etwa in dem Sinne, daß bei Schizophrenen das "Gemachte" unmittelbar erlebt, in der drogeninduzierten Psychose hingegen eher auf "Gemachtes" aufgrund der Veränderung bestimmter psychischer Fähigkeiten geschlossen wird.

Depersonalisation, Ich-Anderes-Abgrenzung
Im Halluzinogenrausch können die Ich-Umwelt-Beziehungen, das Ich- und Körpererleben und das eigene Tun, Denken und Fühlen u.ä. entfremdet sein. In der Literatur sind derartige Ich-Störungen ausführlich beschrieben (BECKER 1949, S. 422 ff, WEYL 1951, S. 45 ff, SAVAGE 1955, S. 9 ff). Bei BERINGER (1927, S. 74, Hervorhebung durch die Autoren) findet sich hierzu die folgende sehr charakteristische Äußerung einer Versuchsperson: "Während dieses Erlebens ist jede geistige Fähigkeit tot, *ich fühle mich geradezu identisch mit dem Objekt.*" An anderer Stelle spricht BERINGER (1927, S. 69) auch von "abnormen Verschmelzungserlebnissen" bzw. vom "Fallen der Subjekt-Objekt-Schranken".

So wird die Umwelt fremd, unwirklich und traumhaft erlebt. Eigene Aktivitäten werden als automatenhaft empfunden, sprachliche Äußerungen sind entfremdet: "Es scheint so, als ob eine zweite Instanz redet oder denkt" (Vp 1, 37 Jahre). Handlungen verlieren den Charakter des "ich tue", statt dessen "wurde es getan" ("der Mund... bewegt sich ohne mein Zutun"; Vp 2, 37 Jahre).

Formales Denken, Intentionaler Bogen, Gestaltzerfall

Die Störungen der Denkvorgänge wurden häufig unter den drei obengenannten Begriffen subsummiert. Ein Fehlen der integrativen Zusammenschau, d. h. der Fähigkeit der Verkettung von Einzelelementen zu einer Ganzheit wurde bemerkt. CONRAD (1958) spricht vom Gestaltzerfall, wie er vor allem bei der beginnenden Schizophrenie auftritt, bei dem Erlebnisse bis hin zu unkenntlichen Bruchstücken zerfallen. Diese bruchstückhafte Wahrnehmung wird auch in den experimentellen Psychosen erlebt und erinnert zudem an andere vergleichbare Zustände, beispielsweise an Träume oder temporale Dämmerattacken (vgl. OEPEN et al., in diesem Band). KARL JASPERS beschrieb bereits 1913 derartige Zustände der *Fragmentierung* wie folgt: "... das Seelenleben [ist] gleichsam in lauter einzelne Stücke zerfallen, indem nur zufällige und für das Individuum gewohnte und leichte einzelne Akte des Gegenstandsbewußtseins ohne jede Beziehung zu früheren und späteren Akten auftreten" (JASPERS 1973, S. 497).

Ich-Verlust

Mit Ich-Verlust wird in der Regel das Vorliegen all der o.g. Erscheinungen in mehr oder weniger starker Ausprägung und damit ein insgesamt schwerwiegendes Syndrom bezeichnet. Denken, Wahrnehmen und Erleben wird nicht mehr als zu mir gehörig, Welt nicht mehr als von mir unabhängig, Zeit nicht mehr als existent und Bewegungen als gemacht erlebt. Derartige Zustände gehen meist mit schweren Erregungszuständen und Angst einher.

Ein psychotischer Kontroll- bzw. Ich-Verlust ist bei keiner unserer Vpn aufgetreten. Bedingt durch die Testsituation mit relativ einfachem, technischem Setting wurde der psychedelisch bzw. psychotomimetisch introversive Zustand häufig unterbrochen und an der weiteren Entfaltung gehindert.

Zur Begründung der nosologischen Spezifität der Ichstörungen für schizophrene Psychosen wird häufig deren Vorhandensein bei Schizophrenen gegenüber deren Nichtvorhandensein bei experimentellen Psychosen angeführt. Erwähnt wird immer wieder der "erhaltene reflektierende Ich-Rest" (LEUNER 1962) bei experimentellen Psychosen als Beleg für die Unterschiedlichkeit derartiger Zustände zu schizophrenen Psychosen. Andererseits gibt es Berichte über die phänomenologische Nichtunterscheidbarkeit von Ich-Störungen (insbesondere Depersonalisation) bei experimentellen und endogenen Psychosen (GUTTMANN und MACCLAY 1936, FISCHMAN 1982). Das "Experimentum crucis" dieser These wäre die Applikation von Drogen an eine gesunde Person ohne deren Wissen. Ein solches "Experiment" wurde vom CIA im Rahmen eines Auswahlverfahrens für einen bestimmten Auftrag durchgeführt, in dem man Personen ohne deren Wissen LSD verabreichte. Eine Person fand man beispielsweise zusammengekauert unter einer Autobahnbrücke; nach Abklingen der Drogenwirkung berichtete die Person, daß sie die vorbeifahrenden Autos für Monster gehalten hatte. Neben dem beschriebenen Wissen um die Umstände spielt sicherlich die Dosierung des Halluzinogens eine wichtige Rolle: Es ist beschrieben, daß gerade bei mittlerer Dosierung die Versuchspersonen zu einer gewissen Introspektion und Reflexion fähig sind, mit steigernder Dosierung kann diese Fähigkeit jedoch verloren gehen. Dieses Beispiel verdeutlicht, daß es sich bei dem "reflektierenden Ich-Rest" eher um ein Epiphänomen handelt (HERMLE et al. 1988). Entsprechend argumentierte WINTERS (1975), daß die Unterschiede hinsichtlich des "reflektierenden Ich-Restes" bei schizophrenen Psychosen und Modellpsychosen ein Epiphänomen darstellen: Wer Drogen appliziert bekommt, der weiß um die Ursache der bei ihm eintretenden Veränderungen, wer an einer endogenen Psychose leidet, der weiß um diese Ursache nicht.

Es ist keineswegs leicht, die Bedeutung des Ausdrucks "Ich-Rest" bei einem bestimmten Autor nachzuvollziehen. Es kann damit gemeint sein, daß eine

Person subjektiv erlebt, daß sie sich unter Kontrolle hat, es kann aber auch damit das Wissen um die Ursache einer beeinträchtigten oder verlorenen Kontrolle gemeint sein, etwa der Gedanke "all das, was ich jetzt erlebe, ist durch eine Substanz in mir erzeugt und wird nach Abklingen von deren Wirkung auch wieder verschwinden". Unklar sind weiterhin die Beziehungen des Kontrollverlustes zur Affektivität: Macht der Kontrollverlust Angst oder ist die Angst Ursache des Kontrollverlustes? Man kann weiter fragen, ob zur Erklärung von Angst und Kontrollverlust überhaupt ein zugrundeliegender Morbus herangezogen werden muß oder ob es sich bei beiden nicht vielmehr um eine "einfühlbare" Reaktion auf die krankheitsbedingten Veränderungen des Erlebens handelt, denen sich der Patient passiv ausgeliefert fühlt.

Nicht nur die Patienten, sondern auch psychopathologisch erfahrene Ärzte haben Mühe, über gestörtes Ich-Erleben adäquat zu sprechen, wie die aufgezeigten Beispiele deutlich machen. Es bedarf weiterer klinischer, experimenteller sowie allgemein psychopathologischer Forschung zur Präzisierungder Theorie als auch der Möglichkeiten der Beschreibung dieser ebenso häufigen wie unverstandenen Symptome.

Zusammenfassung: Ichstörungen bei meskalininduzierten Modellpsychosen werden sowohl anhand im Rahmen eigener Untersuchungen erhobener Selbstschilderungen als auch anhand bislang unpublizierter Meskalinrausch-Protokolle von KURT BERINGER aus den dreißiger Jahren hinsichtlich einer Reihe möglicher Beschreibungskategorien diskutiert. Die Einordnung unter etablierte psychopathologische Konzepte erweist sich dabei als schwierig (es mangelt an klaren Kriterien der Zuordnung), was auf die mit diesen Konzepten verbundenen Probleme der allgemeinen Psychopathologie hinweist. Die bis heute kontrovers diskutierte Frage der nosologische Spezifität von Ichstörungen wird erörtert.

Ichstörungen in Experimental Psychoses

Summary: *Ichstörungen* (disorders of the experiencing self) in mescal induced experimental psychoses are described and discussed. The descriptions were obtained from our own research in this field as well as by using unpublished material of KURT BERINGER, one of the fathers of research in experimental psychoses. Several possible categories for description are presented and it is hard to select valid ones as there are few, if any distinguishing criteria. This points to problems of general psychopathology. The question whether *Ichstörungen* are of any nosological specificity must, however, remain unsolved.

References

Aghajanian, G.K. (1982): Neurophysiologic properties of psychotomimetics. In: Hoffmeister, F., Stille, G. (eds.): Handbook of experimental pharmacology **55**/III. Berlin, Heidelberg, New York, S. 88-109.

Avenarius, R. (1976): Der Verlust der Ich-Umwelt-Balance im Beginn der endogenen Psychose. Nervenarzt **47**, S. 482-487.

Becker, A.M. (1949): Zur Psychopathologie der Lysergsäurediäthylamidwirkung. Wien. Z. Nervenheilk. **2**, S. 402-439.

Beringer, K. (1927, 1963): Der Meskalinrausch. Monograph. Neurol. Psychiatr. H. **49**. Springer, Berlin, Heidelberg.

Beringer, K.: Nicht publizierte Rausch-Protokolle (Beringer-Materialien).

Charalampous, K.D., Walker, K.E., Kinross-Wright, J. (1966): Metabolic Fate of Mescaline in Man. Psychopharmacologia **9**, S. 48-63.

Conrad, K. (1958): Die beginnende Schizophrenie. Thieme, Stuttgart.

Fischer, S. (1929): Zeitstruktur und Schizophrenie. Zeitschrift für die gesamte Neurologie und Psychiatrie **121**, S. 544-574.

Fischman, L.G. (1982): Dreams, Hallucinogenic Drug States and Schizophrenia: A Psychological and Biological Comparison. Schizophrenia Bulletin **9**, S. 73-94.

Guttmann, E., Maclay, W.S. (1936): Mescalin and Depersonalization. Journ. Neurol. Psychopathol. **83**, S. 193-212.

Harrington, A. (1987): Medicine, Mind, and the Double Brain. Princeton University Press, Princeton (Mass.).

Heimann, H. (1961): Ausdrucksphänomenologie der Modellpsychosen. Psychiat. Neurol. **141**, S. 69-100.

Hermle, L., Oepen, G., Spitzer, M. (1988): Zur Bedeutung der Modellpsychosen. Fortschr. Neurol. Psychiat. **56**, S. 48-58.

Huber, G. (1957): Die coenästhetische Schizophrenie. Fortschr. Neurol. Psychiat. **25**, S. 491-520.

Jaspers, K. (1973): Allgemeine Psychopathologie. 9. Aufl. Springer, Berlin.

Kety, S.S. (1972): Toward hypotheses for a biochemical component in the vulnerability to schizophrenia. Seminar in Psychiatry **4**, S. 233-238.

Leuner, H. (1962): Die experimentelle Psychose (Springer-Monographie 95). Springer, Berlin, Göttingen, Heidelberg.

Melges, F.T., Tinklenberg, J.R., Hollister, L.E., Gillespie, H.K. (1970): Temporal disintegration and depersonalization during marihuana intoxication. Arch. Gen. Psychiat. **23**, S. 204-210.

Mullen, D.E. (1986): The Mental State and States of Mind. In: Hill, P., Muray, R., Thorley, A. (eds.): Essentials of Postgraduate Psychiatry, S. 3-36. Grune and Stratton, London. Orlando, New York, San Diego, Boston, San Francisco, Tokyo, Sydney, Toronto.

Oepen, G., Fünfgeld, M., Harrington, A., Hermle, L., Botsch, H. (1988): Right hemisphere involvement in mescaline-induced psychosis. Psychiat. Res. (in print).

Payk , Th.R. (1979): Mensch und Zeit, Chronopathologie im Grundriß. Hippokrates, Stuttgart.

Peters U.H. (1984): Wörterbuch der Psychiatrie und medizinischen Psychologie. Urban und Schwarzenberg, München, Wien, Baltimore.

Savage, C. (1955): Variations of ego-feelings induced by d-lysergic acid diethylamide (LDS-25). Psychoanal. Rev. **42**, S. 1-16.

Schneider, K. (1980): Klinische Psychopathologie. Thieme, Stuttgart, 12. Aufl.

Weyl, B. (1951): Versuch einer psychopathologischen Analyse der LSD-Wirkung. Diss. Freiburg.

Winters, W.D. (1975): The continuum of CNS excitatory states and hallucinosis. In: Siegel, R.K., West, L.J. (eds.): Hallucinations. New York, S. 53-70.

Ichstörungen: In Search of a Theory

M. Spitzer

1. Ichstörungen: An Extensional Introduction

Schizophrenics frequently hallucinate, report delusions, behave in a strange way, react emotionally inadequately and think illogically or in a completely confused way. All these symptoms are pretty well understood within the framework of psychological theories of perception, emotion, thinking, or behavior. The fact that there is not one but many theories about these phenomena shows at least that it seems to be easy for patients as well as for clinicians to talk about the phenomena, i.e. conceptualize perceptual, thought-related, affective or behavioral problems or processes.

There is, however, another group of symptoms which are regarded as belonging to the core of schizophrenic manifestations and which in German are called "*Ichstörungen*". There is no equivalent term in British and American psychiatric literature: the literal translation would be "I-disorders" but there is no such term in English.

As there is no term to indicate what we are talking about, we shall first quote some utterances of patients which in our opinion fall into the category of "Ichstörungen" (i.e. we want to delineate roughly the scope of the German concept of "Ichstörungen").

(a) "I feel that it is not me who is thinking."
(b) "My thoughts are not thought by me. They are thought by somebody else"
(c) "Feelings are not felt by me, things are not seen by me, only by my eyes"
(d) "This (thing, event) directly refers to me."
(e) "There is an immediate relationship between this (object, event) and me."
(f) "My thoughts can influence (things, events). This (event) happens because I think it"
(g) "To keep the world going, I must not stop thinking/breathing, otherwise it would cease to exist."
(h) "My experience has changed somehow. It is not real somehow such as I myself am somehow not real."
(i) "Things do not feel real. There is something between me and the things and persons around me, something like a wall of glass between me and everything else."
(j) "Time has disappeared. Not that it is longer or shorter, it's just not there; you could say there are bits of time, small pieces, shaken and mingled, or you could also say that there is no time at all."

From an extensional point of view[1], that is regarding the phenomena described in German as "Ich-Störung", a number of seemingly unrelated terms have been used in the Anglo-American literature to conceptualize the utterances mentioned above: some of these overlap with the German "Ichstörungen" and some delineate only an aspect of it: "depersonalization", "derealization", "loss of control", "passivity phenomena", "delusions of reference", "experience of breaking down or violation in the unity of the self", "disturbed ego-boundaries" (to mention only a few).

With regard to the utterances mentioned above, statement (h) probably would be regarded as expressing depersonalization, statement (i) as expressing derealization. Statement (c) would, according to some psychiatrists at least, probably be regarded as evidence for both. The utterances (a) and (b) would, by most clinicians, be regarded as Schneiderian first rank symptoms, i.e. as phenomena of the "being made" (disturbed "mine-ness") which by some authors are called "passivity phenomena" (cf. MULLEN 1986) or "inner-outer confusion" (cf. MELGES and FREEMAN 1977). With respect to (a), (b) and (c) most Anglo-American psychiatrists would speak of control and loss of control, thus delineating a concept which comes close to the Schneiderian approach of "Gemachtes". Nowadays many psychiatrists, following DSM-III, would choose to call statements (a) to (j) *delusions* (of influence, control, unreality etc.), thus regarding the phenomena in a completely different way.[2] With respect to statement (i) sometimes the term "ego boundaries" ("Ich-Grenzen") is mentioned.

This last term is vaguely defined, especially because it refers to the "ego", thus leading to the question of whether a hypothetic, intrapsychic entity (FREUD's Ego), the sick person, or the experiencing subject (the I, i.e. the mental center of experience) is meant. Because we do not refer to certain intrapsychic entities (which are thought to interact with other such entities producing a symptom) we avoid the term "ego", which is too close to Freudian theory, in what follows.

Even in German psychiatry there is - contrary to what one would expect - no theory of this "Ich", which is regarded as being somehow disturbed or disordered when there are *Ichstörungen* present. German textbooks, in case they contain a reference to the term "Ich" at all, sometimes refer to the "Ich" in terms of "the Person", but clearly "Ichstörungen" are not regarded as being the same as "Persönlichkeitsstörungen" (personality disorders).[3] At least some authors (cf. FELDMANN 1958, SCHNEIDER 1980) emphasize that one has to differentiate between the "I" that thinks, feels, experiences etc., and the "I" that can be con-

1 Every concept can be differentiated in terms of its extension and its intension: the extension contains all objects within the scope of that concept, and the intension is its meaning. The extension of the concept of a bachelor, to give an example, is simply all bachelors; the intension of that concept is "being an unmarried man".

2 It is important to note that the different "descriptive" concepts (e.g. "delusion of being controlled" versus "passivity phenomenon") run parallel with different approaches regarding the development of the phenomena: the terms "passivity phenomena", "loss of control" and the Schneiderian concept of "das Gemachte" refer *directly* to the *immediate experience* of the patient. The terms "delusion of being controlled" and "delusion of reference" may be interpreted as the patient's inferences with respect to his altered perceptual or emotional experience (cf. MAHER, this volume). Thus, the first *mental* event of the schizophrenic experience, so to speak, would be, in the second case, a disturbance regarding perception, emotion or formal thought, which is explained by the patients in a delusional way. In the first case, however, one would regard these utterances as a direct reflexion of the patients' experience that somehow has changed.

3 We agree with BLANKENBURG (this volume), that with some exceptions there has been little research in Ichstörungen within the last years.

sidered to be a certain person. But nevertheless no clear concept of the Ich in "Ichstörungen" has been established in the field of psychiatry. Therefore, it is not surprising that "Ichstörungen" themselves are also not very clearly defined. Perhaps this is the reason for the fact that Anglo-American psychiatry, although rooted in many concepts of German origin, did not adopt the concept of *Ichstörungen*.

2. KURT SCHNEIDER's "Non-Theory" of Ichstörungen

KURT SCHNEIDER, among others, emphasized the importance of Ichstörungen in the diagnosis of schizophrenia: "Among the basic features of experience certain disorders of the I-experience are of the utmost specificity for schizophrenia..." (SCHNEIDER 1980, p. 120).[4] However, with regard to the possibility of a *theory* of the "Ich" that is disturbed when "Ichstörungen" are present, KURT SCHNEIDER was sceptical. He did not even try to find a theoretical framework that could help towards making sense of what the "Ich" is that is disturbed in "Ichstörungen". The reason for this probably is that so many before him had failed in developing psychological theories of the "Ich". Thus, although his avoidance of "theoretical constructions" (SCHNEIDER 1957, p. 489), combined with a high competence for clinical practice, made him famous, his lack of a theoretical foundation for emphasizing his first-rank-symptoms is as striking, as his very few statements on the "Ich" are confusing.

SCHNEIDER states, "that the I-experience is not a matter of recognizing, evaluating or mirroring one's own personality, but *something formal*"[5] (SCHNEIDER 1980, p. 122, his italics). Although one would expect an explanation of that *form*, this is exactly what SCHNEIDER does not give. He rather states that there are five "formal criteria of consciousness of the I" ("formale Kriterien des Ichbewußtseins"; cf. SCHNEIDER 1980, p. 122). We will later focus on details of these "formal criteria" and see whether they help towards finding a theory of the disturbed I, and begin with the general notion of "formal criteria" with regard to the I.

First of all it should be noted that SCHNEIDER uses the - nowadays quite modern - concept of a criterion in a strange and misleading way: his five formal criteria refer to "I-experiences", but an experience is (a) neither a criterion nor (b) something formal.

Ad a) Criteria in psychology and psychopathology are used to provide *objective* clues to certain facts or events that are regarded as not directly observable. The DSM-III, for instance, extensively uses criteria for the diagnosis of mental disorders because these disorders cannot be seen directly. Thus the notion "criterion" in the field of psychopathology means "objective criterion" and thus refers to intersubjectively verifiable statements about facts or events to which there is no such direct intersubjective access.[6] However, all 5 "criteria" of

4 Translated by the author (M.S.) like the other quotations from German.

5 This statement reminds one strikingly of KANT's "I think", the so called "transcendental apperception"; cf. *Critique of Pure Reason*, § 16.

6 Criteria are not only used on the "diagnosis-level" but also on the "symptom-level" as the definition of the term delusion IN OLTMANNS (1988, p. 5) demonstrates.

SCHNEIDER are formulated in the subjective perspective (he refers to certain experiences of the patients), and thus they cannot be "objective" in the sense of "intersubjectively accessible".

Ad b) SCHNEIDER does not explain why he uses the term "formal" with respect to the experiencing I. He just uses it, adding that "the criteria of the I-experience can hardly be described unambiguouosly even with respect to undisturbed psychic life" (SCHNEIDER 1980, p. 122). So SCHNEIDER neither gives an explanation of what he means by "form" nor the form of what entity he has in mind.

Let us turn to the five criteria themseves: SCHNEIDER refers to KARL JASPERS who had already stated four criteria of the consciousness of I, and gives the following criteria of the I-experience ("Kriterien des Ich-Erlebens"):

1. Demarkation between me and the out-there, other (not me) ("Abgrenzung gegenüber außen und anderen")
2. The experience of unity in the present moment ("Erlebnis der Einfachheit im Augenblick")
3. The experience of one's continuing identity across time ("Erlebnis der Identität im Zeitverlauf")
4. The experience of mine-ness ("Erlebnis der Meinhaftigkeit")
5. The Experience of one's own existence ("Daseinserlebnis").

First we want to emphasize that SCHNEIDER stated the 5 "criteria" for practical reasons and that he derived them from clinical practice. However, two questions remain to be clarified: what does SCHNEIDER mean by these characteristics, and what do they characterize? - It seems quite obvious that SCHNEIDER does not intend to give features of the personality, and that the 5 "formal criteria" do not refer to constructs in personality-research nor to other concepts that have been proposed in the field of empirical psychology in the thirties, forties, or fifties of this century. We will proceed with the discussion of SCHNEIDER's "formal criteria" and will see the form of what they describe and what kind of description they represent. Before that, however, a look at CHRISTIAN SCHARFETTER's work on Ichstörungen will give us further clues for solving the problem of Ichstörungen.

3. CHRISTIAN SCHARFETTER: a Step into the Right Direction and a Methodological Misunderstanding

CHRISTIAN SCHARFETTER is on of the few authors who tried to describe "Ich-störungen" in detail. He refers to five basic dimensions (identity, demarcation, consistency, activity and vitality), disorders of which he also characterizes as syndromes of the first order. From these five basic dimensions he distinguishes the more complex functions "self-assessment" and "self-confidence", and even more complex features such as "deliberateness", "maturity", "relative freedom", "self-possession" and "autonomy". According to SCHARFETTER, schizophrenics show a disturbance of the five basic functions.

The work of SCHARFETTER et al. (1982) on the dimensions mentioned above contains some methodological drawbacks and a basic misunderstanding. Consideration of his work nevertheless offers hints for our own efforts to construct an adequate methodological approach and theoretical framework for the problem of "Ichstörungen".

SCHARFETTER et al. (1982) speak of "phenomenological constructs" in regard to their "dimensions of the I". First we will show that the concept of a "phenomenological construct" is either trivial or vaguely defined (sometimes even contradictory). Describing the development of the constructs, SCHARFETTER writes: "The individual stages of the construct's development are shown by the example of the dimension I-vitality ... On the symptom-level we shall comprise verbalised experience ('I've ceased to live'), observable behavior (e.g. stupor, catatonic hyperventilation, self-mutilation in order to sense oneself) and delusion as the interpretation of the experience of oneself and the world (in our example the delusion of hypochondria, delusion of the end of the world , delusion of being poisoned). We shall group these in the first step of reduction and consider them as a syndrom of first order that stands for a dimension of consciousness of the I: I-vitality. We shall proceed in the same way for the dimensions 2 to 5. These five dimensions shall be comprised as the global construct 'consciousness of the I'" (SCHARFETTER et al. 1982, p. 262). Thus the concept of a "phenomenological construct" is used for a scientific method which is common to all empirical sciences (according to their own view of what they are doing): science proceeds from empirical data to producing more and more general hypotheses which are then tested. Therefore the subtitle of SCHARFETTER's work "Empirical studies on a phenomenological construct" is redundant (empirical *and* phenomenological), and the concept of a phenomenological construct is trivial.

From the fact that SCHARFETTER et al. emphasize phenomenology in addition to empiricism we may assume that they might mean something non-trivial. But what do they mean? - A construct is used within a certain frame of reference in order to explain certain empirical data. Within psychology, "hypothetical constructs" are often mentioned in order to emphasize the epistemological status of constructs. As DREVER and FRÖHLICH (1972, p. 169) put it: "Constructs in a narrower sense refer to those hypothetical conditions or processes that cannot be inferred directly but only from assumed causes, effects, or large classes of indicators (e.g. behavior or actions)." Therefore, if constructs are used to explain certain empirical facts, they will already have been constructed with regard to this material. Then it is not clear what the term "phenomenological" denotes in combination with the term "construct". If it means a special way of constructing (i.e. constructing "closer" to experience, whatever that may mean) the term becomes contradictory, as construction is always a process that involves more than just empirical facts. Thus the concept of a "phenomenological construct" is either trivial or ill-defined.

With regard to scientific method, SCHARFETTER et al. obviously misunderstand their own procedure: They pretend to conduct *empirical* statistical research in the dimensions mentioned above. What SCHARFETTER and his co-workers are doing, however, is in fact not the validation of certain constructs by subjecting them to empirical analysis. Instead, they are searching for statistical means to express the dimensions they take for granted. This can be shown by the following statement: "Phase I, which tested how useful classical methods of test-theory are and found them to be of limited use for this area of reference, demanded the improvement of the instruments and the search for better methods" (SCHARFETTER et al. 1982, p. 265). SCHARFETTER et al. do not, as they clearly state[7] in their work, empirically validate a construct referring to ego-psychopathology, but rather search for the adequate method that will express the dimensions they hold to be essential for the experiencing I.

This can also be shown by another passage of SCHARFETTER et al. (1982, pp. 66-67): "As we stopped evaluating on the basis of classical test-theory we also gave up standardized methods of testing as regards further empirical studies of

7 "A construct on the Ego-psychopathology of the schizophrenic syndrome is introduced and its empirical testing is reported" (SCHARFETTER et al. 1982, p. 262).

patients. So clinical experience shows that free talking with its flexibility and natural development rather contributes to a thorough exploration... Certain items ... have been categorized into a dimension on grounds of a *certain step of interpretation* which connected, so to speak, raw result with its respective layer by way of the intentional sense of the result" (SCHARFETTER et al. 1982, pp. 66-67, our italics). SCHARFETTER et al. thus do *not*, as they pretend to do by using the terms "empirical" and "phenomenological", carry out their research in a "space free of theoretical basic assumptions", but rather do have certain assumptions without stating them: it is not clear, what is meant by the "interpretation" of a person's statement by means of his or her intentional sense, i.e. it is not clear on what assumptions and theories the interpretation is based.

It should be noted, however, that SCHARFETTER et al. take for granted that there is a need for interpretation of the patients' utterances: "Another difficulty arises from the fact that the grouping of items into dimensions is not based on intercorrelations of the items concerned in the sense of empirical syndromes (clusters) but rests on semantic similarities of the content of experiences and on interpretation" (SCHARFETTER et al. 1982, p. 267). The authors also talk about a need for a "complex model, which combines semantic relations or relations of sense ["Sinnzusammenhänge"] with empirical [i.e. statistical] relations" (SCHARFETTER et al. 1982, p. 267).

As we will see, they are right in assuming that there must be a model that serves as a guideline for the interpretation of the patients' utterances. SCHARFETTER et al. are also right in their attempt to interpret empirical data (i.e. the utterances of patients) according to a certain theory. However, as we have shown, SCHARFETTER's work is confused because of a basic misunderstanding with regard to his own method: what he does *not* give is an empirical validation of certain dimensions of the experiencing I. He is rather searching for an adequate method to express these dimensions out of what patients are saying. In short: SCHARFETTER et al. are right in what they are doing (i.e. they interpret the utterances of patients according to a theory about the I) but wrong in what they think of what they are doing (i.e. they think to get the theory from the data).

When speaking of the experiencing I SCHARFETTER says that this is "a construct made of different theories" (SCHARFETTER 1983, p. 31). It may have been this assumption that lead to the misconception: the experiencing subject is *not* a "construct" of empirical data or of different theories; the experiencing subject is rather a structure which is at work in every experiencing person. Like perception, thinking or emotion, the experiencing I does not need to be a construct because first of all, it is simply there. This does not mean, however, that a proper description of this structure at work is also at anybody's disposal. So, how is this structure to be described? Are there theories about that structure at all, and what kind of theories?

4. The Framework of Transcendental Philosophy

4.1 An Analogous Example

To give an example of what it might mean to describe a structure that is "at work" in every experiencing person and what kind of profit one might get out of it, let us outline the process of research on aphasia as an example.

We all use language without thinking about its structure and without having to think about it. Nevertheless, there has been a lot of research on the structure of language which has resulted in theories of grammar, reference etc., i.e. in theories about the structures of language. Disorders of language are well-known for more than a hundred years and have been defined according to certain organic lesions. The application of linguistic theories to the field of aphasia, however, has resulted in new definitions and clearer differentiations between the subgroups of this disorder. Thus, theories, developped by linguists have been successfully applied to the field of language disorders resulting in practical consequences in dealing with aphasic patients. Vice versa, research in aphasia nowadays provides interesting questions for linguists.

The remainder of this article is based on the idea that the relation between Ich-Störungen and philosophical theories of experience (we will concentrate especially on transcendental philosophy) could correspond the relation between aphasia and linguistic theories of language.

4.2 Conditions of the Possibility of any Kind of Experience

SCHNEIDER's five "formal criteria" may sound rather strange to an empirical psychologist, and SCHARFETTER's work on five "dimensions" of the I would probably simply be regarded as having methodological flaws. For a philosopher, however, the given characteristics are a somehow vague description of what we might call *transcendental features of experience*. What does the term "transcendental" mean, what kind of "features" do we mean, and what kind of evidence is it that leads us to detect these features?

First of all, we are inclined to ask psychologists or psychiatrists not to associate forms of meditation with that term, and we also ask the philosopher to be as tolerant as possible with our usage of "transcendental". We shall use this term to refer to statements about the structure of experience and, from a methodological point of view, to refer to the kind of knowledge that is represented by such statements.

KANT gave the term "transcendental", which had already been used within scholastic philosophy to denote the *most general* features of things, this specific meaning: "... the word 'transzendental' ... does not refer to anything beyond experience but rather to something that (a priori) precedes it, which, however, is not determined to anything more than to render experience possible" (KANT 1783/1976, p. 144). Thus KANT says that the word 'transzendental' does refer to experience in a special sense: it refers to *something to which one has to refer to before (in a systematic sense) experience takes place, something dealing with the possibility of any experience.*

Rather than interpreting KANT at this point of our argument (which would indeed be a good idea but would go far beyond the scope of this paper) we want to give a short systematic outline of what can be said about our experience in a sense so basic, i.e. "transcendental", that there is no way of experiencing any difference of content that would count as a clue to what we will say (i.e.: we will not say anything empirical).[8]

4.3 Some Transcendental Features Relevant to Psychopathology

(a) Experience is always an experience of *something*. This simply means that experience has a determinate content, resp. is qualitatively specified.

This statement could be questioned by claiming that there are experiences in which the experiencing subject is not able to give any specification of what he or she has experienced. However, if that is really so we could ask on what basis the subject can claim that there has been an experience at all: if there is an answer to this question, there will be some qualitative determination; if there is no answer, the claim must be questioned.

The psychopathological relevance, i.e. the relevance of this feature for interpreting utterances of patients, is not clear. SCHNEIDER states that schizophrenic or deeply depressed patients, when claiming that they do not live any more, should not be taken seriously. Nevertheless, he not only mentions these experiences under the heading "Daseinserlebnis" (experience of existence) but also adds exactly this feature to the other four which had already been proposed by JASPERS. So SCHNEIDER was at least vague with regard to this feature. On the contrary, it seems to be clear to SCHARFETTER that vitality ("Ich-Vitalität") is among the basic features of the experiencing I, and he would take statements about not living anymore in a quite literal sense as expressions of immediate experiences of patients. However, up to now the question of how to interpret these statements has remained unanswered.

(b) Experience is always the experience of *something else*, i.e. there is a distinction between the experiencing *subject* and the experienced *object*.

One should not, as JASPERS (1973, pp. 289-290) has done, refer to something like a "basic separation of subject and object" because that concept is misleading. Objectivity should rather be conceptualized as the ultimate achievement of a subject in the following sense: when I look at the white, rectangular paper in front of me I do not only abstract from the prevailing yellow component of the light (being reflected from the paper because of the electric light) and also from the appearance of the angles (being not rectangular as I am looking from an oblique angle), but I also abstract that it is I who is watching. Thus I conceive the

---

8 Once again we ask the philosopher for tolerance: we know about the problems of terminology within this field and about the problems of not confounding psychological, epistemological or even logical statements. Nevertheless, we feel that the attempt is worth being made, and thus we prefer to outline the argument without any constraint, and we shall see how far we can get without getting stuck on terminology. What we should say is that we could also refer to the "ontology of the subject" as outlined in the work of WOLFGANG CRAMER (see also UEHLEIN, this volume).

object as something completely independent of my experience of it (and exactly that is the meaning of objectivity: objectivity is not "just there" but achieved by the subject which not only abstracts from color and point of view but also abstracts from his or her act of experiencing).

(c) There is a *unity* of experience.

Experience is not fragmented and does not represent a jumble of nothing but qualities, but there is always a synthesis at work that leads to a unified experience. We do not experience colors, lines, or patterns but we rather experience (see) a landscape for instance.

(d) We experience *time*.

One could argue that the experience of time is a wholly empirical matter. However, in a strict sense, time in the empirical sciences presupposes the experience of time or, as one could also say, presupposes time in every experience: experiencing subjects are not in the same way "just in time" as stones or trees. In every experience there is not only a synthesis with regard to different qualities but also with regard to different points of time. We experience time in somehow synthesizing point t_1 and t_2, thinking them both together to establish the relations of "former" or "later". These relations are not "just there", they have to be made or constructed or synthesized by the experiencing subject.

(e) The experiencing subject is *identical* throughout the different experiences.

It is not so easy to tell what kind of identity is meant with this notion. One can speak of a logical, a philosophical, or a psychological concept of identity. When clinicians refer to identity, they almost always have in mind a certain set of personality-features, memories or character dimensions, i.e. the psychological concept of identity. According to this concept, a person can acquire, lose or change his or her identity. In logic, identity is a binary relation which in its strong form holds only for an entity with regard to itself. In a philosophical framework, identity refers to the identic subject as a presupposition of different experiences (or one could say: of difference in general). If there were no such an identical subject, the notion of difference would simply make no sense.[9] Philosophical identity of a subject of experience accounts also for the synthesizing of points of time and the connection of later and former.

(f) My experience is *my* experience.

It seems trivial to state that my experience is *my* experience. However, not for philosophers, but for psychiatrists, this triviality, like the trivialities mentioned before, becomes a feature of the experiencing I that might be disturbed.

It is indeed hard to tell what the term "my" denotes when we talk of "my experience". STRAWSON has convincingly shown, that one presupposition of this mine-ness is that there are other subjects to which the experience could be ascribed, i.e. that the mine-ness of experience presupposes (otherwise not meaning

9 In this sense the strive for identity (identity versus diffusion of roles) may be mentioned as the main conflict in adolescence which is solved when a stable synthesis out of drives and needs has been achieved (cf. ERIKSON).

anything) the existence of other subjects capable of experiencing, thus leading to a "transcendental" foundation of intersubjectivity.[10]

The empiricist will find all the statements mentioned above rather trivial.[11] However, if he had a look at what patients say (e.g. at the statements a - j above), he would find that some of the basic features of experience just mentioned are changed in schizophrenics: Mine-ness (of any experience), Objectivity (in the specified sense of "being experienced by me as something completely independent of me and my experience of it"), Unity (of experience), Identity (of the experiencing subject during different experiences), and Time (as experienced by a subject in creating a synthesis) may be disturbed.

The combination of the concept of synthesis, identity, unity and mine-ness to describe a structure-at-work in any experience is one of the main points in the work of KANT as can be seen in the following quotation: "Therefore the notion 'all the ideas I get from experience belong to me' means that I unite them in one self-consciousness or at least that I am able to unite them. Although this notion is not yet consciousness of the synthesis of these ideas it presupposes, however, that this synthesis is possible which is to say that it is only because I can comprehend these ideas in one consciousness that I call them as a whole my ideas. Otherwise I would have a self as multicoloured and varied as I have ideas of which I am conscious" (KANT, Criticism of Pure Reason B 134). This quotation shows, that we do not refer just to some symptoms and try to give a theoretical superstructure but rather refer to transcendental philosophy, which is in fact able to provide a theoretical framework for the description not only of experience but also of disturbances of experience.

If disturbances of Mine-ness, Identity, Unity, Time, Objectivity, and Me-not-me-differentiation occur, the patients of course will hardly be able to describe them, because the disturbances are so basic that there is no comparable experience within the scope of variation of normal experience (normal experience does not, by definition, vary with regard to the features we assume to be disturbed). Clinicians having no idea what kind of structure may be basic to *every* kind of experience, will not be able to describe the disturbances of experience in the right way. Thus, it might have been the lack of an adequate theory which lead to the description of all these disturbances as "delusion".

5. Ichstörungen: Consequences Regarding Data and Scientific Method

5.1 Applied Transcendental Philosophy?

Can there really be something like an empirical application of transcendental philosophy? Especially philosophers will shake their heads and insist, that by definition transcendental theory cannot be applied empirically. We do not agree.

10 Quite similar thoughts can also be found in the work of HUSSERL (cf. the *Cartesian Meditations* as well as the third volume of the *Phenomenology of Intersubjectivity*) as opposed to purely empiristic conceptions of the "other" (cf. CARNAP).

11 He may also have objections some of which are easily be refuted while others are more intricate and cannot be discussed here: We surely have to *learn* a lot to experience the way we do, but we *cannot learn to experience*. We neither can learn to have a unified experience and the adult blind who has been operated and sees only colors and patterns until he touched the thing needs must have a unity of touch in order to do this. Nor can I learn that my experince is *mine*. Regarding time, we want to stress that some *synthesis* has to take place. We do not refer to learning what time it is nor to the "time-sense" that tells us how long a certain period was.

In other fields of research, the application of "pure" theories is regarded as quite normal and the interpretation of facts according to such pure theories is also nothing one worries about. The reader should think for example of pure mathematics and its application in physical science. NEWTON and LEIBNIZ had to invent infinitesimal calculus and by this invention the description of movement leading to a whole theory of movement became possible. In fact, without a theoretical framework no such interpretation would have been possible. It was not necessary (and would have been deleterious) for NEWTON to think of a variety of features of the apple falling off the tree to compare this event with the moon circling round the earth and the earth round the sun. He must have had a theory telling him what he was *not* to think about. In this sense, the psychiatrist, who is always confronted with a variety of utterances by patients about a lot of things, must have a theory which tells him what he should regard as a reflexion of basic changes in the experience of the patient (which are happening, as it is agreed upon at least by JASPERS, SCHNEIDER, SCHARFETTER and their followers) and what constitutes all the secondary explanations, inferences and personally influenced interpretations of the patient. With regard to disturbances of the experiencing I, transcendental philosophy may be an adequate frame of reference.

As we see there is in principle no reason not to apply pure theory. On the contrary, we would like to suggest, that one has to apply pure theory in order to describe utterances and behavior to obtain the right kind of data. But what exactly does it mean to apply transcendental philosophy to utterances of patients? Why do we have to apply it? - Let us turn to the second question first.

5.2 The Need for Interpretation and its Consequences

Why should one use such a theory of the experiencing I (the "Ich") to conceptualize the patient's utterances? Why not call them simply delusions? - The answer to this question is another question: why do we not refer to *everything* strange in what patients say as a delusion? Why do we, for instance, consider certain utterances to be clues, hints or proofs of hallucinations? What patients say is at face value something really bizarre, so why is it not a delusion? The answer to this question is that the clinician has something like a theory of "normal" perception in mind, which runs like this: there is an "outer" object which in the process of perception gains an "inner" representation. So if the patient speaks of "outer" things or events without such things or events present, something is wrong.

It is such a theory that is the basis for the notion of a hallucination as defined in most textbooks. The point here is, that the theory does not have to be true, and that hallucinations need not be like perceptions, but *that there has to be some sort of theory* that allows to differentiate between "delusions in the field of perception" (i.e. hallucinations) and delusions of different content. By the same token we are able to delineate "delusions" in the field of emotion (i.e. emotional disturbances) or in the field of thought (i.e. thought disorder): The utterances (k) "I feel so sad that there is almost no feeling at all" and (l) "I find it hard to concentrate; I can hardly think" thus are not to be described as bizarre delusions but as valid descriptions of the patient's experiences in the field of emotion and thought.

To summarize so far: the clinician deals with patients that say strange things. One could stop differentiating at this point and say that these patients have "delusions". If the clinician does not stop short here, he should be aware of the fact that he does not simply describe but does *interpret* the utterances according to certain theories or assumptions regarding the entire mental field. So if he speaks of hallucinations, thought disorder and emotional disturbances, why should he not speak of a disturbance regarding the experiencing I? - The fact that this field or structure is even more basic than the others mentioned is not a counterargument, but could be interpreted as a hint that we are right: hallucinations, thought disorder and disturbed affect are not regarded as essential to schizophrenia and are not symptoms of first rank according to SCHNEIDER; certain DSM-III-"delusions" (which, according to the theory proposed here, should be classified as Ichstörungen) are! The only problem is that the patients do not have a referential framework to describe them without using metaphors that are misleading, especially if clinicians do not have such a theory as well. (What in fact has led to the present situation of having listed Ichstörungen under the headline of delusions.)

There are no uninterpreted "facts" which are "just data". As this consideration regarding method belongs to the core of thoughts within the field of philosophy of science that do not need a discussion any more, we do not go deeper into the argument here.[12]

If we adopt transcendental philosophy as our interpretive framework, we find ourselves in a position where we can begin to classify changes in the basic features of the experiencing I. It is not clear if we then should speak of different "symptoms" of an "I-disturbance" syndrome or whether some of the "symptoms" always occur together. One approach to this classification is the attempt to establish correlations between changes in these dimensions in order to find such an "I-disturbance syndrome". Such a syndrome should include disturbed mineness ("control"), identity, unity ("fragmented experience"), out-there-ness ("inner-outer confusion") as well as desintegration of time ("temporal desorganization"). As MELGES and coworkers (MELGES et al. 1970, MELGES and FREEMAN 1977, FREEMAN and MELGES 1977, 1978) have shown, such correlations indeed exist and are highly significant. However, we regard this approach only as the weakest possibility of how to "apply" features of experience that are a result of "pure" theory. With regard to the problem of interpreting the utterances of patients in the context of a theoretical framework, another application of the transcendental theory of experience - a much stronger one - is possible: the theory is not employed to give hints for possible correlations (as between time desintegration and inner-outer confusion) but rather is used as a means for making sense of what the patients are saying (see below). Thus the fields of delusions, hallucinations, and Ichstörungen can be clearly differentiated.

Looked upon from a more statistical point of view, the argument can be put like this: a symptom in psychiatry is almost always more than the affirmation or negation of a single question. So the answer to "Do you see things that are not there?" will give a first hint to whether a patient is hallucinating but some

12 The need for interpretation of the patients' utterances was already emphasized by SCHARFETTER. However, SCHARFETTER did not say how (or according to what theory) this interpretation should come about. He also did not clarify that interpretation is essential for the generation of data in the field of psychiatry (as in any scientific field).

patients will say "yes" without hallucinating and others will say "no" while hallucinating. In short: the well trained clinician will use a broad spectrum of clues and hints - ranging from answers to questions to the observation of spontaneously occuring behavior - to conclude whether hallucinations (or any other symptom) are present. The problem that more questions always mean more possibilities of disagreement among clinicians is well known as partial incompatibility between reliability and validity: just one question would be most reliable but does not match the scope of a symptom as a whole and therefore is hardly valid; with the combination of many questions the validity increases with regard to the whole symptom but the reliability decreases. To avoid the dilemma of reliable but useless and less reliable but clinically useful statements about a patient, there have to be theories of how to group and interpret utterances in the right way.

It remains to be tested, however, if all the features of experience mentioned above always occur together or if some may occur just on their own. Such a test is not, as might be expected, easy to perform because it is not simply a matter of correlation since the data are not independent of the theory that is to be tested. To give an example: somebody who barely states that he has the idea of being controlled could not only have a "slight form" (or whatever one may call it) of an Ichstörung but also no Ichstörung at all but a delusion. Careful examination should reveal if there are any disturbances in his way of experiencing and this examination will include other questions referring to other features of the experiencing I. So if it finally is concluded that the patient has an Ichstörung there will, by definition, be correlations between "control" and other features. If is is concluded that the patient has just a delusion, no such correlations will be found, again by definition! The only way to advance in such a situation seems to be a very careful investigation of possible relations to other criteria that lie beyond the scope of Ichstörungen. Thus for instance one could look for neuropsychological changes that go parallel with Ichstörungen (indeed an approach that has not been followed or at least not been followed very far as I see).

So in the long run there are consequences with regard to method that promise new insights into the symptomatology of the schizophrenic syndrome. At least some advantages, however, can be stated already at present.

5.3 Getting More Detailed Descriptions

First of all it should be stated again that the psychiatrist deals with utterances of patients referring to their own mental activity. A psychiatrist does not see or hear a hallucination and probably the patient also does not hear or see it. The patient has a certain experience and tries to communicate it. In the case of hallucinations he uses the vocabulary of perception and thus tries to tell the clinician what is wrong with him. As every clinician will know, on careful examination most hallucinations (to mention only one example) turn out not to be like perceptions, but somehow different.[13] So patients as well as clinicians use *metaphors* of perception to talk about disturbances regarding certain sense modalities. In the same way patients and clinicians may have no difficulty in talking about emotions, formal thought or behavior. However, when patients

13 For this reason JASPERS thought that most hallucinations should be conceptualized as pseudo-hallucinations (cf. SPITZER 1987, 1988).

have to talk about their immediate experience there seems to be a shortage or even a lack of descriptive language: the fact that my thoughts are mine is so obvious and trivial to everybody that the experience of one's thoughts as not his own can only be referred to by the metaphor of broadcasting, inserting, or being controlled by somebody else. A disturbance of the immediate experienced relation to objects or events as "being there" and "happening without my experience of them" in most cases is referred to by the patients quite well, but the clinicians introduce such misleading concepts as "ego-boundaries" and their disintegration to refer to it because they lack another framework. Thus, they do *not* refer to the experiencing subject. Disturbances of time are often not asked for by the clinician; the fragmentation of the unity of experience is presumably in most cases referred to as a bizarre delusion, and the concept of identity is only referred to in its psychological sense. Thus instead of referring to the experiencing subject, there is rather some reference to a hypothesized intrapsychic entity that functions in a certain way according to the Freudian theory. (We already mentioned that the term "ego" is often used in an unclear way.)

Therefore, one argument why it is better to describe the schizophrenic experience with a theory of Ich-Störungen in mind is that one gets a more detailed and more adequate description of the disturbed experience of a schizophrenic patient when applying the concepts derived from transcendental philosophy.

Summing up what has been said so far, we are of the opinion that a basic diagnostic conceptual change needs to be made in the approach to schizophrenia: the concept of "Ichstörungen" should be substituted for the unclear category of experiential changes that presently are classified as delusions. The "deluded" talk of the patient is in fact a reflection of his or her inadequate, metaphoric effort to inform us of basic disturbances in his or her immediate experience. In short: Ichstörungen are not just delusions.

What in the German psychopathological tradition is called "Ich-Störung" is referred to in the contemporary Anglo-American tradition as contentual thought disorder, which can be seen, for instance, in the DSM-III-R: "Certain delusions are observed far more frequently in schizophrenia than in other psychotic disorders. These include, for instance, the belief or experience that one's thoughts, as they occur, are broadcast from one's head to the external world so that others can hear them (thought broadcasting) that thoughts that are not one's own are inserted into one's mind (thought-insertion); that thoughts have been removed from one's head (thought-withdrawal); or that one's feelings, impulses, thoughts or actions are not one's own, but are imposed by some external force (delusions of being controlled)." According to the German tradition, utterances of patients indicating phenomena of the kind mentioned do not reflect delusions (i.e. "false personal believes based on incorrect inference about external reality"; DSM-III-R, p. 395), but rather the patients' attempt to explain what their immediate experiences are like. That patients will use certain metaphors, for instance broadcasting or insertion of thoughts (or in other times and cultures the spread or making of one's own thoughts by Gods or Demons) should not lead to the labelling of these experiences as delusional (i.e. in principle *false* ones), otherwise the question arises why these delusional contents do occur so often. If one interprets these utterances as delusions which just do have a certain bizarre content, one has no answer to this question. Delusions of reference or delusions of being controlled are often regarded as the most important symptoms especially in schizophrenics. In fact, we would argue that the utterances of patients (for example a - g) should not be called delusions (i.e. false or at least inadequate descriptions of reality) but rather as the patients' attempts to refer to their immediate experience which has somehow changed. Thus "control" or "reference" do not refer to certain "themes" of delusions, as for instance "jealousy", "being loved", "querulance" etc., but they are the direct though metaphorical expression of experiences that reflect a deformation of basic features of the experiencing I.

If one considers these phenomena not as delusions at all but as Ichstörungen (i.e. symptoms wich are regarded as belonging to the core of schizophrenia), it is not surprising that they occur so often.

Transcultural psychiatry gives a further argument: delusions of reference or delusions of control are transculturally "delusional" symptoms in schizophrenics with the highest number of occurrence having a frequency of about 70 % while other "themes" of delusions are in a lower range (cf. MURRAY 1987). We think that this difference clearly indicates that "control" or "reference" do not denote certain "themes" (i.e. matters of content), but do reflect changes in immediate experience occuring in the course of schizophrenia.[14]

MULLEN (1986, pp. 26-27) probably comes closest to us: he refers to "Ichstörungen" under the headline "Passivity phenomena (disturbances of ego-boundary)" thus indicating, that he is dealing with Meinhaftigkeit (mine-ness) and the immediate experience of the self and of the world as distinct from the self. He does not speak of delusions and rather regards broadcasting and thought control or thought insertion as phenomena of I-pathology or me-pathology. MULLEN is also one of the few who discuss the genesis of delusions from these experiences, thus trying to give a theory of the relation between Ichstörungen and delusions[15]: "In more florid form there can be the experience of one's own thoughts being shared and participated by every one around. This experience may lead to delusions of explanation. One of my patients described a complicated plot whereby a neighbour who was a BBC journalist, would nightly broadcast her every secret thought to the nation and this explained why everybody knew about them and shared them." (MULLEN 1986, p. 26).

Not only delusions but also disorders of time should be described more carefully. Although in the current psychiatric literature there is little interest for disturbances of *time* in schizophrenia, there has been such interest in the past. Time-fragmentation or temporal desintegration (opposite to the lengthening or shortening of time occuring in manic-depressive illness) has been mentioned as frequently happening in schizophrenics. One could even say that the more psychiatrists have payed attention to disturbances of the experience of time, the more they have got the impression that this symptom might even be a necessary condition of the diagnosis of schizophrenia. So FISCHER as early as 1929 has made the assumption that probably every schizophrenic does experience a certain fragmentation of time.[16]

The older German psychiatric literature contains many descriptions of disturbances of time. More recently, MELGES and FREEDMAN (1977) have emphasized the fact that disturbances of time in patients who are not temporally desoriented (as patients with organic brain disorders) are common in acute mental illness. The authors even propose a genetic modell of symptom formation of delusions with temporal desintegration as the start. Their correlations of temporal desintegration with other first rank symptoms (i.e. roughly: Ichstörun-

14 cf. my contribution on Ichstörungen, this volume.

15 Such theories of a somehow disturbed I in the beginning of delusions can be said to have almost a tradition in German psychopathology although there has never been done much of empirical research within that field (cf. BLANKENBURG, this volume, and my contribution on Ichstörungen, this volume).

16 for details see SPITZER 1985, chapter 5.

gen) are of great interest for our discussion but nevertheles have to be regarded with great care with regard to our argument on method stated above.

There has not been much research in Ichstörungen, either conceptually or empirically. If the present contribution should lend a hand to the improvement of this situation, it would have achieved its aim.

Summary: An argument is proposed to regard certain utterances of schizophrenics which sound very bizarre not as delusions, as current psychopathology (e.g. DSM-III) does, but as Ichstörungen (disorders of the experiencing I). Ichstörungen have been given broad attention to by the German psychopathologists KARL JASPERS and KURT SCHNEIDER and have been investigated by SCHARFETTER in recent years, but nevertheless there is no theory of what they are about and what features they describe. We propose that transcendental philosophy (i.e. a theory of general features of any experience) is the adequate conceptual framework to make sense of the patients' disturbed mine-ness of experience, disturbed capacity to differentiate between me and not me, experience of fragmented identity, time and unity of experience.

Ichstörungen - auf der Suche nach einer Theorie

Zusammenfassung: Bestimmte Äußerungen Schizophener, die fremdartig und nicht nachvollziehbar klingen und Veränderungen des eigenen Erlebens betreffen, sollten nicht als Wahn (wie beispielsweise im DSM-III), sondern als "Ichstörungen" bezeichnet werden. Den Ichstörungen wurde innerhalb der deutschen Psychopathologie von KARL JASPERS und KURT SCHNEIDER große Bedeutung beigemessen. Empirische Untersuchungen wurden in jüngerer Zeit u.a. von SCHARFETTER durchgeführt. Dennoch gibt es bis heute keine Theorie der Ichstörungen, die zu explizieren vermag, was mit "Ich" gemeint ist und welche Eigenschaften als gestört beschrieben werden. Nach unserer Auffassung stellt die Transzendentalphilosophie (als Theorie der Strukturmomente von Erfahrung überhaupt) den adäquaten begrifflichen Rahmen zur Beschreibung pathologisch veränderter Erfahrung dar, d.h. zur Beschreibung von Erlebnissen gestörter Meinhaftigkeit der Erfahrung, gestörter Fähigkeit zur Abgrenzung "Ich - Anderes" sowie von Erlebnissen fragmentierter Identität, Zeit oder Einheit der Erfahrung.

References

AMERICAN PSYCHIATRIC ASSOCIATION (1987): Diagnostic and Statistical Manual of Mental Disorders, 3rd. Ed., revised (DSM-III-R). Washington DC.

BLANKENBURG, W. (1988): Zur Psychopathologie des Ich-Erlebens. (this volume).

CARNAP, R. (1979): Der logische Aufbau der Welt. Ullstein, Frankfurt a.M.

CRAMER, W. (1975): Grundlegung einer Theorie des Geistes. Klostermann, Frankfurt a.M.

DREVER, J., FRÖHLICH, W.D. (1972): Wörterbuch zur Psychologie. 7. Ed. dtv., München.

ERIKSON, E.H. (1966): Identität und Lebenszyklus. Suhrkamp, Frakfurt a.M.

Feldmann, H. (1958): Zur phänomenologische Strukturanalyse der Störungen des Ichbewußtseins. Archiv für Psychiatrie **198**, pp. 96-102.

Freeman, A.M., Melges, F.T. (1977): Depersonalization and Temporal Disorganization in Acute Mental Illness. American Journal of Psychiatry **134**, pp. 679-681.

Freeman, A.M., Melges, F.T. (1978): Temporal Disorganization, Depersonalization and Persecutory Ideation in Acute Mental Illness. American Journal of Psychiatry **135**, pp. 123-124.

Fischer, S. (1929): Zeitstruktur und Schizophrenie. Zeitschrift f.d.ges. Neurol. Psychiat. 121, pp. 544-574.

Husserl, E. (1973): Zur Phänomenologie der Intersubjektivität, vol. III (Ed.: I. Kern), Husserliana XV, Nijhoff, Haag.

Husserl, E. (1973): Cartesianische Meditationen und Pariser Vorträge, (Ed.: S. Strasser), Husserliana I, Nijhoff, Haag.

Jaspers, K. (1973): Allgemeine Psychopathologie, 9. Ed. Springer, Berlin.

Kant, I. (1783/1976). Kritik der reinen Vernunft. Meiner, Hamburg.

Maher, B.A. (1988): Language Disorders in Psychoses and Their Impact on Delusions. (this volume).

Melges, F.T., Tinklenberg, J.R., Hollister, L.E., Gillespie, H.K. (1970): Temporal Disintegration and Depersonalization During Marihuana Intoxication. Arch. Gen Psychiat. **23**, pp. 204-210.

Melges, F.T., Freeman, A.M. (1978): Temporal Disorganization and Inner-Outer Confusion in Acute Mental Illness. American Journal of Psychiatry **134**, pp. 874-877.

Mullen, P.E. (1986): The mental state and states of the mind. In: Hill, P., Murray, R., Thorley, A. (eds.): Essentials of Postgraduate Psychiatry, pp. 3-36. Grune and Stratton, London, Orlando, New York, San Diego, Boston, San Francisco, Tokyo, Sydney, Toronto.

Murray, R. (1986): Schizophrenia. In: Hill, P., Murray, R., Thorley, A. (eds.): Essentials of Postgraduate Psychiatry, pp. 339-379. Grune and Stratton, London, Orlando, New York, San Diego, Boston, San Francisco, Tokyo, Sydney, Toronto.

Oltmanns, T.S. (1988): Approaches to the definition and study of delusions. In. Oltmanns, T.S., Maher, B.A. (eds.): Delusional Beliefs, pp. 3-11, Wiley, New York, Chichester, Brisbane, Toronto, Singapore.

Scharfetter, C. (1983): Schizophrene Menschen. Urban und Schwarzenberg, München.

Scharfetter, C., Brauchli, B., Weber, A. (1982): Ich-psychopathologie des schizophrenen Syndroms. Nervenarzt **53**, pp. 262-267.

Schneider, K. (1957): Primäre und sekundäre Symptome bei der Schizophrenie. Fortschr. Neurol. Psychiatr. **25**, pp. 487-490.

Schneider, K. (1980): Klinische Psychopathologie, 12th ed. Thieme, Stuttgart.

Spitzer, M. (1985): Allgemeine Subjektivität und Psychopathologie. Haag und Herchen, Frankfurt a.M.

Spitzer, M. (1987): Pseudohalluzinationen. Fortschr. Neurol. Psychiatr. **55**, pp. 91-97.

Spitzer, M. (1988): Halluzinationen. Springer, Berlin, Heidelberg, New York, London, Paris, Tokyo.

Uehlein, F.A. (1988): Bewußtsein und Selbstbewußtsein. (this volume).

Zur Psychopathologie des Ich-Erlebens Schizophrener

W. Blankenburg

1. Einleitung: Die basalen Ambiguitäten des Ich-Erlebens und Kurt Schneiders Konzeption der Ichstörungen

Welches Interesse hat die Psychopathologie am Ich-Erleben?[1] Der vorgegebene Rahmen für diese Erörterungen ist begrenzt. In anderem Zusammenhang habe ich mich mit normalen und pathologischen Abwandlungen der Subjektivität des Subjekts befaßt (Blankenburg 1987b).[2] - Hier soll in erster Linie von den schizophrenen Ich-Störungen (im engeren Sinne des Wortes) die Rede sein. In seiner *Klinischen Psychopathologie* schrieb Kurt Schneider:

> "Unter den Grundeigenschaften des Erlebens sind gewisse Störungen des *Ich-Erlebnisses* von größter schizophrener Spezifität und zwar meinen wir jene Störungen der Ichhaftigkeit oder Meinhaftigkeit, die darin bestehen, daß die eigenen Akte und Zustände nicht als solche *eigene*, sondern *von andern* gelenkte und beeinflußte erlebt werden... Ihre Erfassung wird dadurch erschwert, daß die normal-psychologischen Kriterien des Ich-Erlebnisses kaum eindeutig beschreibbar sind ..." (Schneider 1955, S.134).

Welches sind die normalpsychologischen Kriterien des Ich-Erlebens? Was heißt in diesem Zusammenhang überhaupt "Ich-Erleben"? Das Wort "Erleben" ist nicht mit Leben gleichzusetzen, aber auch nicht mit Wahrnehmung oder Vorstellung. Wir nehmen unser Ich nicht wahr, wie wir einen Tisch oder einen Stuhl oder einen anderen Menschen wahrnehmen. Wir haben es uns nicht

---

1 Das Problem, dem wir hier begegnen, bekundet sich schon im sprachlichen Ausdruck: Wenn von "Ich-Erleben"(="Erleben *des* Ichs") die Rede ist: im Sinne eines Genitivus subjectivus oder objectivus? Offenkundig ist beides gemeint, obschon sich nicht beides *zugleich* vergegenwärtigen läßt. Beides gehört sich ausschließenden Seins- und Zeitigungsweisen an. Dies bedeutet, daß es sich um einen jener "zwittrigen" Sachverhalte handelt, die für eine an der Subjekt-Objekt-Relation orientierte, zweiwertige Logik nicht faßbar sind. Ob dies mit einer mehrwertigen (polykontexturalen, nichtaristotelischen) Logik eher möglich ist (Günther 1978, Mittenauer 1980), ist eine interessante, nachgehenswerte Frage, die hier offenbleiben muß. Die genannten Autoren sprechen (wie der ganz anders denkende V.v. Weizsäcker) von einem "Grundverhältnis".

2 Dies geschah im Rahmen einer interdisziplinären japanisch-deutschen Tagung in Nagoya 1986 mit dem Thema *Das Selbst in östlicher und westlicher Sicht*. Die eigenen Ausführungen hierzu konzentrierten sich auf das Verhältnis zwischen einem voregologischen "Von-Selbst-Sein" (d.h. einer vorreflexiven, naturwüchsigen Spontaneität) und einem egologisch strukturierten (reflexiven) Selbstsein; mit anderen Worten: zwischen einer anonymen Spontaneität der Natur und einer ichhaften Spontaneität i.S. einer konstituierenden Subjektivität (vgl. dazu Blankenburg 1987b).

gegenüber. Einerseits *sind* wir unser Ich. Andererseits können wir *darüber* sprechen, fast wie über einen "Anderen", "Fremden". Identität und Differenz zeigen sich in Bezug auf unser Ich eigentümlich ineinander verschränkt. Bei allen anderen Wahrnehmungen setzen wir das Wahrgenommene als bereits existent voraus. Ist aber unser Ich ein "Ich", ohne daß es - zumindest mitunter - *sich* "weiß" (nicht nur: *von* sich weiß)? Ist das Ich etwas, was schlicht vorhanden ist, was sich lediglich in bestimmten ("reflexiven") Momenten außerdem auch noch wahrzunehmen vermag? Oder bringt es zugleich *mit* der Wahrnehmung seiner selbst (durch einen Akt, den Fichte "Tathandlung" nannte) sich allererst hervor? Die Erfahrung zeigt, daß wir auf uns selbst als bereits vorhandene reflektieren können; so zum Beispiel in der Form von Selbstbeurteilungen, wenn wir sagen: "Ich tauge nichts" oder "Ich war mal wieder in Form" o.ä. Aber es gibt noch eine andere - *unmittelbarere* - Form des "Um-sich-Wissens" und damit zugleich eines Wissens um die Urheberschaft seelischer Akte wie auch um die Grenzen des eigenen Ichs.

Kimura (1986) unterscheidet (in Fortsetzung früherer Erörterungen über "Identität und Differenz als Momente des Selbstseins" (1984), an Arbeiten von M. Nagai anknüpfend) zwischen einer *sukzessiven* (d.h. nachfolgenden) und einer *simultanen* Reflexion. Erstere sei die Form der Reflexion, die jeder Mensch kenne, der über sich nachdenke; die an zweiter Stelle genannte, beschwöre dagegen etwas herauf, was als ein Widerspruch in sich selbst angesehen werden könne. Aus dieser zuletzt genannten Reflexivität leiten Kimura und Nagai die schizophrenen Ich-Störungen ab.

Die sukzessive Reflexion bezieht sich auf einen mehr oder weniger feststehenden Inhalt (im Sinne von Selbstbeurteilungen): "Ich bin so und so ...". Daß ein solches Reflektieren nicht gemeint ist, betonte auch Schneider: "Zuerst muß man hier beachten, daß es sich beim Ich-Erlebnis nicht um das Erkennen, Bewerten, Bespiegeln der eigenen Persönlichkeit handelt, sondern um etwas Formales." - Was ist mit diesem "Formalen" gemeint ?

Was Kurt Schneider unter "formalen Kriterien" des Ich-Erlebens verstand - er bevorzugte den Begriff "Ich-Erlebnis" gegenüber dem (mit mehr Äquivokationen belasteten) Begriff "Ich-Bewußtsein" - geht aus seiner Aufzählung derselben hervor.

Vier Kriterien übernahm er von Jaspers:

1. Ich-Bewußtsein im Gegensatz zu Außen und Anderen,
2. Tätigkeitsgefühl ("Vollzugsbewußtsein" bei Jaspers),
3. Bewußtsein der Identität im Zeitverlauf,
4. Bewußtsein der Einfachheit im Augenblick.

Von sich aus fügte Schneider hinzu:

5. Existenzbewußtsein; eine Ergänzung, die Jaspers in der 4.Auflage seiner *Allgemeinen Psychopathologie* unter dem Titel "Daseinsbewußtsein" übernahm.[3]

---

3 Scharfetter (1982, 1985) entwickelte in neuerer Zeit eine (nur zum Teil sich daran anschließende) Konzeption von fünf verschiedenen Dimensionen bzw. Modalitäten des "Ichs". Er bezeichnet sie als "Konstrukt", obwohl sie phänomenologischen Analysen entstammt (vgl. dazu die Kritik von Spitzer 1985). Die Verwendung des Begriffs "Konstrukt" spiegelt die auch sonst in der Literatur zu findende Ambitendenz wider, das "Ich" entweder als vorfindlichen Erlebnistatbestand oder aber als theoretisches Konstrukt zu fassen. In dieser Zwiespältigkeit manifestiert sich nicht nur ein methodologisches Problem, sondern auch eine in der Sache selbst begründete Ambiguität. (Können wir doch fragen: Inwieweit ist unser "Ich" etwas schlicht *Vor*findliches, inwieweit ist es das, wozu wir es erst "machen" [sei es aus uns selbst heraus, sei es gesellschaftsbestimmt]). Ob die Verwendung von phänomenologisch Gefundenem als "Konstrukt" für empirische Untersuchungen gemäß der Kritik von Spitzer (1985) in *jedem* Fall auf den Versuch hinauslaufen muß, zuvor versteckte "Ostereier" durch ein entsprechend generiertes Forschungsdesign dort wieder zu finden, wo sie zuvor versteckt wurden, möchte ich bezweifeln.

2. "Vollzugsbewußtsein", "Meinhaftigkeit" und "Interpenetranz"

Bei der Durchmusterung dieser fünf Kriterien werden für Schneider im Hinblick auf differentialdiagnostische Verwertbarkeit in erster Linie Veränderungen im "Tätigkeitsgefühl" relevant.

Er bevorzugt den Terminus Erlebnis der "Meinhaftigkeit"[4], weil man bei einem Gefühlserlebnis, auch bei manchen Denkerlebnissen, wohl kaum von "Aktivität" reden könne. Jaspers hatte von "Vollzugsbewußtsein" gesprochen. Fraglich ist, was größere Beachtung beansprucht: Aktivität/Passivität[5] oder die Frage der Mirzugehörigkeit Es ist fraglich, ob das, was wir als "schizophrene" Ich-Störungen kennen, allein vom Begriff der "Meinhaftigkeit" her zureichend anzugehen ist, ebenso wie das Stichwort "Aktivität" zu kurz greift. Als ein weiteres Kriterium soll daher das Erleben - nicht der Richtung, Stärke (Dynamik) oder Zugehörigkeit, sondern - der *Unmittelbarkeit* des gespürten Wirkens genannt werden. Es ist das, was Schizophrene veranlaßt, ihr Erleben in die Nähe von "Magie" oder "Fernsteuerung" zu rücken bzw. mit einem von daher genommenen Vokabular zu beschreiben.

Gemeint sind die bekannten Klagen Schizophrener darüber, daß ihnen bestimmte Bewegungen, Handlungen, Impulse, Gefühle, Gedanken usw. "gemacht" würden, - daß sie es nicht selber seien, die dies alles steuerten, sondern fremde Mächte oder sogar bestimmte Personen.

So sagte mir ein Patient noch vor wenigen Tagen, alle seine Handlungen, Gefühle und Gedanken würden nicht nur ständig "kontrolliert", sondern auch "geführt". Sie würden ihm abgenommen, ihm "gemacht", und zwar in erster Linie von einer Frau (deren Stimme er halluziniert). Er selbst könne darauf keinen Einfluß nehmen. Der Patient erlebt dies zwiespältig: einerseits sei es für ihn entlastend und tröstlich, daß ihm alle Verantwortung für seine Handlungen, Gefühle, Gedanken usf. abgenommen werde, zumal dies auf eine sehr wohlwollende Weise geschähe; andererseits erlebe er es aber nicht nur als fremdartig, sondern zugleich auch als entmündigend und entmächtigend. - Manchmal habe er dagegen das Gefühl, er könne nicht nur die Gedanken anderer lesen, sondern auch unmittelbar lenken; ein "ganz eigentümliches Gefühl", wie er selbst feststellt.

Wenn man zu einem adäquaten Verständnis der Veränderungen, die wir als "schizophrene Ich-Störungen" bezeichnen, kommen will, ist es daher vernünftig, nicht nur die von den Patienten geschilderten Phänomene des "Gemacht-Bekommens" zu berücksichtigen, sondern auch die - selteneren - eines abnormen "*Machen*"-Könnens (d.h. das von starker subjektiver Evidenz getragene Gefühl, z.B. den Straßenverkehr, das Wetter oder das Verhalten anderer Menschen unmittelbar zu steuern oder sogar "zu machen"). Dann zeigt sich, daß nicht die "Meinhaftigkeit" und nicht die Stärke oder Schwäche des Aktivitätsgefühls, nicht

4 Bei Gruhle (1932, S. 188ff) findet sich der Begriff "Ichgehalt". Neben "Ichstörung" spricht er auch von "Ichlähmung". Unter Zugrundelegung des topologischen Konzepts von Lewin haben Conrad (1958) und - differenzierter - Kisker (1960) die Ich-Störungen Schizophrener als "Wandlungen der Selbstverfügbarkeit" analysiert. Glatzel (1981) interpretierte sie unter den Gesichtspunkten einer "Interaktionalen Psychopathologie". - Wichtig ist, darauf hinzuweisen, daß ein Fehlen "erlebter Ich-Qualität" und ein Ausbleiben "reflektierter Ich-Zuschreibung" sich keineswegs stets decken müssen (Janzarik 1988). Zu den typischen "Ich-Störungen" Schizophrener gehört allerdings (im Gegensatz zu den uncharakteristischen Entfremdungssyndromen), daß beides gleichsinnig ausbleibt.

5 Zu erinnern ist hier an Berze (1914) und an all jene Konzeptionen, die in der Schizophrenie vornehmlich eine Intentionalitätsstörung sehen (vgl. Mundt 1984, 1987, 1988).

Macht oder Ohnmacht ("Entmächtigungsgefühl"[6]) das allein Entscheidende sind, sondern darüber hinaus ganz wesentlich die *Unmittelbarkeit* der vom Patienten gespürten Art des "Wirkens": "Sein" und "Wirken" konfluieren für ihn miteinander.

In der akuten Psychose kommt es sogar vor, daß ein Patient glaubt, das Fortbestehen der Welt hänge von ihm ab, z.B. davon, ob er selbst weiter atme, dies oder jenes tue usw. Der maximalen Enteignung der Intentionalität als eigener steht hier ein Omnipotenzerleben gegenüber, das sich als Kehrseite der absoluten Selbstentmächtigung darstellt. Von manischen Größenideen unterscheidet es sich durch die *Unmittelbarkeit,* mit der erlebt wird, alles in der Außenwelt Begegnende gleichsam "magisch" steuern zu können, oft auch durch das Fehlen bzw. die Abspaltung eines dazu kongruenten Affektes (d.h. eines entspr. Größengefühls). Der Autor (BLANKENBURG 1962) hat von einem "Transitiv"-Werden des "ist" - seltener des "bin" - für das eigene Erleben des Patienten gesprochen: sowohl des Seins des (z.B. als bedrohlich) Begegnenden als auch des eigenen Seins. PAUL FEDERN beschrieb dies (1926/1952) als ein Durchlässigwerden der "Ich-Grenzen" (vgl. dazu BENEDETTI 1987). SCHARFETTER (1985) unterscheidet im Rahmen seiner Differenzierung von fünf Ich-Dimensionen bzw. "-Konstrukten" (s. Anm. 3) unter anderen "Ich-Aktivität" und "Ich-Demarkation".

3. "Vollzugsbewußtsein", "Meinhaftigkeit", "Interpenetranz": Inhalt oder Form des Erlebens oder Verschränkung von beidem?

Den Begriff der "Meinhaftigkeit" - GRUHLE sprach von "Ichgehalt" - setzte KURT SCHNEIDER an die Stelle des Begriffs einer Störung des "Vollzugsbewußtseins" (JASPERS), weil nicht alle in Betracht kommenden seelischen Regungen den Charakter einer Aktivität trügen. Offenkundig wurde dieser Terminus durch HEIDEGGERS Konzeption einer "Jemeinigkeit" des Daseins (1927, S. 41 ff., 187 ff., 221, 240, 263, 278ff, 297ff) angeregt.

Aber gegen die Bedeutung der "Meinhaftigkeit" kann man einwenden, daß beim Gefühl des "Machen-" und "Beherrschen"könnens (das nicht weniger zu den Ichstörungen gehört als das des "Gemacht"bekommens) nicht nur kein Daniederliegen (vielmehr eine Steigerung) des Tätigkeitkeitsgefühls vorliegt, sondern auch keine Beeinträchtigung (vielmehr eher eine Erweiterung) der "Meinhaftigkeit", obgleich die Zueinandergehörigkeit beider Veränderungen des Erlebens ganz offenkundig ist. In beiden Fällen zeigt sich der Ich-Umwelt-Bezug in einer charakteristischen Weise qualitativ verändert. Nicht die Richtung, nicht wer von beiden als mächtiger erlebt wird, nicht einseitig die Meinhaftigkeit im Erleben ist betroffen, sondern die Grenze zwischen "mein" und "dein" (bzw. der Außenwelt) ist das Entscheidende, aber auch nicht *nur* die Grenze, sondern die Art und Weise, *wie* sie überschritten wird. Man könnte versucht sein, hierfür den

6 Vgl. BINSWANGER (1957), CONRAD (1958) KISKER (1960) u.a. GLATZEL (1971) hebt am "Entmächtigungserlebnis" auf die "radikale Alternativlosigkeit als Ausdruck einer "rigide[n] und hinsichtlich ihrer thematischen Relevanz fixierte[n] Situationsdefinition" ab.

Begriff der "*Interpenetranz*"[7] zu verwenden. Dies war es, wie gesagt, was den Autor (vgl. BLANKENBURG 1962) vor langer Zeit davon sprechen ließ, daß von Schizophrenen mit Ichstörungen (freilich zumeist nur in bestimmten Bereichen) das Intransitivum "sein" *transitiv* erlebt werde. Das Verhältnis zwischen "sein" und "wirken" hat sich für sie (partiell) verändert. Die Charakterisierung dieser Veränderung als eines Durchlässigwerdens der "Ichgrenzen" (FEDERN) erweist sich somit, wie schon WEITBRECHT (1973) einräumte, gegenüber derjenigen eines Verlusts der "Meinhaftigkeit" letztlich als die treffendere. Was allerdings "Ichgrenzen" sind, wie sie sich konstituieren und wodurch sie sich abwandeln, ist bis heute noch wenig geklärt.[8]

Der Autor (BLANKENBURG 1962) hat hierfür, den Begriff einer "transzendentalen Organisation"[9] geprägt. Damit war keine theoretisch hypostasierte Instanz gemeint, sondern das durch *deskriptive* Analysen herauszuarbeitende Gefüge der Bedingungen der Möglichkeit der Erfahrung (im Sinne KANTS) unter Einbeziehung schizophrenen Erlebens. Das Problem des Hinüberwechselns von der Reflexion auf die "Möglichkeit" zum Konstatieren der "Wirklichkeit" psychotischer Erlebnisweisen und vice versa - wie auch des Verhältnisses beider zueinander - ist hier nicht zu erörtern.

SPITZER (1985, 1988) ist der Auffassung, die "Meinhaftigkeit" seelischer Abläufe (z.B. von Gedanken, Gefühlen usw.) werde gar nicht "erlebt", sondern *gehöre zur Struktur* der erfahrenden und denkenden Subjektivität. Er kritisiert an SCHNEIDER, daß dieser (entgegen seiner eigenen Behauptung, wonach die Ich-Störungen nichts Inhaltliches, sondern nur etwas Formales beträfen) das "Meinhafte" in seinen weiteren Ausführungen gerade nicht als "formal", sondern als "erlebte" Qualität auffasse. Demgegenüber vertritt er selbst sehr entschieden die These, daß wir es dabei mit einem Strukturmerkmal zu tun hätten. Handelt es sich bei dieser Gegenüberstellung: "erlebter Inhalt" *oder* "formale Struktur" (Struktur *oder* Gegenstand des Erlebens) um eine echte Alternative? Ich meine, daß dem nicht so ist, daß es vielmehr etwas *Drittes* gibt.

Die These von SPITZER (1985): "Alle meine Gedanken sind meine Gedanken, sonst wären sie überhaupt nicht" (SPITZER 1985, S. 210), mit der er den transzendental-formalen Charakter des Ich-Bezugs begründet, entspricht KANTS Ausführungen zur "transzendentalen Apperzeption":

"Das: *Ich denke*, muß alle meine Vorstellungen begleiten *können*; denn sonst würde etwas in mir vorgestellt werden, was garnicht gedacht werden könnte ..." (KANT, B131/132). Daß dies unserer traditionellen Auffassung entspricht, steht außer Frage. Für uns ist aber wichtig, wie es *für* denjenigen sich ausnimmt, der diese Gedanken "hat". Daß Zwangsgedanken kein Gegenargument hergeben, ist mit Recht oft genug hervorgehoben worden. Sie drängen sich uns zwar auf. Aber dennoch sind *wir* es - wenn auch unfreiwillig-, die nicht aufhören können, sie zu denken. Sobald ein Patient sagt, die Gedanken, zu denen er sich zuvor nur zwanghaft gedrängt fühlt, würden ihm "eingegeben", ihm "gemacht" oder von anderen "gelenkt", ändern wir die Diagnose. Dennoch: Gibt es hinsichtlich der "Meinhaftigkeit" von Gedanken nicht schon bei Gesunden - wenn auch noch so feine - graduelle Unterschiede im Sinne eines Mehr oder Minder? Eindrucksvoll sind transkulturelle Vergleiche zwischen fernöstlichem und euro-

---

7 Wie ich im nachhinein feststelle, verwendet LUHMANN (1988) diesen Begriff neuerdings mit ganz anderer Bedeutung im Rahmen systemtheoretischer Überlegungen.

8 Das Konzept der zwölf "Ego functions" von BELLAK et al. (1973) führt im Hinblick auf die schizophrenen Ichstörungen meines Erachtens nicht entscheidend über die Konzeption von FEDERN (1952) hinaus.

9 Vgl. auch BLANKENBURG 1965a, 1971, wo sich die eingehendsten Analysen der mit diesem Terminus bezeichneten Strukturen finden. Wenn der Terminus später nicht mehr verwendet wurde, so nicht aus sachlichen Gründen, sondern weil er zu mißverständlich ist.

päischem Selbst- bzw. Ich-Erleben (vgl. Anm. 2). Die typischen schizophrenen Erlebnisse eines "Gemachtbekommens" überschreiten freilich dieses Spektrum gradueller Unterschiede, welches wir bei Gesunden finden. Von daher ist es zu verstehen, daß SCHNEIDER die von ihm gesuchte *qualitative* Differenz zwischen Nichtschizophrenem und Schizophrenem besonders an den "Ichstörungen" glaubte festmachen zu können. Aber gerade dieses Symptom erlaubt in anderen Kulturen, in denen das Erleben von Verhexung, Anhexung, "bösem Blick", Besessenheit, von magischem Beeinflußtwerden und Beeinflussenkönnen endemisch ist, keineswegs eine so klare und eindeutige Abgrenzung wie bei uns.[10]

Inwieweit alles Denken "Denken eines Ich" ist, wird nicht erst in unserem Jahrhundert kontrovers diskutiert. Die Bedeutung, die dem "ego" im "ego cogito" DESCARTES' zuzusprechen ist, war schon früh ein Gegenstand von Auseinandersetzungen. Von LICHTENBERG stammt die Bemerkung, statt "ich denke" könne man ebensogut sagen "es denkt" - wie man sage, "es blitzt". F.v.BAADER ging so weit, dem "cogito ergo sum" DESCARTES' ein "cogit*or* ergo sum" entgegenzuhalten. Hierbei kann einem jener eindrucksvolle Traum C.G. JUNGS (1962, S. 326) einfallen, in dem er sich - sein gesamtes Sein - von einem Yogi meditiert erlebte: "Ich erschrak zutiefst und erwachte an dem Gedanken: Ach so, das ist der, der mich meditiert. Er hat einen Traum, und das bin ich". In einer poetischen Form finden wir Ähnliches in dem berühmten Schmetterlingstraum des Dschuang Dsi.

Reicht die Akzentuierung der Einzigartigkeit der Erfahrung des "Ich denke" auch bis DESCARTES zurück, so kulminierte sie doch erst in der Transzendentalphilosophie um 1800. Nicht nur in der Philosophie, auch in der Dichtung fand die "Manifestation des Selbstbewußtseins im 'Ich bin'" mannigfaltigen Niederschlag (vgl. UEHLEIN 1982). Aufschlußreich ist in dieser Hinsicht der von WUTHENOW (1974) herausgegebene Band "Das erinnerte Ich". Entsprechende Kindheitserinnerungen wurden wichtig. Ein besonders eindrucksvolles Beispiel bietet die bekannte Selbstschilderung JEAN PAULS (1826/28, S. 53), in der das erste Aufblitzen des "Ich bin ein Ich" als eine im "verhangenen Allerheiligsten des Menschen vorgefallene Begebenheit" gefeiert wird. Der "Deus absconditus" wurde vom "Ego absconditus" abgelöst; so wie später die Proklama- tion vom "Tod Gottes" durch die vom "Tod des Subjekts" abgelöst wurde (vgl. BLANKENBURG 1987).[11]

In unserem Jahrhundert spielt die Frage, ob jedem Denken ein Ich zugrunde liege oder ob das "Ich" erst ein Produkt der durch das Denken (und andere Faktoren) bedingten Zweiteilung alles für uns Seienden in "Ich" und "Welt" sei - das Denken also hinter diese Dichotomie zurückreiche und daher gerade nicht rein ichlicher Natur sein könne -, eine nicht unerhebliche Rolle; dies nicht erst unter dem Motto "Tod des Subjekts" (vgl. NAGL-DOCEKAL und VETTER 1987), sondern bereits in der älteren Phänomenologie, z.B. im Briefwechsel zwischen ALFRED SCHÜTZ und AARON GURWITSCH (GRATHOFF 1985).

Die Mehrzahl der heutigen Auffassungen steht in einer klaren Gegenposition zur Transzendentalphilosophie FICHTES und des frühen SCHELLING ("Das Ich als Prinzip der Philosophie") wie auch zur transzendentalen Egologie HUSSERLS. Es ist die alte (schon in Indien gestellte) Frage nach dem Denker des Denkens, die hier in skeptischer Version neu aufgegriffen wird. Daß ein Denken nicht ohne Gedachtes vorstellbar ist, ist evident. Aber ist das Zurückführen jedes Denkens auf einen Denker - "Ich" genannt - ebenso evident? Könnte es

10 Es ist, von daher gesehen, zweifhaft, ob die von KURT SCHNEIDER betonte Trennschärfe der Ich-Störungen (als "Symptome 1. Ranges") eine so universelle Gültigkeit beanspruchen kann, wie es nach seinen Formulierungen den Anschein hat. Gehört es am Ende zur Eigenart der westlichen Bewußtseinsentwicklung, daß sich schizophrenes Erleben von ihr signifikanter abhebt als von einem weniger *ich*zentrierten Bewußtsein, wie es z.B. im asiatischen Kulturkreis begegnet (vgl. WULFF 1967). Inwieweit transkulturelle Differenzen tatsächlich auf (soziokulturell oder biologisch bedingte) Unterschiede der Erkrankung, inwieweit sie nur auf die unterschiedliche Abhebbarkeit von den jeweiligen (soziokulturell bedingt unterschiedlichen) *Normal*verfassungen zu beziehen sind, muß vorerst offen bleiben. Es ist bis heute nicht endgültig geklärt, ob die Unterschiede in der Art der Erkrankung als solcher zu suchen sind oder ob dafür eher Unterschiede in der Bewußtseins- bzw. Selbstbewußtseinsbildung der Gesunden verantwortlich zu machen sind.) Transkulturelle, epidemiologische Untersuchungen der WHO (vgl. HÄFNER 1987, SARTORIUS et al. 1987, ZUBIN 1987) sprechen eher für letzteres. Im DSM-III spielen die Ichstörungen eine relativ geringe Rolle. - Zur angedeuteten differentialdiagnostischen und anthropologischen Fragestellung wäre aus der älteren Literatur vor allem auf Devereux zu verweisen, aus der neueren auf DITTRICH (1985).

11 Über eine ähnliche Selbstentdeckung des "Ichs" bei einem Kleinkind unseres Jahrhunderts berichtet WYRSCH (1956, S. 51).

sich dabei vielleicht nur einen Rückschluß bzw. eine Art Rückprojektion handeln?[12] Ist am Ende die These KANTS: "Das stehende und bleibende Ich macht das Korrelatum aller unserer Vorstellungen aus" (KANT A 123) an eine bestimmte soziokulturelle Entwicklungsstufe der Menschheit gebunden? Daß KANT dieses Primat dem "Ich" nicht nur in erkenntnistheoretischer, sondern auch in anthropologischer Hinsicht einräumte, zeigen die bekannten Worte zu Beginn der "Anthropologie in pragmatischer Hinsicht" (1798, S. 127): "Daß der Mensch in seiner Vorstellung das Ich haben kann, erhebt ihn unendlich über alle andere auf Erden lebenden Wesen".

Ist nach alldem die Gegenüberstellung von Erlebnis*inhalt* und formaler "Struktur der erfahrenden und denkenden Subjektivität" (SPITZER) eine echte Alternative? Ich meine: Nein. Die Gegenüberstellung von "Form" und "Inhalt" ist in Frage zu stellen. Der Rückschluß auf eine rein formale (apriorische) Struktur entspricht einem Reflexionsstandpunkt, der meines Erachtens die dynamische Dialektik des Selbstverhältnisses nicht hinreichend berücksichtigt. Statt dessen könnte gerade in einer *andersartigen Verschränkung* von Form und Inhalt das Spezifische dieses Erlebens zu suchen sein. - Der Satz "Alle meine Gedanken sind meine Gedanken, sonst wären sie überhaupt nicht" ist kein apriori gültiger Satz, sondern ein Postulat, dessen Gültigkeit - wie das Erleben Schizophrener (aber nicht *nur* Schizophrener) zeigt - begrenzt ist.

4. Grundsätzliche Überlegungen zum Ich-Bezug

Führt die Reflexion auf ein transzendentales "Ich" erkenntnistheoretisch notwendigerweise zu einem Solipsismus, zumindest zu einem Perspektivismus - und auf der psycho(patho)logischen Ebene: zum Narzißmus oder gar zum Autismus? Dies wäre der Fall, wenn die Subjektivität des menschlichen Subjekts in nichts anderem bestünde als einer vorgegebenen (als gegeben hinzunehmenden) Bezogenheit von allem Begegnenden einschließlich seiner selbst auf sich selbst. Dies ist jedoch nicht der Fall: Die Subjektivität des Subjekts besteht weder in diesem einzigen Sachverhalt der Selbstbezogenheit noch ist sie ausschließlich eine vorgegebene. Sie erweist sich vielmehr als "aufgespalten" in zwei einander polar entgegengesetzt ausgerichtete Komponenten (BLANKENBURG 1987a,b): Diese bestehen darin, daß einerseits in der Tat jedes Subjekt an seine eigene Vorgegebenheit gebunden ist (z.B. an seinen Standort, an das Milieu, in dem es aufgewachsen ist, an seinen genetischen Code, d.h. seine mitgebrachte Anlage). Diese Vorgegebenheiten machen die Faktizität und die Kontingenz des menschlichen Daseins aus.

Gäbe es nur diesen *einen* Aspekt der Subjektivität des Subjekts, wäre am Solipsismus - zumindest am Perspektivismus - menschlichen Erlebens gar nicht zu zweifeln. Wir wären gänzlich darin gefangen. Wodurch unterschiede sich dann noch die "condition humaine" des seelisch Gesunden vom Autismus eines Schizophrenen? Sie unterscheidet sich davon, weil zur Subjektivität des Subjekts

12 Vgl. NAGL-DOCEKAL und VETTER (1987); ferner aus der sehr umfangreichen Diskussion um den Stellenwert des Subjekts, des "Ich" und des "Selbst": HAUG 1985, HENRICH 1982, HOLENSTEIN 1986, CRAMER 1987, SANCHEZ 1986, die Autoren der sog. "Postmoderne" einerseits, der Systemtheorie (z.B. LUHMANN 1988, DELL 1986) andererseits. Im Hinblick auf unser Thema ist aus der älteren Literatur der in seiner Art originelle Versuch über das "Sichselbstverstehen" von GÜNTHER (1934) von Interesse.

- in komplementärer Gegenläufigkeit - noch etwas anderes als Subjektbezogenheit gehört: die Fähigkeit, sich selbst zu bewegen, quasi sich von sich selbst wegzubewegen, z.B. sich auf andere zu beziehen und sogar sich in andere "hineinzuversetzen" und bis zu einem gewissen - wenn auch noch so geringen - Grade sich selbst zu verändern.

Der Standort, an dem ich stehe, bleibt nicht mein Standort. Ich kann ihn - und zwar für mich selbst durchsichtig - verändern. Ich kann alsdann auf ihn zurückschauen, kann ihn mit anderen Stand orten vergleichen und somit *relativieren*. Die Standortgebundenheit menschlicher Sicht wird partiell aufgehoben durch die Fähigkeit, Standorte zu verändern. Somit wird auch die Relativität menschlicher "Standpunkte" -im wörtlichen und im übertragenen Sinn- noch einmal relativiert durch die Fähigkeit, sie zu verändern. Im "übertragenen" Sinn meint: Dies gilt für die gesamte Subjektivität, insoweit damit die Gebundenheit an die Faktizität der Vorgegebenheit des eigenen Seins zum Ausdruck gebracht wird. Es gilt also (freilich in einem sehr viel geringeren Umfang) auch für menschliche Eigenschaften: In dem Maße, in dem es gelingt, Eigenschaften der eigenen Person selbstdurchsichtig zu verändern, gelingt ein Stück Überwindung der Subjektivität des Subjekts. Die Relativität (und damit Subjektivität) der menschlichen Existenz kann zwar nicht rückgängig gemacht werden, aber sie kann noch einmal relativiert und dadurch partiell aufgehoben werden. Die wechselseitige Relativierung entgegengesetzter Determinanten ist ein entscheidender Kunstgriff der Natur, durch den Evolution (auf verschiedensten Ebenen) möglich wird.

So wie der Mensch die Standortbezogenheit seiner Sicht in *dem* Maße zu relativieren vermag, wie er seinen Standort autonom und selbstdurchsichtig zu verändern vermag, so ist er auch in anderen Bereichen in der Lage, seine Subjektivität (d.h. seine ausschließliche Subjektbezogenheit) ein Stück weit zu relativieren und sogar aufzuheben. Selbsttätige und zugleich selbstdurchsichtige (reafferente) Veränderung von Vorgegebenheit ist es, wodurch dies möglich wird.

Die autonome und reflexive Steuerung der Bewegung - deshalb liegt die Betonung auf *Sich*bewegen und *Sich*verändern - ist notwendig, weil nur sie Selbstdurchsichtigkeit ermöglicht, die als eine Voraussetzung für jegliches Transzendieren angesehen werden muß. Dafür liefert bereits die Wahrnehmungsphysiologie und -psychologie eindrucksvolle Belege. Dort erledigt das Reafferenzprinzip (v. Holst), was auf höheren Stufen der Organisation des Menschen von "ihm selbst" (mittels eines Sich-selbst-Durchsichtigwerdens autonomer Spontaneität) zu leisten ist. Nur dann ermöglichen Bewegen und Verändern die Überwindung der Subjektivität des Subjekts (d.h. der Subjektbezogenheit und Selbstbefangenheit) wenn sie *als* eigene, autonome (und damit potentiell selbstdurchsichtige) in den Dienst des Transzendierens gestellt werden. Oder setzen sie schon ein Transzendieren-Können voraus? Hierbei dürfte es sich um einen jener Zirkel handeln, die es nicht zu vermeiden, sondern in die es auf die rechte Weise hineinzukommen gilt.[13]

Was hat das alles mit schizophrenen Ichstörungen zu tun ? Gerade dies: der Verlust an (sich selbst durchsichtig werdender, und in diesem Sinne "reafferenter") Spontaneität ist es, was die - aus welchen Gründen auch immer entstandenen - schizophrenen Ichstörungen kennzeichnet. Es geht hier nicht um eine kausale Erklärung, sondern nur um eine Klärung der Funktionsabwandlung derselben. Spontaneität ist dabei nicht in einem naturalistischen, sondern in einem *transzendentalen* Sinn zu verstehen. Andernfalls böte sich wiederum als

13 Schon E. Straus (1963, S. 960f) vermerkte kritisch: "das Mein ist kein Urphänomen des reinen Bewußtseins, das der Welterfahrung vorangeht ...". Das "Mein" erscheine zwar bei Husserl als ein "Urdatum"; doch würden dabei "dem absoluten Bewußtsein offenbar Charaktere zugeschrieben, die von dem Menschen, als empirischem Subjekt, geborgt" seien. In Abhebung von Heidegger fügte er hinzu: "Die Individuation ist ein natürliches Verhältnis zur Welt; sie ist nicht in der Jemeinigkeit des Seins des Daseins, das sich zu seinem Sein verhält, begründet. Mit dem 'ich bin', 'ich tue' wird ein Verhältnis zur Welt zum Ausdruck gebracht, das für jeden Sprecher einzig und einmalig ist, und doch ganz allgemein für alle gilt." Dies "für alle" muß freilich - nicht nur im Hinblick auf die Ichstörungen Schizophrener - in Frage gestellt werden.

Gegenargument an, auf ein Durchlässigwerden der Ichgrenzen in umgekehrter Richtung (d.h.in der Richtung des Gefühls eines omnipotenten Machenkönnens) zu verweisen.

5. Klinische Relevanz

Wenn wir uns jetzt erneut der alltäglichen Erfahrung, die wir mit Schizophrenen machen, die unter Ichstörungen leiden, zuwenden, werden uns nicht allgemeine Wesensbestimmungen weiterhelfen, sondern in erster Linie eine Differentialphänomenologie (Blankenburg 1965b). Im Gegensatz zu den groben Kontrastierungen allgemeinerer Wesensbestimmungen und Definitionen geht es in ihr gerade um die Grenzphänomene: Was bezeichnen wir "schon" als Ichstörung und was gerade noch nicht? Dazu wird man das "Gemachtbekommen" eines Bewegungsimpulses nicht mit der selbstgesteuerten, natürlichen Bewegung eines Gesunden kontrastieren, sondern fragen, was dieses schizophrene Erleben z.B. von als ebenfalls nichtselbstgesteuert erlebten Bewegungen (z.B. einem Tic, einem Muskelfaszikulieren, oder sog. Einschlafzuckungen u.ä) erlebnismäßig unterscheidet.

Im Rahmen einer elektromyographischen Untersuchung können ja auch Gesunden Bewegungen im wörtlichsten Sinn "gemacht" werden. Denkbar wäre dies bei weiter vorangeschrittener Technik sogar auf leiterfreiem (quasi "drahtlosem") Wege. Wodurch würde sich solche Sensationen vom schizophrenen Erleben des"Gemacht-Bekommens" unterscheiden? Die Qualität des Erlebens bliebe sicherlich eine andere. Daß das "Gemachtbekommen" nicht nur als ein verdeckt beachsichtigtes, sondern auch bedeutungsvolles erlebt wird, gehört offenbar primär zum schizophrenen Erleben. Die "Absichtlichkeit" wird zumeist nicht (i.S. eines Erklärungswahnes, den es daneben freilich auch gibt) erst hintennach erschlossen, sondern in einer sehr unmittelbaren Weise vom Kranken gespürt bzw. "wahrgenommen". Dies wäre gesondert herauszuarbeiten.

Ebenso wäre in einer differenzierenden Analyse herauszuarbeiten, wodurch das Gefühl Schizophrener, "hypnotisiert" zu werden, sich von einer echten Hypnose unterscheidet. Für eine Differentialdiagnose ist dergleichen freilich kaum je erforderlich. Auch der Laie vermag zumeist ohne spezielle Kenntnisse beides auf Anhieb voneinander zu unterscheiden. Aber wodurch vermag er es? Das ist bis heute nicht hinreichend geklärt. Am ehesten ist dies hinsichtlich der notwendigen Differenzierung zwischen "Depersonalisation" und "Ichstörung" geschehen; eine Unterscheidung, die sich allerdings nur zögend durchgesetzt hat und noch bis heute in manchen Lehrbücher unterbelichtet ist, obwohl sie nicht geringe differentialdiagnostische Bedeutung besitzt. In befriedigender Weise wird dagegen zwischen Zwangsphänomenen (wie auch Drang- bzw. Durchbruchshandlungen) und Ichstörungen unterschieden. Dagegen lassen die Differenzierungen zwischen magischem Aberglauben (z.B. auch zwischen Beeinflussungserlebnissen bei sog. "Tonbandstimmenhörern", wie wir sie beobachteten) und schizophrenen Ichstörungen noch zu wünschen übrig. Mag auch die Differentialdiagnose in den meisten Fällen , aufgrund des intuitiven klinischen Gesamteindruckes leicht sein, so gibt es doch Ausnahmen. Dies gilt unter anderem auch für religiös erlebtes "Geführtwerden". Auf diesem Felde kommen Fehldiagnosen in beiderlei Richtungen vor. Eine Darstellung der einschlägigen Kasuistik würde ein weiteres Ausholen erforderlich machen und mehr Raum beanspruchen.

Mit dem hier Ausgeführten soll lediglich darauf aufmerksam gemacht werden, daß wir (trotz gegenteiliger Beteuerungen) auf dem Gebiet der Psychopathologie - speziell auch auf demjenigen der Ichstörungen - bis heute nicht davon sprechen können, "die Ernte" sei "eingebracht". Es bleibt noch genug zu tun.

Bevor wir schließen, ist in Anbetracht des hohen diffentialdiagnostischen Wertes, der den Ichstörungen von Schneider beigemessen wurde, kurz zu erörtern, inwieweit bei den übrigen "Symptomen 1. Ranges" Veränderungen des Ich-Erlebens beteiligt sein können.

"Symptome 1.Ranges" sind für Schneider bekanntlich: "Gedankenlautwerden, Hören von Stimmen in der Form von Rede und Gegenrede, Hören von Stimmen, die das eigene Tun mit Bemerkungen begleiten, leibliche Beeinflussungserlebnisse, Gedankenentzug und andere Gedankenbeeinflussungen, Gedankenausbreitung, Wahnwahrnehmung, sowie alles von andern Gemachte und Beeinflußte auf dem Gebiet des Fühlens, Strebens (der Triebe) und des Willens" (Schneider 1955, S. 146).

"Alles von andern Gemachte und Beeinflußte auf dem Gebiet des Fühlens, Strebens (der Triebe) und des Willens" (das Erleben eines abnormen, unmittelbaren Selbst-"Machen"-Könnens nennt Schneider eigentümlicherweise nicht) gehört per definitionem zu den Ichstörungen; dies wird man auch im Hinblick auf "Gedankenentzug und andere Gedankenbeeinflussungen" sagen müssen, die er gesondert aufführt. Auch "Gedankenlautwerden" und "Gedankenausbreitung" sind ohne eine Veränderung des Ich-Bezuges nicht denkbar. Hier ist auf zwei verschiedene Arten die *Privatheit* seelischen Lebens aufgehoben. Bei ersterem ist dies nur in Bezug auf das eigene Erleben der Fall, bei letzterem auch im Verhältnis zu den anderen Menschen (bzw. zur "Öffentlichkeit"). Daß beides - in unterschiedlicher Weise - eine Veränderung der "Ichgrenzen" voraussetzt, ist offenkundig. Die Frage, was es für den Gesunden bedeutet, daß er seine Gedanken nicht gleichzeitig hört, ist bisher wenig erörtert worden, wäre aber im Hinblick auf das veränderte Erleben Schizophrener von Interesse. Beim "Hören von Stimmen, die das eigene Tun mit Bemerkungen begleiten" (Kommentarstimmen) handelt es sich ganz offensichtlich um ein vom Ich-Erleben abgespaltenes Reflektieren, das den Ich-Bezug unschwer erkennen läß, aber ihn nicht als solchen aktualisiert. Das Ich taucht wie bei autistischen Kindern in der "dritten Person" auf ("Jetzt tut er" das und das ...). An die Konzeption der Ich-Anachorese von Winkler (1954) sei hier nur erinnert (das Fehlen einer psychodynamischen Brisanz des Inhalts ist prognostisch bekanntlich eher ungünstig zu beurteilen); ebenso an die Bedeutung, die gerade diese Form des Halluzinierens für die Entwicklung der psychoanalytischen Theorie für Freud hatte, worauf Spitzer (1988a, S. 203ff) noch einmal aufmerksam gemacht hat. - Beim "Hören von Stimmen in der Form von Rede und Gegenrede" ist es insbesondere die eigentümliche Form der *Anonymisierung*, auf die hinzuweisen ist. Sie muß aufgrund ihrer Erlebnisqualität unterschieden werden von der derb-drastischen, viel weniger hintergründigen Art, in der Alkoholhalluzinanten Stimmen in Rede und Gegenrede hören. Inwiefern schließlich auch "Wahnwahrnehmungen" - unabhängig davon, ob sie inhaltlich einem "Beziehungswahn" entsprechen oder nicht - eine veränderte Ich-Struktur voraussetzen, hat Spitzer (1988a,b) so eingehend diskutiert, daß es sich hier erübrigt, näher darauf einzugehen.

Zum Schluß muß noch einmal betont werden, daß keineswegs die gesamte Psychopathologie des Ich-Erlebens Schizophrener behandelt werden konnte. Erörtert wurden im wesentlichen "Vollzugsbewußtsein" (Jaspers), "Meinhaftigkeit (SCHNEIDER), "Ich-Aktivität" und "-Demarkation" (SCHARFETTER) als diejenigen Bereiche, in denen sich bei Schizophrenen die spezifischsten Veränderungen finden. Die Ebenen der "Ich-Vitalität", der Ich-Konsistenz" und der "Ich-Identität" blieben außer Betracht. Über (weniger eindeutige) Veränderungen der letzteren habe ich bereits andernorts (BLANKENBURG 1986, 1987b) einiges im Zusammenhang mit transkulturellen Überlegungen zur Diskussion gestellt. Insgesamt bedarf die Psychopathologie des Ich-Erlebens einer eingehenderen Beschäftigung, als ihr mit wenigen Ausnahmen in den vergangenen zehn Jahren zuteil wurde.

Zusammenfassung: 1. Die Frage nach Veränderungen des Ich-Erlebens wird eingegrenzt auf das Problem der "Ichstörungen" (KURT SCHNEIDER). Ein knapp umrissenes klinisches Beispiel illustriert, was gemeint ist. Das Problem der Reflexivität des Subjekts, das darin besteht, daß das "Ich" im Akt des Reflektierens sowohl Subjekt als auch Objekt ist, wird nur kurz angeschnitten, gleichwohl als Schlüssel zum Verständnis von Ichstörungen angesehen.
2. Die historische Frage, ob es sich dabei um eine Störung des Vollzugsbewußtseins (Aktivitätsgefühls) oder der (unhinterfragt als Norm gesetzten) "Meinhaftigkeit" des Erlebens handelt, wird als Alternative nicht akzeptiert. Im Hinblick darauf, daß auch das Erleben des unmittelbaren "Machen"könnens (bis hin zum Omnipotenzgefühl) den Ichstörungen zuzuzählen ist, wird auf ein drittes Kennzeichen - die "Interpenetranz", i.S. eines "Transitiv"werdens des (fremden oder seltener des eigenen) Seins - abgehoben.
3. An dritter Stelle wird die Frage diskutiert, ob Ichstörungen den Inhalt "*oder*" die Form des Erlebens betreffen. These: Sie können als ein Beleg dafür angesehen werden, daß diese Alternative der Realität seelischen Lebens nicht gerecht wird. Sie zeigen vielmehr, daß spezielle Inhalte des Erlebens zugleich einen Wandel der Struktur (Form) desselben indizieren bzw. implizieren können.
4. Dem hohen differentialdiagnostischen Stellenwert, den KURT SCHNEIDER den Ichstörungen einräumte, kann man entgegenhalten, daß er möglicherweise nur für Menschen unserer Kultur gültig ist. Transkulturelle Vergleiche (WULFF), die allerdings nicht unwidersprochen geblieben sind, lassen es möglich erscheinen, daß die differentialdiagnostische Trennschärfe weniger durch die Eigenart schizophrener Erkrankungen, als vielmehr durch die Eigenart der (durch sie besonders tangierbaren) Ichstruktur des von der westlichen Zivilisation geprägten Menschen bedingt ist. Das setzt allerdings voraus, daß die schizophrenen Erkrankungen als *eine* einheitliche, biologisch definierbare Entität angesetzt werden.
5. Veränderungen der Intentionalität (MUNDT), des Vollzugsbewußtseins (JASPERS), der Ich-Grenzen (FEDERN), eine Transitivierung von "ist" und "bin" für den Patienten (BLANKENBURG) markieren das schizophrene Erleben. Sie sagen aber nichts über die pathogenetischen Voraussetzungen desselben aus. Das ist schon eher der Fall, wenn die *Funktions*zusammenhänge herausgearbeitet werden, in deren Rahmen es zu einer Beeinträchtigung der Ichleistungen kommt.

6. Dazu wird kurz auf die Voraussetzungen des Transzendieren-Könnens eingegangen. Sie werden in der Fähigkeit zu relativ selbstdurchsichtiger Selbstbewegung (insbes. Perspektivenbeweglichkeit) gesehen. Diese Fähigkeit ist bei Schizophrenen offenkundig beeinträchtigt. Zu klären, in welcher Weise und mit welchen Konsequenzen (nicht: warum) dies der Fall ist, gehört zu den wesentlichen Aufgaben einer phänomenologischen (gleichwohl dynamischen) Psychopathologie

The Psychopathology of I-Experience in Schizophrenics

Summary: 1. The point in question, changes of self-experience, is narrowed down to the problem of "I-disorders" ("Ichstörungen": KURT SCHNEIDER). An example from clinical practice, described in brief outline, elucidates this point. The problem of the subject's reflexivity - the "I" being both subject and object when reflecting - is only touched on although it is regarded as the key to the understanding of "I-disorders".

2. The historical question whether "I-disorders" are a disturbance of feeling of being active or of the "mineness" of experience (which is without having been scrutinized set up as a norm) is not accepted as an alternative. As regards the point that the experience of immediate capability of "doing something" (which can even amount to a feeling of omnipotence) is also to be regarded as an "I-disorder", a third characteristic is pointed out, namely "interpenetration" in the sense of being (one's own or somebody else's) becoming transitive.

3. Thirdly it is discussed whether "I-disorders" concern the content "or" the form of experience. Thesis: They can be regarded as a proof that this alternative does not grasp the real conditions of inner life. On the contrary, they show that special contents of experience may at the same time indicate or imply a change of its structure (form).

4. As regards the high value for differential diagnosis that SCHNEIDER assigns to "I-disorders", one might advance the objection that this value might be valid only for our 'Western' culture. Transcultural comparisons (WULFF), which have, however, been objected to, show the possibility that the difference as regards differential diagnosis of schizophrenic disorders is not due to characteristics inherent in these disorders, but rather to the peculiar character of persons who have been shaped by Western civilization and who are especially susceptive to these disorders. This comparison, however, presupposes that schizophrenic disorders can be regarded as one homogeneous, biologically definable entity.

5. Schizophrenic experience is marked by changes of intentionality (MUNDT), of consciousness while acting (JASPERS), of the "I-boundaries" (FEDERN), "is" and "am" becoming transitive for the patient (BLANKENBURG). But these concepts do hardly express anything concerning the pathogenetic preconditions of schizophrenia. Only when the correlation of operational factors are worked out, which set the frame for I-disturbances, the preconditions are comprehended.

6. In order to show this, the capability to transcend is briefly discussed. The prerequisite to this faculty is assumed to consist in the ability to move oneself, to change ones perspective and to do this with a certain degree of selftransparency.

This ability is obviously impaired in schizophrenic patients. It is one of the essential tasks of phenomenological (and, at the same time, dynamic) psychopathology, to clarify in what way and to what consequences - but not on what grounds - that inhibition occurs.

Literatur

Bartlett, S.J., Suber, P. (eds.; 1987): Self-Reference. Reflections on Reflexivity. Nijhoff, Dordrecht Boston Lancaster.

Bellak, L., Hurvich, M., Gediman, H.K. (1973): Ego Functions in Schizo-phrenics, Neurotics and Normals. Wiley & Sons, New York.

Benedetti, G. (1978): VIII.Psychotherapeutische Behandlungsmethoden. In: Kisker, K.P., Lauter, H., Meyer, J.-E., Müller, C., Strömgren, E. (Hg.): Schizophrenien. Psychiatrie der Gegenwart, 3. Aufl., Bd.4. Springer, Berlin Heidelberg New York London Paris Tokyo.

Berze, J. (1914): Die primäre Insuffizienz der psychischen Aktivität. Deuticke, Wien Leipzig.

Binswanger, L. (1957): Schizophrenie. Neske, Pfullingen.

Blankenburg, W. (1962): Aus dem phänomenologischen Erfahrungsfeld innerhalb der Psychiatrie. Schw. Arch. Neuro. Psychiat. **90**, S. 412-421.

Blankenburg, W. (1965a) Die Verselbständigung eines Themas zum Wahn. Jb. Psychol. Psychother. med. Anthropol. **13**, S 137-164.

Blankenburg, W. (1965b): Zur Differentialphänomenologie der Wahnwahrnehmung. Nervenarzt **36**, S. 285-298.

Blankenburg, W. (1986): Zur Phänomenologie und Psychopathologie des Ich" Kawai, Nagoya [Vortrag].

Blankenburg, W. (1987a): Halluzination und Wahn in phänomenologisch-anthropologischer Sicht. In: Olbrich, H. (Hg.) Halluzination und Wahn. Springer, Berlin Heidelberg New York Tokyo.

Blankenburg, W. (1987b): Zur Subjektivität des Subjekts aus psychopathologischer Sicht. In: Nagl. Docekal, H., Vetter, H. (Hg.): Tod des Subjekts? Oldenbourg, Wien München.

Conrad, K. (1958): Die beginnende Schizophrenie. Thieme, Stuttgart.

Cramer, K. (1987): Über Kants Satz: Das: Ich denke, muß alle meine Vorstellungen begleiten können. In: Cramer, K. et al. (Hg.): Theorie der Subjektivität. Suhrkamp, Frankfurt a.M.

Dell, P.F. (1986): Klinische Erkenntnis. Verlag Modernes Lernen, Dortmund.

Dittrich, A. (1985): Ätiologie-unabhängige Strukturen veränderter Wachbewußtseinszustände. Enke, Stuttgart.

Federn, P. (1952): Ich-Psychologie und die Psychosen. Huber, Bern.

Frank (1986):

Glatzel, J. (1981): Spezielle Psychopathologie. Enke, Stuttgart.

Grathoff, R. (1985): Alfred Schütz, Aaron Gurwitsch - Briefwechsel 1939-1959. Fink, München.

Gruhle, H.W.: Die Psychopathologie. In: Bumke, O. (Hg.) Handbuch der Geisteskrankheiten, Bd. 9/Teil 5; Die Schizophrenie, Springer, Berlin.

Günther, G. (1978): Idee und Grundriß einer nicht-Aristotelischen Logik. Meiner, Hamburg.

Günther, H.R.G. (1934): Das Problem des Sichselbstverstehens. Duncker, Berlin.

Haug, W.F. (1985): Die Frage nach der Konstitution des Subjekts. In: Braun, K.H, Holzkamp, K. (Hg.) Subjektivität als Problem psychologischer Methodik. Campus, Frankfurt.

Häfner, H. (1987): Epidemiology of Schizophrenia. In: Häfner, H. Gattaz, W.F., Janzarik, W. (Hg.): Search for the causes of schizophrenia. Springer, Berlin Heidelberg New York London Paris Tokyo.

Heidegger, M. (1927): Sein und Zeit. Niemeyer, Halle.

Henrich, D. (1982): Selbstverhältnisse. Reclam, Stuttgart.

Holenstein, E. (1985): Menschliches Selbstverständnis. Suhrkamp, Frankfurt.

Jaspers, K. (1959): Allgemeine Psychopathologie. 7. Aufl., Springer, Berlin Göttingen Heidelberg.

JUNG, C.G. (1962): Erinnerungen, Träume, Gedanken von C.G. Jung, aufgez. und hrsg. von A. Jaffé. Buchclub Ex Libris, Zürich (S. 326), Random House, New York.

KANT, I. (1781/1787/1976): Kritik der reinen Vernunft. Meiner, Hamburg.

KANT, I. (1798/1917): Anthropologie in pragmatischer Hinsicht. Kant's gesammelte Schriften, herausgegeben von der Königlich Preußischen Akademie der Wissenschaften, Bd. VII., Berlin.

KIMURA, B. (1984): Identität und Differenz als Momente des Selbst-seins. Vortrag beim Weltkongreß der Psychiatrie. Abstracts, Wien.

KIMURA, B. (1986): Reflexion und Selbst beim Schizophrenen. Kawai, Nagoya [Vortrag].

KISKER, K.P. (1960): Der Erlebniswandel des Schizophrenen. Springer, Berlin Göttingen Heidelberg.

KRONFELD, A. (1922): Über schizophrene Veränderungen des Bewußtseins der Aktivität. Z. ges. Neurol. Psychiat. **74**, S. 15-68.

LUHMANN, N. (1988): Selbstreferentielle Systeme. In: SIMON, F.B.: Lebende Systeme; S. 47-53. Springer, Berlin Heidelberg New York London Paris Tokyo.

MITTERAUER, B.J. (1980): Das Ich-Kreis-Modell. In: GASTAGER, H.et al. (Hg.): Psychoanalyse als Herausforderung. Festschrift Caruso, Verband der Wissenschaftl. Gesellschaften Österreichs, Wien.

MUNDT, C. (1984): Der Begriff der Intentionalität und die Defizienzlehre von den Schizophrenien. Nervenarzt **55**, S. 582-588.

MUNDT, C. (1988, im Druck): Psychopathologie heute. In: KISKER, K.P., LAUTER, H., MEYER, J.E., MÜLLER, C., STRÖMGREN E. (Hg.): Psychiatrie der Gegenwart, Bd.9. Springer, Berlin Heidelberg New York London Paris Tokyo.

MUNDT, CH., LANG, H. (1987): Die Psychopathologie der Schizophrenien. In: KISKER, K.P., LAUTER, H., MEYER, J.-E., MÜLLER, C., STRÖMGREN, E. (Hg.): Psychiatrie der Gegenwart, 3.Aufl, Bd. 4, Schizophrenien. Springer, Berlin Heidelberg New York London Paris Tokyo.

NAGAI, M. (1981): On the experience of 'thought divulged' in schizophrenics. Jap. Journal of Psychopathology **2**, S. 157-172.

NAGL-DOCEKAL, H., VETTER, H. (1987): Tod des Subjckts? Oldenbourg, Wien München.

SANCHEZ, J. (1986): Über die Selbsterkenntnis des Menschen. Barth, München.

SARTORIUS, N., JABLENSKY, G., ERNBERG, J., LEFF, J., GULBINAT, W. (1987): Course of schizophrenia in different countries: Some Results of a WHO International Comparative 5-Year Follow-up Study. In: HÄFNER, H. GATTAZ, W.F., JANZARIK, W. (Hg.) Search for the causes of schizophrenia, Springer, Berlin Heidelberg New York London Paris Tokyo.

SCHARFETTER, C. (1982): Ich-Psychopathologie des schizophrenen Syndroms. In: JANZARIK, W (Hg.) Enke, Stuttgart.

SCHARFETTER, C. (1985): Allgemeine Psychopathologie. 2. Aufl., Thieme, Stuttgart New York.

SCHNEIDER, K (1955): Klinische Psychopathologie. 4., erw. Aufl. der Beiträge zur Psychiatrie. Thieme, Stuttgart.

SCHNEIDER, K. (1949): Notiz über Ichstörungen und Entfremdungen. Fortschr. Neurol. Psychiat. **17**, S. 343-347.

SPITZER, M. (1985): Allgemeine Subjektivität und Psychopathologie. Haag und Herchen, Frankfurt/Main.

SPITZER, M. (1988a): Halluzinationen. Springer, Berlin Heidelberg New York London Paris Tokyo.

SPITZER, M. (1988b): Untersuchungen zum Wahnproblem. Habilitationsschrift, Freiburg.

UEHLEIN, F.A. (1982): Die Manifestation des Selbstbewußtseins im konkreten "Ich bin". Meiner, Hamburg.

WEITBRECHT, H.J. (1973): Psychiatrie im Grundriß, 3. Aufl., Springer Berlin Heidelberg New York.

WINKLER, W.Th. (1954): Zum Begriff der "Ich-Anachorese" beim schizophrenen Erleben. Arch. Psychiat. **192**, S. 234-240.

WULFF, E. (1967) Psychiatrischer Bericht aus Vietnam. In: PETRILOWITSCH, N. (Hg.): Beiträge vergleichender Psychiatrie, Akt. Fragen Psychiatr. Neurol. vol. **5**, S. 1-84. Karger, Basel New York.

WYRSCH, J. (1956): Das Ich. Merkmal der psychischen Akte, Kap. VI; In: Zur Geschichte und Deutung der endogenen Psychosen. Thieme, Stuttgart.

Was sind Quasi-Indikatoren? Eine Einführung in Castañedas Theorie der Subjektivität

H. Pape, U. Leisinger

1. Zur Semantik und Syntax des Bewußtseins

Eine Reihe philosophischer und psychopathologischer Beiträge dieses Sammelbandes thematisieren das "Ich" in seinem doppelten Bezug sowohl auf sich selbst wie auf das "Ich" von anderen. Die ursprüngliche Selbstbezogenheit, so kann vielleicht z.B. der Beitrag von UEHLEIN verstanden werden, weist über sich selbst hinaus bzw. steht in Zusammenhang mit dem Bezug auf anderes und andere. Diese Konzeption erscheint mir problematisch, nicht zuletzt deshalb, weil unklar ist, auf welcher Ebene die verschiedenen reflexiven und nicht reflexiven Formen des Bezugs auf ein Ich statthaben.

Ist beispielsweise Selbstbewußtsein auch ohne Sprache möglich? Wenn die Antwort auf diese Frage "ja" lautet, dann stellt sich weiter die Frage, ob eine Darstellung des Selbst etwa durch geistige Bilder möglich ist und wie sie gegebenenfalls aussähe.

Vielleicht ist es nützlich, wenn man diese Fragen einfach offenläßt, einen ganz anderen Problemansatz erprobt und das Problem der Reflexivität und der Verschränkung von Selbstbewußtsein und Bewußtsein-von-etwas im Lichte des Sprechens über sich und Gegenstände der Erfahrung (d.h. über Selbstbewußtsein und Bewußtseinsinhalte) neu überdenkt. Für diesen Versuch erscheint CASTAÑEDAS Ansatz interessant, weil hier bestimmte sprachliche Strukturen herausgearbeitet werden, die unser Erfahrungsbewußtsein und Selbstbewußtsein darstellen.

Ein altes Vorurteil seitens der empiristischen und (älteren) sprachanalytischen Philosophen lautet, daß mein Hinweisen, die deiktische Bezugnahme auf meine gegenwärtigen Erfahrungen subjektiv und damit trügerisch ist. CASTAÑEDAS Entdeckung der *Quasi-Indikatoren* - d.h., soviel sei kurz vorweg gesagt, die Entdeckung der besonderen Verwendungsweise bestimmter Pronomina in abhängiger, z.B. in indirekter Rede - hat dieses Vorurteil in gewisser Hinsicht widerlegt und daher Konsequenzen für unser Verständnis von Sprache, Geist und Erkenntnis. Wir sind nämlich schon in der Umgangssprache in der Lage, das Subjektive unserer Urteile durch Quasi-Indikatoren zu *objektivieren*:

Quasi-Indikatoren stellen den subjektiven Gehalt der Äußerung einer Person aus der Perspektive einer anderen Person dar.

Wie geht das vor sich? Was können Philosophie, Psycho-Linguistik und Psychatrie aus dieser Entdeckung der sprachlichen Darstellung von Subjektivität lernen? Um diese Fragen beantworten zu können, müssen wir sowohl die syntaktischen und semantischen Eigenarten als auch den theoretischen Hintergrund genauer kennenlernen, von dem aus CASTAÑEDA die Quasi-Indikatoren entdeckt und entwickelt hat.

Wir werden deshalb im ersten Schritt die semantischen und syntaktischen Eigenarten dieser Gruppe von Ausdrücken untersuchen. Wenn Sie dann mit dem linguistischen Mechanismus der Quasi-Indikation einigermaßen vertraut sind, werden wir auf den sprach*philosophischen*, nämlich semantischen und ontologischen Hintergrund eingehen können. Diesen hat CASTAÑEDAS Theorie der Quasi-Indikatoren und ebenso seine Ontologie der Gestaltungen durch die Einführung einer Theorie der Subjektivität ergänzt. Die Behandlung abgestuft starker Identitätsrelationen geht - wie im dritten und letzten Schritt gezeigt werden soll - in die Ontologie der Gestaltungen ein, die eine Verallgemeinerung der Einsicht ist, daß die Quasi-Indikatoren autonom sind und nicht auf die objektiven Bezeichnungsweisen von Einzeldingen zurückgeführt werden können. Wir werden uns in diesen einführenden Bemerkungen auf Darstellung und vorsichtige Interpretation der Quasi-Indikation beschränken und von einer kritischen Diskussion absehen.

1.1 Indikatoren

Bevor wir uns den Quasi-Indikatoren zuwenden, sollen kurz einige Merkmale von *Indikatoren*, soweit sie für das Verständnis der Quasi-Indikation notwendig sind, referiert werden.

Termini wie "ich", "hier", "jetzt" haben die Eigenschaft, daß sie je nach Verwendungssituation anderes bezeichnen: "ich" verändert seine Bedeutung mit jedem Wechsel der Person, die "ich" äußert, "hier" mit jeder meßbaren Veränderung im Raum und "jetzt" sogar mit jedem Anlaß, zu dem es verwendet wird.

Indikatoren[1] sind solche benennenden Ausdrücke wie "ich", "hier", "jetzt", die eine Beziehung zwischen singulären Termini und den von ihnen bezeichneten Gegenständen herstellen, wobei die Beziehung abhängig ist von der je besonderen Situation ihrer Verwendung. Logische Analyse der Sprache, d.h. der Versuch natürliche Sprachen auf logische und somit allgemeingültige Elemente zu reduzieren, hat gezeigt, daß Indikatoren (anders als viele andere Gruppen von sprachlichen Ausdrücken) aus dem Kontext nicht herausgelöst werden können, ohne die betreffende Äußerung zu entstellen. Auf weitere Eigen-

1 Die Terminologie ist in der Literatur nicht einheitlich. So spricht CHARLES S. PEIRCE von "indices", BERTRAND RUSSELL von "egocentric particulars" und KARL BÜHLER von "Deixis". Der Terminus "Indikator" hat sich, in Anschluß an RUDOLPH CARNAP und NELSON GOODMAN ebenso durchgesetzt wie das Merkmal der Kontextabhängigkeit in der Definition von Indikatoren.

schaften sowie auf Castañedas Definition der Indikatoren soll an geeigneter Stelle (vgl. 3.3) eingegangen werden.

1.2 Quasi-Indikatoren

Quasi-Indikatoren stehen in abhängiger, sehr häufig in indirekter Rede. Charakteristisch ist, daß Quasi-Indikatoren in einer irreduziblen Beziehung zu einem Ausdruck in direkter Rede stehen, der im selben Satz im übergeordnetem Satzteil, dem Antezedens, vorkommt. So ist in

(1.) Helmut Pape glaubt, daß er (selbst) der Erstautor des Beitrags "Was sind Quasi-Indikatoren?" ist.

"Helmut Pape" das Antezedens in direkter Rede (*oratio recta*) für den Quasi-Indikator "er" in abhängiger, hier in indirekter Rede (*oratio obliqua*). Diese syntaktische Eigenschaft ist für Quasi-Indikatoren definitorisch: Ohne ein Antezedens außerhalb der abhängigen Rede, auf das von dort aus Bezug genommen wird, kann man nicht von einem Quasi-Indikator sprechen. Dieses syntaktische Charakteristikum hängt unmittelbar mit der wichtigsten sprach- und bewußtseinstheoretischen Funktion des Quasi-Indikators zusammen: Wir verwenden Quasi-Indikatoren, um einer Person als bewußtem und denkendem Subjekt das kennzeichnende Hinweisen auf etwas, das Vollziehen einer *indexikalischen Bezugnahme*, zuzuschreiben. Das indexikalische Gegenstück zu (1.) ist also die Äußerung Helmut Papes

(2.) Ich bin der Erstautor des Vortrags "Was sind Quasi-Indikatoren?".

Wichtig ist hier, daß (2.) Wahrheitsbedingung für (1.) ist: Nur wenn es der Fall ist, daß ich, Helmut Pape, (2.) tatsächlich geäußert oder gedacht habe (oder denken werde), kann (1.) wahr sein. Quasi-Indikatoren sind also ein Mittel für die Darstellung des kontextabhängigen indexikalischen Sprechens - aus der Perspektive einer anderen Person und abhängig von der Selbstzuschreibung in der ersten Person Singular.[2]

2 Die Struktur der Quasi-Indikation ist nicht an eine bestimmte Partikel (etwa ein Pronomen) im Satz gebunden. So könnte man den Satz (1.) auch wiedergeben durch

(1a.) Helmut Pape glaubt von sich, der Erstautor von "Was sind Quasi-Indikatoren?" zu sein.

(1a.) enthält allem Anschein nach keine den Quasi-Indikator repräsentierende Partikel. Dennoch haben auch solche Sätze eine quasi-indexikalische Struktur: In dem Aufsatz "Über die Grundlagen der Kommunikation: Referenz" hat CASTAÑEDA argumentiert, daß in diesen Fällen anaphorische Ausdrücke - wie in unserem Beispiel "von sich" - eine implizite quasi-indexikalische Rolle spielen können. Die Rekonstruktion der impliziten quasi-indexikalischen Funktion läßt sich durch eine Analyse nachweisen, die eine Eigenschaft postuliert, die wir *a* nennen wollen. Sie besteht darin, eine Selbigkeitsrelation "ist identisch mit" zwischen Bestandteilen eines oder mehrerer Sätze zu schaffen. So kommt z.B. *a* dem Ausdruck "von sich" zu. Denn *a* besteht darin, daß durch "von sich", das Präfix "Helmut Pape" mit dem zweiten Ausdruck in der abhängigen Rede, also "Erstautor von 'Was sind Quasi-Indikatoren?'" identifiziert werden kann. Die quasi-indexikalische Eigenschaft *a* bedeutet also in diesem Fall nichts anderes, als daß eine Person sich auf irgendeine Weise mit irgendeiner kontingenten Eigenschaft als "dieselbe" versteht. Der Satz (1a.) ist nämlich nur richtig, wenn in unserem Beispiel Helmut Pape glaubt, was er mit

(1b.) Ich bin derselbe wie der Erstautor von "Was sind Quasi-Indikatoren?"

Der Versuch, Quasi-Indikatoren im Sinne der logischen Analyse auf Kontextunabhängiges zu reduzieren, scheitert. Die einzig mögliche naheliegende Einsetzung "Helmut Pape" statt des Quasi-Indikators "er (selbst)" führt zu

(3.) Helmut Pape glaubt, daß Helmut Pape der Erstautor des Beitrags "Was sind Quasi-Indikatoren?" ist.

Gegenüber dem eindeutigen Beispielsatz (1.) ist (3.) mißverständlich: Es bleibt offen, ob Helmut Pape weiß, daß er mit dem Autor des Artikels identisch ist, oder ob es vielleicht sogar mehrere Personen mit dem Namen "Helmut Pape" gibt. Quasi-Indikatoren sind folglich stets kontextabhängig und damit zugleich nicht im logischen Sinne analysierbar. Auf die Darstellung und Darstellbarkeit durch Indikatoren und Quasi-Indikatoren kann erst in Abschnitt 4 näher eingegangen werden.

2. Logische Analyse und das Problem der Erfahrung

Um die Bedeutung von CASTAÑEDAS Entdeckung der Quasi-Indikation abzuschätzen, lohnt es sich, dem Zusammenhang zwischen logischer Analyse der Sprache, Indikatoren und Quasi-Indikatoren nachzugehen. 1963 erschien in *Mind* ein Aufsatz von BAR-HILLEL mit dem Titel *Indexical Expressions,* der damals viel Beachtung fand. Der Aufsatz endet mit einem sehr merkwürdigen Beweis. BAR-HILLEL führt eine *reductio ad absurdum,* die sich nicht gegen irgendeine spezielle These oder Theorie, sondern die Möglichkeit einer "Phänomenologischen Sprache" überhaupt wendet.

BAR-HILLEL definiert den Terminus indexikalischer Ausdruck (*indexical expression*) als ein sprachliches Zeichen, das "token-reflexive"[3] ist, also nur dann eine Bedeutung hat, wenn es verwendet wird. Das bedeutet: indexikalische Ausdrücke bezeichnen nur dadurch ein Objekt, daß es ein Verwendungsereignis gibt, auf das sie reflexiv bezogen sind, und sie bezeichnen nur dann ein Objekt, wenn die Bezugnahme vom Verwendungsereignis ausgehend verstanden wird. Also bezeichnet das Vorkommnis von "dies" in meiner Behauptung

(4.) Dies ist ein zu langer Text

zunächst einmal sich selbst, also jenes "dies" im obigen Satz, sodann bezeichnet es den ganzen Satz (4.). Wir haben es, gemäß dieser Analyse, bei den Indikatoren also mit Zeichen zu tun, deren bezugnehmende Funktion über das Verwendungsereignis (*token*) an die jeweilige Situation ihrer Verwendung gebunden ist. Für eine phänomenologische Sprache gilt nun nach BAR-HILLEL, daß alle ihre Sätze indexikalische Ausdrücke enthalten, die nicht elimimierbar sind.

BAR-HILLEL entwickelt aus diesen Annahmen eine Art logischer Hölle - nämlich eine Hölle für einen Philosophen, der eine Sprache allein durch kontextunabhängige logische Eigenschaften analysieren möchte:

Jeder Satz einer durch Indikatoren beherrschten phänomenologischen Sprache ist logisch gesehen ein *Ereignis*, keine Aussage (im Sinne der Aussagenlogik), also *sui generis*. Logische Beziehungen bestehen nur zwischen Aussagen, nicht zwischen Ereignissen. Mithin kann kein Satz einer phänomenologischen Sprache in logischem Zusammenhang mit anderen Sätzen stehen.

---

ausdrücken kann.

3 Der Ausdruck "token-reflexive" geht auf HANS REICHENBACH zurück.

Diese Situation ist für jeden Versuch, die Sprache allein auf logische und semantische Strukturen zurückzuführen, insofern prekär, weil man guten Grund hat anzunehmen, daß unsere Umgangssprache genau das ist: eine phänomenologische Sprache, in der alle Sätze im Bereich eines expliziten oder impliziten indexikalischen Ausdrucks eingebettet sind. Dann aber sind alle Sätze dieser Sprache auf den Kontext ihrer Verwendung bezogen, und wenn wir sie tatsächlich als Ereignisse behandeln müssen, dann läßt sich das Instrumentarium logischer Analyse nicht anwenden - zumindest ist die Sprache nicht mehr unabhängig von den Situationen ihrer Verwendung für eine Analyse zugänglich. Denn Ereignisse stehen weder in logischen Beziehungen zueinander noch haben sie eine innere logische Struktur. Also, so argumentiert BAR-HILLEL, muß in irgendeinem Sinne die logische Semantik grundlegender sein, wenn überhaupt eine allgemeingültige Theorie der Sprache möglich ist.[4]

BAR-HILLELS merkwürdiger Kampf gegen das Gespenst einer phänomenologischen Sprache ist Symptom eines Wandels in der Sprachphilosophie und Bewußtseinstheorie, der damals schon angebrochen war und gegen den BAR-HILLEL sich beunruhigt zur Wehr gesetzt hat. Die "Überwindung der Metaphysik durch logische Analyse der Sprache" (CARNAP) sollte mit "Ich", "Subjektivität" und "Seele" ebenso kurzen Prozeß machen wie mit "Sein" und "Nichts". Was zu Ende ging, war das Zeitalter des Paradigmas rein logischer Analyse in der angelsächsischen Philosophie. Über dieses "Golden Age of Pure Semantics" hat DAVID KAPLAN 1978 mit einer gewissen Trauer geschrieben:

"Wir entwickelten eine nette, homogene Theorie, wobei die Sprache, die Bedeutungen und die Entitäten in der Welt jeweils auf ziemlich bequeme und reibungslose Weise ordentlich voneinander getrennt und aufeinander bezogen wurden. ... Jede Bezeichnung (designator) hat sowohl eine Intension als auch eine Extension. Sätze haben Wahrheitswerte als Extensionen und Propositionen als Intensionen, Prädikate haben Klassen als Extensionen und Eigenschaften als Intension, Termini haben Einzeldinge als Extensionen und Individualbegriffe als Intensionen und so weiter. Die Intension eines Satzzusammenhangs ist eine Funktion der Intensionen der Teile und das gleiche gilt für die Extension. ... Diese Theorie ist von großer Schönheit und Kraft." (KAPLAN 1979, S. 385)

Die volle Bedeutung der These CASTAÑEDAS von der Autonomie der Indikatoren und Quasi-Indikatoren und des Vorschlages, daß ihre Verweisungsstruktur eine Logik der Subjektivität bildet, wird erst deutlich vor dem Hintergrund des Modells der reinen logischen Semantik der analytischen Philosophie. CASTAÑEDA entwickelt mit der Theorie der Quasi-Indikatoren und der Ontologie der Gestaltungen einen nicht-logischen Typ der Analyse der natürlichen Sprachen und des Bewußtseins, der das von BAR-HILLEL aufgeworfene Problem der beunruhigenden Dominanz pragmatischer und phänomenologischer Elemente in den natürlichen Sprachen überwand.

CASTAÑEDA hat jedoch nicht nur gezeigt, daß es in unserer Sprache mit den Indikatoren und Quasi-Indikatoren logisch irreduzible Formelemente gibt, sondern er führt zugleich den Nachweis, daß Quasi-Indikatoren ein zwar im klassischen Sinne *nicht-logisches*, sehr wohl aber *allgemeingültiges* Mittel der Darstellung der indexikalischen Bezugnahme sind. Mit der Entdeckung der Quasi-Indikatoren war nachgewiesen, daß es neben den Indikatoren noch eine

4 Positiv formuliert würde BAR-HILLEL ungefähr das folgende Programm vertreten: Wir müssen zunächst zwischen einer Sprache, ihrer Bedeutung und den ontologischen Entitäten unterscheiden können, bevor wir uns auf die verwirrende und beunruhigende Situation einlassen, daß unsere Sprache schon immer von Personen relativ zu Situationen gesprochen wird. BAR-HILLELS Argumentation gegen die Möglichkeit einer phänomenologischen Sprache ist bei näherem Hinsehen nichts anderes als eine uralte philosophische Argumentationsstrategie: Dasjenige, was in der Erfahrung offenkundig vorliegt, ist der bloße Schein, den die philosophische Erklärung (bei BAR-HILLEL die Angabe einer logischen Tiefenstruktur) hinter sich läßt. Der Glaube, daß die formallogische Analyse der Sprache die unveränderliche Struktur der Wirklichkeit hinter dem trügerischen Schein der Sprache entdeckt, hat eine offensichtliche Tendenz zu einem Platonismus, wie er wohl in WITTGENSTEINS *Tractatus* am deutlichsten spürbar wird.

weitere Gruppe von Ausdrücken (oder bestimmter Verwendungsweisen von Ausdrücken) gibt, die sich nicht auf eine semantische Funktion von Intensionen zu Extensionen zurückführen läßt. Denken wir nun wieder an den Ansatz des "Golden Age" zurück, daß sich alle Elemente einer Sprache semantisch sauber auf logische Funktionen, die Extensionen mit Intensionen verknüpfen, zurückführen lassen sollten! Man kann ermessen, welchen Umschwung es bedeutete, als CASTAÑEDA in seinem 1967 veröffentlichten Aufsatz *Indicators and Quasi-Indicators* behauptete, daß es nicht nur prinzipiell unmöglich ist, Indikatoren sinnerhaltend durch andere, logisch "ordentliche" singuläre Termini zu ersetzen, sondern daß es sogar eine weitere Gruppe von Pronomina in abhängiger Rede wie "er", "sie", "es" gibt, die dazu benutzt werden, unseren Gebrauch von Indikatoren darzustellen, und die ebenfalls nicht auf das Standard-Instrumentarium einer logischen Semantik reduzierbar sind.[5]

3. Ontologische und bewußtseinstheoretische Bedeutung der Quasi-Indikatoren

Kommen wir auf die eigentliche systematische Frage zurück: In welchem Sinne ist die mit Quasi-Indikatoren mögliche Darstellung von indexikalischen Bezugnahmen sowohl ontologisch wie bewußtseinstheoretisch von grundlegender Bedeutung?

Der Zusammenhang wird klar, wenn man beachtet, daß CASTAÑEDA hier auf vier miteinander zusammenhängende Thesen eingeht:

a) auf die zu einer philosophischen Mode ausgeuferte Semantik möglicher Welten (vgl. 3.1).
b) auf die Möglichkeit einer Privatsprache als Ausdruck unseres Denkens (vgl. 3.2),
c) auf die strikt allgemeine Bedeutung des nicht reduzierbaren Mechanismus der singulären quasi-indexikalischen Bezugnahme (vgl. 3.3), woraus sich übergreifend
d) die ontologisch und semantisch konstitutive Rolle der Subjektivität ableiten läßt (vgl. 5.).

Im folgenden werde ich kurz den systematischen Zusammenhang darlegen, den ich zwischen b), c) und d) sehe, wobei ich mich insbesondere auf c), die wichtige Entdeckung der Rolle der Quasi-Indikatoren und deren Auswirkung auf Semantik und Ontologie am Beispiel der Eigennamen, konzentrieren werde. Diese Überlegungen werden uns, so hoffe ich, bis zu dem Punkt führen, an dem wir sehen können, daß die Semiotik und Semantik der Subjektivität unserer Sprache zur Ontologie der Gestaltungen führt.

---

5 Entdeckungen von dieser Tragweite werden häufig mit großer Zurückhaltung aufgenommen. Die Fülle von Implikationen, die sich aus der Quasi-Indikation für das Verständnis von Sprache und Erkenntnis ergeben, macht verständlich, warum sie erst mehr als zehn Jahre später allgemein anerkannt war.

3.1 Mögliche Welten

Doch zunächst einige wenige Worte zum Punkt (a). Die Ontologie der Gestaltungen gibt der rein formalen Semantik möglicher Welten ontologische Tiefe, statt eine Konkurrentin der Semantik möglicher Welten zu sein. Es geht dabei vor allem um die sogenannten Einstellungsaussagen (*propositional attitudes*). Dies sind epistemische, deontische und perzeptuelle Sätze vom Typ "X glaubt (meint usw.), daß p", die einer Person Aussagen relativiert durch ein kognitives Verb zuschreiben. In diesen Fällen konstruiert die Semantik möglicher Welten Alternativbeziehungen zwischen möglichen Welten, um die abweichenden logischen Eigenschaften, die durch den Bezug zur Weise der Erfahrung einer Person entstehen, erklären zu können. Dagegen spricht die Ontologie der Gestaltungen von verschieden starken Selbigkeitsrelationen zwischen Eigenschaften, die durch diese Selbigkeitsrelationen zu Objekten verbunden werden. So sind die Eigenschaften, durch die wir Shakespeares Gestalt Hamlet denken nur miteinander *konsoziiert*, was eine relativ schwache Selbigkeitsrelation ist, da ihre "Bündelung" davon abhängig ist, daß Shakespeare sie auf diese Weise gedacht hat. Sie schließt z.B. aus, daß der Schauspieler, der in einer Aufführung Hamlet ist, nämlich konsoziiert ist mit "Hamlet", alle Eigenschaften der fiktiven Gestalt Hamlet hat - wie eine Erfindung Shakespeares zu sein, in soundsovielen Inszenierungen auf verschiedene Weisen interpretiert worden zu sein usw.

Nehmen wir ein Beispiel für eine stärkere Selbigkeitsrelation! Wenn ich über meinen Hund Hamlet spreche, so nehme ich an, daß alle Eigenschaften, die ich ihm wahrheitsgemäß zuschreibe, auch für den Hund Hamlet gelten, den jemand anders beschreibt. Diese Selbigkeitsbeziehung zwischen den verschiedenen Weisen, wie wir ein materielles Objekt beschreiben, nennt CASTAÑEDA *Konsubstantiation*. Die Selbigkeitsbeziehung eines objektiven physikalischen Objekts überträgt also Eigenschaften auf alle Weisen, in denen uns dieses Objekt gegeben ist, ist also im Unterschied zur Konsoziation transitiv. Ansonsten haben Konsubstantiation und Konsoziation viele logische Eigenschaften wie Kommutativität, logische Geschlossenheit und Vollständigkeit gemeinsam. CASTAÑEDA lehnt die Semantik möglicher Welten auch deshalb ab, weil er glaubt, mit seiner Ontologie der Gestaltungen und den verschiedenen Arten von Selbigkeitsrelationen eine Alternative zur Hand zu haben, die allen Arten von Phänomenen gerecht werden kann, ohne sie gewaltsamen Reduktionen zu unterwerfen. Doch kann ich auf diesen Punkt nicht weiter eingehen.

3.2 Das Privatsprachenargument

Mit der These (b) ist behauptet worden, daß sich CASTAÑEDAS Entdeckung der Quasi-Indikatoren und die zentrale, ja konstitutive Rolle, die er der Subjektivität beimißt, in der Auseinandersetzung mit WITTGENSTEINS *Privatsprachenargument* (Privat Language Argument) entwickelt hat. Im Privatsprachenargument geht es - kurz zusammengefaßt - um die Frage, ob es möglich ist, daß jemand in einer Sprache denken kann, die nur ihm allein zugänglich, für jeden anderen jedoch prinzipiell unverstehbar ist. Nach WITTGENSTEINS Argumentation kann es eine solche Privatsprache nicht geben: Wenn das "Denken" des sogenannten Privatus für alle anderen prinzipiell unverstehbar ist, ist es notwendigerweise auch ihm selbst unverständlich. Jedes Denken und jede Sprache, die ein einzelner versteht, kann im Prinzip auch von anderen nachvollzogen werden (PEARS 1987, vgl. auch CASTAÑEDA 1967b)

In seiner Opposition gegen einige der Argumente aus einem ganzen Bündel von Überlegungen, das in den fünfziger Jahren unter dem Titel "The Private Language Argument" gehandelt wurde, stand CASTAÑEDA fast allein da. 1984 hat er seine philosophische Entwicklung, die durch das Privatsprachenargument ausgelöst wurde, einmal wie folgt beschrieben:

"Ich bin auf den Bereich der indexikalischen Referenz nicht von der mengentheoretischen Semantik her gestoßen. Mein zentrales philosophisches Interesse war bereits auf die Struktur der Erfahrung konzentriert, einschließlich der erfahrungshaften Rolle der Sprache. Also war ich sehr an den Rollen der Indikatoren - und Quasi-Indikatoren - in der Erfahrung interessiert. In den späten Fünfzigern beschäftigte ich mich eingehend mit Privatsprachen. Da die damals üblichen Angriffe auf Privatsprache typischerweise Diskussionen von Empfindung enthielten, formulierte ich eine Grundlage für solche Diskussionen unter dem Titel "Schmerzpostulate". Diese enthielten das verwirrende Pronomina "er (selbst)", z.B. in dem von mir hier vorgeschlagenen Axiom der Unkorrigierbarkeit von Schmerz:

(S.Un) Wenn X glaubt, während er sich seinen geistigen Prozessen zuwendet, daß er (selbst) Schmerzen hat, dann weiß X, daß er (selbst) Schmerzen hat.

Dies "er (selbst)" erwies sich dann als der Quasi-Indikator der dritten Person, der Zuschreibungen der Bezugnahme in der ersten Person darstellt. In den frühen Sechzigern ging ich von den Quasi-Indikatoren zu den Indikatoren über. Mein Ziel war es, einen phänomenologischen Umriß ihrer natürlichen syntaktischen und semantischen Eigenschaften herzustellen. Ich stieß auf eine Form direkter Bezugnahme. Der Begriff der indexikalisch perspektivischen Eigenschaften wurde damals eingeführt. In den späten Sechzigern ging ich zur Theorie der Gestaltungen über, einer epistemischen (doxastischen) Ontologie, die eine natürliche Semantik einschließt, gemäß der alle echten singulären Termini direkt referentiell sind: sie beziehen sich auf individuelle Gestaltungen" (CASTAÑEDA 1984, S. 6).

3.3 Direkte Referenz

Diese kleine biographische Skizze stammt aus einem Aufsatz, in dem CASTAÑEDA Einwände gegen DAVID KAPLANS Theorie der direkten Referenz entwickelt. Der Begriff der direkten Referenz wird von KAPLAN und CASTAÑEDA jeweils verschieden gefaßt. Nach KAPLAN bedeutet die direkte Referenz der Indikatoren, daß wir uns mit ihnen direkt auf physikalisch reale Individuen beziehen, die wir vor uns haben. Nach CASTAÑEDA aber können sich Indikatoren nur auf in der Erfahrung gestaltete Entitäten beziehen. Also auf jene individuellen Gestaltungen, die als Produkt der indexikalisch markierten Eigenschaften zu unserer Erfahrung des so gegebenen Objekts werden. Nach CASTAÑEDA ist die Bezugnahme mit Hilfe von Indikatoren sowohl unmittelbar als auch strikt:

"Die unmittelbare Bezugnahme durch einen Indikator besteht darin, daß er in einem gegebenen Kontext eine Entität, auf die sich ein Sprecher bezieht, ohne die Vermittlung einer anderen Bezugnahme bezeichnet; die strikte Bezugnahme eines Indikators besteht darin, daß er in einem gegebenen Sprechakt das bezeichnet, worauf der Sprecher allein sich bezieht, ohne jemand anderem irgendeine solche Bezugnahme zuzuschreiben" (CASTAÑEDA 1981, S. 149f).

Wir benötigen also für die Bezugnahme mithilfe von Indikatoren keine anderen singulären Termini; ein Indikator drückt nicht aus, daß jemand über einen Mechanismus der singulären Bezugnahme verfügt, sondern er vollzieht diese Bezugnahme, gleichgültig, ob er in direkter oder indirekter Rede gebraucht wird. Oder in CASTAÑEDAS Worten:

"Indikatoren besitzen eine vollziehende Funktion: einen Indikator richtig zu verwenden, heißt vorauszusetzen und, im Falle von 'ich', 'hier' und 'jetzt' sogar festzulegen, daß ein indexikalischer Gegenstand in genau der Erfahrung gegenwärtig und als in ihr enthalten anzusiedeln ist, die in der Äußerung des Teils der Sprache verkörpert wird, der den betreffenden Indikator enthält" (CASTAÑEDA 1984, S. 24).

Im Unterschied zu REICHENBACHS Charakterisierung der Indikatoren als "token-reflexive" - die BAR-HILLEL lediglich aufgenommen hatte - findet CASTAÑEDA mit der vollziehenden Funktion der Indikatoren eine Erklärung dafür, daß man Indikatoren zwar durch Quasi-Indikatoren darstellen, jedoch nicht durch Quasi-Indikatoren oder Beschreibungen analysieren kann.

Selbstverständlich gibt es wahre Beschreibungen, die Indikatoren charakterisieren, sagen wir einmal die komplexe Eigenschaft "ist ein Ausdruck, der sich singulär auf Entitäten bezieht, die durch seine Verwendung in der Erfahrung angesiedelt werden". Doch diese Beschreibung - und denkbare speziellere für die einzelnen Indikatoren - vollziehen nicht, was sie da beschreiben. Also selbst wenn eine Beschreibung eines oder aller Indikatoren richtig ist, bleibt ihre besondere semantische und pragmatische Funktion, der Sprache den Weg über die Erfahrung zur Realität zu bahnen, unangetastet.

4. Zur Darstellung und Darstellbarkeit durch Indikatoren

Das Enthaltensein von Indikatoren in der Erfahrung ist von anderen Sprachphilosophen als die Kontextabhängigkeit der Aussagen beschrieben worden, die durch sie an die Situationen ihrer Verwendung gebunden werden. Eine Aussage wie z. B. Max Meyers Bekundung am 16. 7. 1988 um 13:30 im Raum 204 gegenüber Susanne Schulz

(5.) "Ich will Dich hier und jetzt küssen",

ist abhängig von der Kenntnis der Situation, um überhaupt von anderen Verwendungen derselben Aussage durch andere Personen in anderen Situationen unterscheidbar zu sein, und geht daher sozusagen mit der Situation verloren. Wie eine Handlung ist diese Aussage nicht als dieselbe, sondern nur als ein zweites Exemplar (*token*) eines allgemeinen Typs (*type*) wiederholbar.

Genau dies ist der Grund, warum für BAR-HILLEL die Möglichkeit einer phänomenologischen Sprache problematisch war: Will man natürliche Sprachen im wesentlichen mit Hilfe der formalen Logik sowie der Verwendung einer Reihe von semantischen und syntaktischen Regeln, Schlußregeln und

Einsetzungsregeln verstehen, so zeigt sich die Unmöglichkeit eines solchen Vorhabens, denn die Ableitungsverhältnisse, die wir auf logisch-semantischer Grundlage zwischen wahren Aussagen darstellen können, basieren alle darauf, daß es gleichgültig sein muß, unter welchen Umständen eine Aussage behauptet wird. Anders formuliert: Die logische Rekonstruktion einer natürlichen Sprache, die zunächst einmal ausgeht von einer quantifizierten Logik erster Stufe, unterstellt, daß die Gültigkeit von Aussagen vom Kontext ihrer Verwendung unabhängig ist oder unabhängig gemacht werden kann, ohne daß sich der Sinn der formalisierten Aussagen dadurch entscheidend verändert. Natürliche Sprachen sind jedoch kontextabhängig.

Betrachten wir die Eigenschaften der Darstellung durch einen Quasi-Indikator noch einmal, jedoch in dieser zweiten Annäherung etwas genauer. Versuchen wir, die Aussage (5.) mit Hilfe von Quasi-Indikatoren darzustellen. Dann lautet sie

(6.) Max Meyer sagte am 16. 7. 1988 in Raum 204 zu Susanne Schulz, daß er sie damals dort küssen wollte.

Konzentrieren wir uns zunächst auf das "er" in (6.). Warum soll es etwas anderes bedeuten als "Max Meyer" oder als der Indikator "er" in "Da kommt er ja"? CASTAÑEDA nennt in *Über die Phänomen-Logik des Ich* vier Charakteristika der besonderen Rolle des Pronomens "er (selbst)". Sie gelten entsprechend auch für die Verwendung von "er" in unserem Beispielsatz (6.):

(i) Das Pronomen "er (selbst)" wird nicht verwendet, um eine demonstrative Bezugnahme derjenigen Person auszudrücken, die den Satz (6.) äußert;

(ii) es bezieht sich nicht direkt auf die Person Max Meyer, sondern indirekt, indem es sich auf den Ausdruck "Max Meyer" zurückbezieht, der folglich sein Antezedens ist;

(iii) es steht in abhängiger Rede, während sein Antezedens außerhalb der abhängigen Rede steht zu der "er (selbst)" gehört, es steht also bei Fällen mit einem Präfix, das in der übergeordneten Rede steht, die es unmittelbar umschließt;

(iv) es wird verwendet, um Max Meyer Bezugnahmen in der ersten Person zuzuschreiben, wenngleich die zugeschriebenen Bezugnahmen nur implizit (oder dispositional) sein können, da ja Max Meyer nicht auch im selben Augenblick das denken oder behaupten muß, was er gemäß der Proposition (5) glaubt.[6]

Mit CASTAÑEDAS Worten: *Wir können den Quasi-Indikator benutzen, um jemand anderem Selbstbewußtsein zuzuschreiben.* Dies ist der entscheidende Punkt: Die Darstellung von situativ relativierten Indikatoren, z. B. von "ich",

6 Die Eigenschaften (ii) und (iii) treffen auch auf andere anaphorische Konstruktionen zu. Im Beispielsatz

(6a.) Es war Richard Schmidt, von dem ich glaubte, daß er gerade zur Tür hereinkommen sei.

schreibe ich mit "er" natürlich Richard Schmidt keine Bezugnahmen in der ersten Person mit "ich" zu. Gleichwohl zeigt (6a.) die syntaktischen Merkmale (ii) und (iii). Entscheidend ist hier, daß im Unterschied zu (6a.) in (6.) "er" verwendet wird, um darzustellen, was jemand anders dachte oder sagte, indem er einen Indikator, nämlich das Pronomen der ersten Person benutzt hat.

"dich", "hier", "jetzt" in Satz (5.), gelingt nur dann, wenn es zutrifft, daß die betreffende Person selbst die korrespondierende Proposition denkt oder äußert. Aus diesem Grund wird z.B. der Indikator "dich" in (5.) zwar in indirekter Rede (6.) durch "sie" wiedergegeben, ist aber dennoch kein Quasi-Indikator.

In den Bereich der Darstellbarkeit von Indikatoren fallen also nur jene deiktisch verwendeten Ausdrücke, welche die im Antezedens erwähnte Person sich selbst zuschreibt. In einem strengen Sinn, der durch die vollziehende Funktion der Indikatoren festgelegt wird, gibt es nur drei Indikatoren, die stets jeder sich selbst zuschreiben muß, der überhaupt einen propositionalen Gehalt erfährt, denkt, bezweifelt, wahrnimmt usw. Wir finden alle drei auch in unserem Beispielsatz (5.), nämlich "ich", "hier", "jetzt":

Antezendens in *direkter Rede in (6.)*	*Indikator in (5.)*	*Quasi-Indikator in (6.)*
Max Meyer	ich	er
16. 7. 1988, 13:30	jetzt	damals (dann)
Raum 204	hier	dort

5. Quasi-Indikatoren und die Ontologie der Gestaltungen

Quasi-Indikatoren sind, zusammengefaßt, Weisen der Bezugnahme, die aus nichts anderem als komplexen nicht-trivialen Selbigkeitsaussagen bestehen. Aus diesem Grund sind sie eine bestimmte Form von Gestaltungen: An sich selbst zu glauben, insofern man derselbe ist wie der Autor eines Vortrages, ist eine individuelle Gestaltung der eigenen Person. In diesem Sinne schreibt Castañeda 1981 in der "Einleitung" zu seinem fast 20 Jahre älterem Aufsatz "Indikatoren und Quasi-Indikatoren":

"Einige wichtige Unklarheiten von 'Indikatoren und Quasi-Indikatoren' hängen mit der Tatsache zusammen, daß ich 1965 keine ontologische Theorie zur Verfügung hatte ... Statt individuelle Gestaltungen einzuführen, ... mußte ich damals auf den dunklen Begriff der Weisen der Bezugnahme zurückgreifen. Folglich sind die Weisen der Bezugnahme die Vorläufer der individuellen Gestaltungen" (Castañeda 1982, S. 148).

Zusammenfassung: Bei Quasi-Indikatoren handelt es sich um eine irreduzible semantische Struktur. Sie dienen dazu, auf die Bewußtseinszustände anderer Personen Bezug zu nehmen. Logische Analyse der Sprache zeigt, daß die Indikatoren "ich", "hier" und "jetzt" situations- bzw. kontextabhängig sind. Quasi-Indikatoren sind entsprechene Partikel in abhängiger Rede, wie z.B. "er", "dort" und "dann", die den subjektiven Gehalt der Äußerung einer Person aus der Perspektive einer anderen Person darstellen; sie objektivieren das Subjektive von Urteilen, schreiben Personen Selbstbewußtsein zu.

On Quasi-Indicators. Introduction into CASTAÑEDA's Theory of Subjectivity

Summary: Quasi-indicators are of an irreducible semantical structure and are used to refer to mental events of other persons. Indicators like "I", "here", and "now" necessarily depend on context and situation as can be shown by logical analysis of language. Quasi-indicators are the respective particles "he", "there" and "then" used in oratio obliqua. They represent the subjective content of a person's utterance from the perspective of another person and thus objectify the subjective aspect of statements and ascribe self-consciousness to persons.

Literatur

BAR-HILLEL, Y. (1954): Indexical Expressions. Mind **63**, S. 359-379.

CASTAÑEDA, H.-N. (1967a): Indicators und Quasi-Indicators. American Philosophical Quarterly **4**, S. 85-100, (dt. in CASTAÑEDA 1982).

CASTAÑEDA, H.-N. (1967b): Private Language Problem. In: The Encyclopedia of Philosophy, Vol. 6, S. 458-466.

CASTAÑEDA, H.-N. (1968): On the Phenomeno-logic of the I. Proceedings of the XIVth International Congress of Philosophy **3**, S. 260-266, (dt. in CASTAÑEDA 1982).

CASTAÑEDA, H.-N. (1981): Einführung zu Indikatoren und Quasi-Indikatoren. In: CASTAÑEDA 1982.

CASTAÑEDA, H.-N.(1982): Sprache und Erfahrung. Eingeleitet und übers. von H. PAPE, Suhrkamp, Frankfurt.

CASTAÑEDA, H.-N. (1984): Direct Reference, Realism, and Guise Theory. In: WETTSTEIN, H., PERRY, J. (eds.): On the Philosophy of David Kaplan.

KAPLAN, D. (1979): Dthat. In: FRENCH, UEHLING & WETTSTEIN (eds.): Contemporary Perspectives in the Philosophy of Language, University of Minnesota Press, Minneapolis, S.383-400.

PEARS, D. (1987): Wittgenstein's Philosophy of Language. In: GREGORY, R.L.: The Oxford Companion to the Mind, S. 811-813, Oxford und New York.

REICHENBACH, H. (1947): Elements of Symbolic Logic. New York und London.

UEHLEIN, F.A. (1988): Bewußtsein und Selbstbewußtsein. (Beitrag in diesem Band).

Persons, Egos, and I's: Their Sameness Relations

H.-N. Castañeda

> *"There are also dreams in which MY EGO appears together with other persons, who when the identification is resolved, again, reveal themselves to be my ego. ... I may also give my ego multiple representations in my dream, either directly or by means of identification with other people. ... That ONE'S EGO should appear in the same dream several times or in different forms is fundamentally no more surprising than that IT should appear, in conscious thoughts, many times and in different places or in different relations: as, for example, in the sentence: 'When I think what a healthy child I was'."*
>
> FREUD, The Interpretation of Dreams (1900/1938, p. 349)

1. Introduction

This is an inquiry into the nature of what we, whether in dreams or in waking experience, think as "I". What does one refer to internally, *de dicto*, when one uses assertively a sentence containing an inflection of the first-person pronoun? What sort of entity that referent is? How does such a referent relate to the person calling himself or herself "I"? Consider for example FREUD's wishful self-assuring statement:

(1) Sometimes I think what a healthy child I was!

We shall say that a token of a form of the first-person pronoun used to make a thinking singular reference strictly or internally denotes an *I* [ein *Ich*]. This is a neutral piece of terminology. It leaves open that an *I* be nothing at all even in the most liberal conception of referent. We are, thus, inquiring into the constitution of *I*'s, if there be such, the roles they play in experience, and the ontological structures enveloping them. These ontological structures may, again, be such as to determine the annihilation of all *I*'s. This topic is of the greatest intrinsic importance. It is, of course, of special value in attempting to understand FREUD's, as well as other philosophers and psychiatrists', views of the ego or the self. Indeed the above passage from FREUD constitutes an excellent initial datum.

2. I and my Ego: Some Questions

2.1 My Ego is Myself

Undoubtedly, FREUD thought that what he called a person's ego [das Ich] is in some sense identical to the person's *I* or *I*'s. Let's reflect on the last sentence of the above passage (the capitals are added to express my emphasis):

(2) That ONE'S EGO [das eigene Ich] should appear in the same dream several times or in different forms is fundamentally no more surprising than that IT should appear, in conscious thinking, many times and in different places or in different relations, as, for example, in a statement (1).

The capitalized pronoun 'IT' refers back to 'one's ego'. The ego that appears as such in the dream is oneself - referred to in the first-person way. It is FREUD's EGO what the pronoun 'I' of example (1) denotes. Hence, as FREUD reveals in (2):

(FI.1) One is (the same as) one's ego.
I am (the same as) my ego.

(FI.1) is a sort of semantic axiom characterizing what FREUD meant by the ego (*das Ich*). But what does 'my' denote in the locution 'my ego'? What sort of sameness is that?

On a conceptually economic interpretation FREUD is being verbose in (2): 'my ego' is simply short for 'I', and 'one's ego' for 'one'. On this interpretation, (2) is a verbose version of:

(2.A) That ONE should appear in the same dream several times or in different forms is fundamentally no more surprising than that ONE should appear, in conscious thinking, many times and in different places or in different relations, as, for example, in statement (1).

There seems to be something right here. A patient must express in the first-person the identifications, brought forth by psychotherapy, that she has executed in her dreams. For instance, Tayra's:

(3) I dreamt that George [my undersexed husband] was anxiously, very tenderly, trying to feed *me*. I kicked him hard at the groin. He groaned, but stopped offering *me* the food. Immediately the food became a liquid column that fell very slowly to the ground, and then vanished. ...
I see now that in my dream *I* was George, and George was ME. In kicking him I was refusing him. Also blaming me for his real refusals.

The first-person pronoun in (3) is crucial. It threads the unity of the person who lives the dream, has the underlying psychological states, and undergoes the ensuing interpretive waking experiences. This first-person overall unity is what FREUD emphatically signals in (2).

2.2 I Cannot be my Ego

Yet the sameness between one's ego and oneself postulated by FREUD's (2) is not the strict identity proclaimed by the verbose interpretation. To begin with, let's ponder his tantalizing statement in the above text:

(4) I may also give my ego multiple representation in my dream, directly, or by means of identification with other persons.

This separates my ego from me. I am like a playwright, my ego a sort of historical personage about whom I write a kind of fable narrated in the first-person way. The personage is carved into different characters in the dream fable. The direct representation of my ego is the first-person character that narrates the story; the indirect representations are the third-person characters. These need not be real persons. Indeed, why should they be ordinary persons, at all, and not, as in genuine fables, animals, or non-existing animated, even inanimate, objects? In any case, there is the internal ego or I of the dream story, the external ego that appears piecemeal multiply manifested in the story, and I that create the story. In some sense, I am my ego. Hence, there is this meta-external ego that composes the dream. There is also the I that interprets the story. Presumably they are all the same. These levels of sameness cry out for elucidation. It is clear, however, that all these samenesses operate within a background of fundamental differences. None of these samenesses is the strict identity of the verbose interpretation.

For FREUD the phrase 'my ego' was really not just a verbose version of 'I'. He meant by 'ego' (das Ich) a special part of a person's mind centering about his/her powers to undergo episodes of consciousness. Each of us has an ego, but one also has other psychic parts. Later on he posited an Id and a super-ego as in some sense parts of oneself, but not of one's ego. Patently:

(5) I am (the whole of) the person H-N. C.

is true, whereas:

(6) My ego is (the whole of) the person H-N. C.

is false.

FREUD is better construed as claiming in passage (2) and its surrounding text that:

(FI.2) One's ego is in some sense (at least) the same as one's thinking part - the part of oneself that enjoys episodes of consciousness.

Perhaps one's ego is more than one's thinking part. Nevertheless, there are many things one is that one's ego is not. In particular:

(FI.2Ph) For every physical property Fness, one may be F but one's ego is not F.

For instance, I weigh 160 pounds, but my ego apparently has no weight. One can be at places where something else in some appropriate relation to oneself is at, e.g., in a law court when one's proxy or one's lawyer is performing his representation function. But one's ego is not the one so related to a lawyer, or what is vicariously present at the law court.

In passage (2) FREUD declares - truly, we suppose - that *he (himself)* was a healthy child. This 'he himself' is a quasi-indicator depicting the first-person of his statement (1).[1] Perhaps there existed an *I* of FREUD's (the whole person) that was a healthy child; yet FREUD's ego was neither a healthy child nor an unhealthy one. (Toward the end of this essay we return to this topic.)

There is an important tension between (FI.1) and (FI.2). I do *not* claim that FREUD in (2) is contradicting himself by holding that a finite whole is the same as one of its proper parts. I want, rather, to pursue the semantic elucidation of the first-person pronoun to ascertain what an *I* is. This elucidation should help us understand FREUD's consistent, and profound, tenets about the ego.

The sense of 'part' in (FI.2) is very special. To be sure, one is also one's id as well as one's super-ego in the sense in which they are one's own psychic components. However, the identification between oneself and one's ego is special. (FI.2) alone can mislead. The ego is not merely the thinking part of oneself, but is that part of oneself that one thinks of as operating in the first-person way. This is precisely what (FI.1) brings forth. The hermeneutic task is to specify in detail the complementarity between (FI.1) and (FI.2).

Patently, (FI.1) and (FI.2) are semantic axioms characterizing what Freud meant by the ego (*das Ich*). They are, though obscure, analytic or logical truths in the logic of the ego. (FI.1) is a bridging principle connecting a person's ego [Ich] with his/her *I*'s [*I c h* s]. (FI.2) connects the ego to the operational powers of thinking, rather than to the psychological context within which those powers function.

2.3 I's and Persons

In the background of FREUD's identifications lie, of course, many identifications which one acknowledges in daily life. For instance, I am (the same as) Hector-Neri Castañeda, the Editor of *Nous*, the Mahlon Powell Professor of Philosophy

1 On quasi-indicators see CASTAÑEDA (1967) and TOMBERLIN (1983).

of Indiana University, the father of Frieda Xmucane Wiebeck. We summarize all these identifications with the master equation:

(*I.3X) There are (infinitely) many unique personal characterizations Xness such that:
One is (the same as) the person X.
E.g., I am (the same as) the person X.

Postulate (*I.3X) is a logical truth in the logic of the embodiment of the *I*'s. It is a pervasive truth prior to psycho-analysis. FREUD assumes and uses it in reporting his cases. On the other hand, each particular truth (*I.3j) that instantiates (*I.3X) is contingent and empirical.

Postulate (*I.3X) is a Pandora's box. To the extent that one thinks oneself the (*I.3X) equations, things look (though just look) clear and calm. Those equations also identify what a speaker refers to as *I* with what others refer to as *the person X.* Yet strict identity must fail here. *What* one thinks, *de dicto*, i.e., the internal content that one thinks, when one thinks in the first-person way is entirely different from what others think in the third-person way. Yet a necessary and sufficient condition of being a person, or being fully a person, is to be able to think of oneself as *oneself*, in the first-person way. Others must perforce think of one in the third-person way. This contrast is enormous and enormously important.

Consider a totally amnesiac person. She cannot forget to refer to herself as *I*. However, for any third-personal characterization Xness whatever, she may fail to know that *she herself* is (the same as) the X one. (Here again, 'she herself' is a quasi-indicator depicting the amnesiac's use of 'I'.) Let's focus on the moment at which, having been transported in a state of coma to a strange place, she first awakes with total amnesia. To be sure when she asks: "Where am I? WHO am I?" she is groping for some true equations of the (*I.3X) type. Patently she is not inquiring whether logical reflexivity holds for her: "Am I I, the same as myself?" For practically every property Fness, she may believe (and think) that some person X - who happens to be the same as she - is F without believing that she herself is F.

To underscore this fact observe that one can refer to oneself demonstratively without making a first-person reference. One can see oneself into a mirror and, without realizing that it is oneself one is seeing, think demonstratively "THAT person looks pitifully tired!" The surprise one experiences at seeing such a pitifully looking person may show on one's face, and seeing it reflected into the mirror one may proceed to think:

(7) That man must be thinking that I am horrified by his thinking that I am pleased by thinking that I am so different from him that I could never look like him.

Then the mirror disappears, and one may never realize that once one thought that one was not oneself. One may of course learn later on that it was oneself one saw in that mirror experience. One may then think:

(8) Once I, without realizing what was happening, saw myself in a mirror with a horrified expression at looking at myself in the mirror, and thought then that I in the mirror, looking intently at me, must be thinking that I was so horrified by my mirror image thinking that I was pleased by thinking that I was so different from what I saw myself looking like that I could never look like that.

Undoubtedly, what one thinks in the original mis-identification experience involves no contradiction. It hinges on a lack of I-integration. What one thinks in the later, recognitional experience need not involve a contradiction. It must for consistency provide an I-identification that corrects, yet respects the earlier lack of I-integration. This is all within normal experience. It merely hints at psychiatric possibilities.

What I strictly think as *I* is not the same as what others think when they refer to me. What the others think is more or less clear: they think of a person (whatever this may be) that has for them certain uniquely differentiating properties. But what do I think as this I that I am and that in principle I can think as having no property other than being currently involved in some experiences? In brief:

(*I.4) Where being F is not simply being myself, all propositions of the form *I am F* are synthetic *a posteriori* in KANT's sense, i.e., not tautological.

The predicate F of any such proposition contains something not contained in the subject. The attributions of experience are additive to what 'I' means. They are empirical, requiring the existence of the experience in question to be true. Let's go over this in some detail.

To attribute some property to an object X, that is, to think something of the form *X is F*, presupposes that the attributer has differentiated and segregated (individuated) that subject of predication from all other individuals. Thus when one thinks something of the form *I am F* one must individuate oneself as an I as the subject of Fness. How does one accomplish this feat?

Compare the case of a physical object. We can differentiate and individuate it as a subject by means of some identifying properties. Suppose that we individuate an object as *the tallest man in Heidelberg in 1986*. Then we can attribute to it all sorts of properties, e.g., we can think "The tallest man in Heidelberg in 1986 was a Swede, was an engineer, was a grandfather, ..." And we can think tautologically, analytically in KANT's sense: "The tallest man in Heidelberg in 1986 was a man, was a very tall person, was in Heidelberg, lived in 1986, ..." This tautological thinking we cannot do with one's *I* or *I*'s, with one*self*. By (*I.4) no property Fness, physical or psychological, can serve to individuate an *I*. The utilization of any such property presupposes that one has already, so to speak, in one's hands a constituted subject of predication - an *I*.

Yet what I think as *I* must be the same as what others think when they refer to me. How is that feasible? What sort of sameness is that? What exactly is an I?

2.4 Main Problems

The task of determining the way in which (FI.1) and (FI.2) complement each other must be carried out in the context determined by the truths conforming to (*I.3X) and (*I.4). We must investigate the the experience of first-person reference. There we can study the living semantics and the pragmatics of first-person language. There we can establish what exactly the *I*'s [*I c h* s] are. (We cannot examine now FREUD's texts to ascertain what he calls a person's ego (das Ich).) We focus on the fundamental *sameness* relations. We attempt to elucidate the general principles (*I.3X) and (*I.4), and the interpretive sameness, illustrated by (3), examples of which psycho-analytic practice aims at finding. We cannot tackle here the corresponding problems of the *individuation* of the *I*'s [*I c h* s], the persons X each one of us is, and FREUD's egos [Ichs].[2] Thus, we not deal with normal lack of I-integration, not even with the trivial case like those illustrated by examples (6) and (7), let alone the exciting psychiatric cases of synchronic *Ichstörung*.

3. Indexical Reference as the Structural Core of Experience

3.1 Subsumption of the Problem of the I's Under Indexical Reference

The problem of the *I*'s is a central piece in the problem of the self. Here we will not consider the self in general. We must, however, generalize our problem in a different direction. Evidently firs-person reference is a special case of indexical reference. Personal pronouns and demonstratives form a unified semantic category. Most discussions of the self or of the I, nevertheless, adopt a type of referential atomism. They deal with the *I*'s in isolation, neglecting the place of THE *I*'s within the general phenomenon of indexicality. I propose to examine this general phenomenon first in order to build an appropriate background, and distill some guidance, for the study of the *I*'s.

3.2 Confrontational Reference to Objects

To live one must deal with objects and persons in one's environment as the individuals they are. One must locate them by confronting them *in propria persona* in some experience, or by connecting them to confronted objects. In confronting an object one places it in present experience thereby constituting it both as present

2 The general ontological and semantical theory from which I am approaching the problems in this paper is Guise Theory. It contains a full account of the different sameness relations discussed here as well as of others. This theory was first formulated in CASTAÑEDA (1974). This is reprinted in PAPE (1982) and in TLE. Guise Theory is discussed in PLANTINGA (1983) and in CLARK (1983), and in CASTAÑEDA's Replies to these authors (CASTAÑEDA 1983). Further discussions appear in articles of ROSENBERG (1986), SMITH (1986), SICHA (1986) and in CASTAÑEDA's Replies (CASTAÑEDA 1986). More recent discussions can be found in KÜNG (1989), HECKMANN (1989), KAPITAN (1989), RAPP (1989), BURKHARDT and DUFOUR (1989), JACOBI (1989) and CASTAÑEDA's (1989) replies to these authors, all in JACOBI and PAPE (1989). Guise Theory has been discussed and developed into an alternative ontology by WILLIAM RAPAPORT in several papers (1978, 1985/86). FRANCESCO ORILIA (1986, 1988) has also developed an alternative.

and as a presented referent. Confrontational perceptual experience is fundamental. Its core is indexical reference, whose sole function is to pinpoint items in experience. In the normal, doxastically default case of perception, we believe that what we are appeared to is physically real. That is, we equate items internal to the experience with items in the external world. Furthermore, in the veridical sub-case our indexical experiential equations are true. Let's consider a visual experience as a model:

The AUSTIN-KÜNNE Datum. Krista is driving us to her summer house perched on a high hill in the Black Forest. The road twists and turns in a long chain of loops; we don't complain, for we are enjoying the beautiful kaleidoscopic landscape. Suddenly Krista makes a very sharp turn left, and, keeping her hands firmly glued to the steering wheel, says:

(21) That tiny white dot on the very right is my house, where I live in July.

As KÜNNE has pointed out[3], Krista's (21) does not imply:

(22) I [Krista] live in a tiny white dot.

This lack of implication of (22) by (21) I have called the AUSTIN-KÜNNE Datum.[4] As I interpret this Datum, it establishes that the property being a tiny white dot is not predicated in (21) of a physical object. We must, however, go on to ask: *What* has that property? Patently, it must be something internal to Krista's perceptual content. If Krista succeeds in communicating her thoughts to her guests that property will also appear instantiated in her guests' perceptual experiences. Still, what is the subject having that property? A new look at (21) furnishes the answer. Statement (21) presents the property of being a tiny white dot as exemplified by what Krista calls "That." Krista's sentence (21) expresses compactly the selfsame statement as is expressed, with its structure more visibly, by the sentence:

(21*) That, which IS a tiny white dot, is my house, where I live in July.

Krista's *that*, as an internal item in her perceptual field, has really the properties it appears to have. In the logic of perception, Krista's statement (21) is equivalent to, but not identical to, Krista's statement:

(23) *That*, which *looks like* a tiny white dot, is my house, where I live in July.

This raises a profoundly important question: What is the meaning of the first, capitalized 'IS' in (21*)? Clearly, it is an equational 'is'. It is short for 'is the same as'. What sort of sameness is this?

---

3 See WOLFGANG KÜNNE (1989). He refers to J. L. AUSTIN (1962), pp. 98, 136.

4 See my reply to WOLFGANG KÜNNE in JACOBI and PAPE (1989). For additional delving into perceptual indexicality see PILOT (1989), PRAUSS (1989), and my replies to these papers in JACOBI and PAPE (1989).

3.3 Identity, Consubstantiation, and Consociation

According to the story, Krista's perceptual experience is veridical. Hence her visual judgment (21), identical with (21*), is true. This helps in determining its truth conditions and the sense of 'IS' in (21*). To be sure (21) may be false. Krista may have confused her house with another, or she may have been joking. No matter. If (21) is true, there exists in the physical world a house where Krista lives, which she sees, and, furthermore, it is really (the same as) what she calls *that*. Thus, (21), or (21*), is a mixed equation of the form:

(21.A)	That which is [looks like] a tiny white dot	*is the same as*	my house, where I live.

This sameness relation is very exciting. Krista's *that* is just an internal part of her perceptual presentational content. Her house is an external object in physical space. They are not strictly identical. By strict identity I mean Leibnizian identity: total unrestricted indiscernibility. The Austin-Künne Datum is a masterful stroke. It differentiates at once between Krista's subjective perceptual *that* and her house, and between strict identity and the subjective-objective sameness of (21).

The Austin-Künne Datum shows further that the sameness proclaimed in (21) is *non-communitarian*. By this I mean that each of the items said correctly to be the same have properties that do not transfer to the other items across the sameness relation. We have already seen how the properties of being a tiny white dot, being a dot, being white, being tiny, possessed by Krista's *that* do not transfer to Krista's house. In fact, later on we learned in confirmation that Krista's July residence is a huge blue three-story house. None of these properties transfers to Krista's visual *that*.

With the sameness posited by Krista in her statement (21) we must compare a homogeneously objective sameness, say, the one in:

(24) Krista's huge blue three-story house is (the same as) the villa Il Ritiro built by Braunschweiger in 1775 where Baron Karl von Falkenberg and Baron Franz von Frankenburg fought a mortal duel for the affections of the Attendant to the Marchesa Francesca di Soavia.

This sameness is communitarian. All the properties of Krista's house mentioned in (24) transfer to the villa *Il Ritiro*, and vice versa. For example, (24) implies each of the following:

(25.1) Krista's blue house was built by Braunschweiger;
(25.2) Krista's huge house is where Von Falkenberg and Von Frankenburg fought for Francesca's Attendant;
(26.1) The villa Il Ritiro is a blue house;
(26.2) The villa Il Ritiro is a huge building, where Krista lives in July.

We must, consequently, distinguish the sameness of (21) from the sameness of (24), and both from strict identity. Both sameness are contingent. Both are epistemologically empirical: they must be known on the basis of experience. The thoroughly objective, existential sameness of (24) we call *consubstantiation*. The paired items that are the same in this sense all belong to the real world in one unitary entity: they constitute one physical substance. The reality of this existential sameness needs in general no experience to obtain. On the other hand, the hybrid sameness of (21) is inherently, ontologically empirical: it is *experiential*. To have an experience is to confront such subjective indexical items through which the external world reveals itself. Thus, Krista's very visual experience creates her visual *that* wrapped up in its apparent *sameness* to a physical object. This subjective-objective sameness includes a component association established by an operation of a finite mind. This is the kind of association a novelist creates who lays it down that the murderer of XXX is XXX's lover. It is the association of John F. Kennedy and the Attorney General of the United States in 1962 in the mind of a person who confuses the Kennedy brothers. This mind-made sameness we call *consociation*.

A full account of the structure of experience and of the world we confront in experience requires other sameness relations. These are copulational relations, that is, forms of predication. Here we cannot go into these matters. We speak of existential or consubstantiational predication to refer to the having of properties by existents *qua* existents. We call consociational the possession of properties by objects through stipulation, or through mental activity, wheter in confused thinking about the world or in literary creation. It does not matter whether the consociated items do not exist. Strict identity, or self-identity is the most pervasive, absolutely reflexive, wholly trivial, and utterly necessary form of sameness valid for everything, whether existing or not[5].

3.4 Perceptual Judgments: This's and That's

To sum up our discussion of demonstrative reference in perception let's outline an analysis of perceptual judgments. Recall Krista's visual judgment:

(21) That tiny white dot is my house, where I live.

The first step in its analysis is:

(21.A)	That which is [looks like] a tiny white dot	*is the same as*	my house, where I live.

This reveals the following components of (21):

(a) The central hybrid sameness proposition:
THAT *IS THE SAME* AS MY HOUSE;

5 On identity and the other sameness relations see the materials mentioned in Note 2.

(b1) The *is*-predication of the subjective element:
THAT IS A TINY WHITE DOT;

(b2) The *looks-like*-predication of the subjective element:
THAT LOOKS LIKE A TINY WHITE DOT

(c) The objective predication of the objective element:
MY HOUSE IS WHERE I LIVE.

Undoubtedly, there are several illuminating theories that can be erected to account for these data. I propose, tentatively, to interpret the copulational relations present in (a)-(c) as follows:

A. The sameness predication in (a) is consubstantiation;
B. The predication in (b1) is consociational;
C. The predication in (b2) is consubstantiational;
D. The predication in (c) is consubstantiational.

By **A** we secure in veridical perception an access to the external world. In veridical perception every subjective *that* [*this*] forms the same substance with the perceived physical individual. Physical objects, when perceived, grow demonstrative tails by means of which the perceivers apprehend them. By **B** we secure a general non-transferability of the properties of the subjective item to the physical objects with which it forms the same substance. The actual manifestations of things in perceptual consciousness are subjective. They may be causallly matched in other persons' perceptions of the same things. Nevertheless, each one has his/her own experiences with his/her own perceptual contents. Thus, consubstantiation is transitive, but consociation is not. It is the combination of **A** and **B** that makes the sameness of (21) non-communitarian. Thus, the ostensive sameness of (21) is, as observed, a compacting of **A** and **B** and **C**. **C** secures the transferability of the *looks-like* properties of the subjective elements to the perceived physical objects. Clearly, *what* things look like is personal; but *that* they look like such and such is an intersubjective matter. **D** secures a wholly objective sameness in the physical world.

3.5 Confrontational Reference to Time and Space: Now's and Here's

Perceptual confrontation with objects is the placing of objects in the world. To place objects in the world is to place them in the causal structure of the world. This involves placing them in the spatiotemporal structure that underlies the causal order. Therefore, to experience a confrontation of objects in the world is to experience a confrontation of the space and the time of the world.

As we have seen, confrontations of objects pivot on demonstrative reference of the *this* [*that*] type. The demonstrative individuals are the subjective protrusions of the perceived physical objects. Clearly, we must have the undergirding subjective protrusions of space and time. These are the internal contents strictly referred to indexically as *here* [*there*] or as *now*. Hence, the same considerations about identity, consubstantiation, and consociation we deployed above about *this*'s and *that*'s apply to *here*'s and *now*'s.

3.6 Confrontational Reference to the Experiencer: The I's

Elsewhere I have argued, siding with SARTRE, against the Fichtean thesis that all consciousness is self-consciousness.[6] The fundamental type of consciousness is non-reflexive, egoless. Furthermore, reflexive consciousness is mounted on a base of unreflective consciousness of objects. This in its turn is mounted on diffuse, inarticulated sensory consciousness. This cumulative hierarchical structure of consciousness is crucial. Of course, unreflective consciousness of objects is, as discussed above, built on third-person indexical reference.

Here we are interested in reflexive, *I*-anchored consciousness. An episode of self-consciousness has as its top echelon a sub-experience of confrontation with the experiencer in *propria persona*. Again, the backbone of this confrontation is indexical reference: reference to oneself in the first-person way. This exhibits the same pattern of indexicality found above in the analysis of Krista's visual demonstrative reference to her house.

An *I* is, thus, strictly speaking, a subjective, experienced item. It presents itself as existing, and as being, like Krista's visual *that*, consubstantiated with a physical individual. Consider this example:

(27) I, who feels at the moment exhilarated, am the author of TSM, an unknown treatise, where he discusses an agent's occasional moral duty to change his moral code.

Its basic logical form is the general pattern of indexicality:

(27.A)	I who feels [seems to feel]...	*am the same as*	the author of TSM, who discusses ...

Again, we have here the following components of (27):

(a) The central hybrid sameness proposition:
I *AM THE SAME AS* THE AUTHOR OF TSM;

(b1) The *is*-predication of the subjective element:
I FEEL AT THE MOMENT EXHILARATED

(b2) The *looks-like*-predication of the subjective element:
I SEEM TO FEEL EXHILARATED

6 See JOHANN GOTTLIEB FICHTE, *Science of Knowledge*, and JEAN-PAUL SARTRE, *Being and Nothingness: An essay on Phenomenological Ontology*. My latest discussion of an Externus-type of consciousness appears in TOMBERLIN 1987.

(c) The objective predication of the objective element:
THE AUTHOR OF TSM DISCUSSES AN AGENT'S MORAL DUTY...

Again, the copulational relations present in (a)-(c) are as follows:

A. The sameness predication in (a) is consubstantiation;
B. The predication in (b1) is consociational;
C. The predication in (b2) is consubstantiational;
D. The predication in (c) is consubstantiational.

Of course there are most important differences between third-person and first-person reference. These have two sources. On the one hand, the role of subject of experience is a fundamental structural element of experience. On the other hand, the role of subject has certain unique and peculiar epistemic features. Let's discuss these features briefly.

3.7 Dimensions of Certainty in Indexical Reference

The epistemological accessibility of reality to a thinker requires that there be in principle a *manifestation* of reality *in* experience. This requires a structure within which the manifestation can occur. That is precisely the experienced space-time structure. This is a network of *now*- and *here*[*there*'s]-positions for experienced *this*'s and *that*'s, and for experienced *I*'s. That network is fundamental for experience. It not only constitutes the framework for indexical items representing objects. It must be accessible in itself. There cannot be uncertainty about these experiential coordinates. This is the first dimension of certainty, *subjective certainty*, of indexical reference.

If we are to gain any access to reality the experienced spatio-temporal framework must *somehow* correspond, must be fastened, to the structure of reality. There must be a certified hook-up between experienced space and time and physical spacetime. This hook-up must make itself present in every experience. Hence, each experienced *now* is underlain by an interval of real physical time, and every experienced *here* or *there* is underwritten by a volume of real physical space. However, this implies logically nothing about the actual geometrical, or causal, nature of physical space or physical time. Nor does it imply that experienced spaces and times have all the same geometry, let alone the geometry of physical space.[7] Physical geometry and specific causal principles are needed to give a precise sense to the above underlined crucial 'somehow'. In any case, here is the second dimension of certainty, *structural objective certainty*, characteristic of

7 These are the fundamental premises behind KANT's view that space and time are forms of perception. He also saw the structural objective certainty of references to perceived time and space. This led him to what I call *Kant's Unifying Hypothesis About Time and Space*. This is the thesis that physical space [time] and all perceptual spaces are one and the same. See Critique of Pure Reason, Transcendental Aesthetics. This hypothesis has been shown to be false. There is an enormous literature on perceptual spaces. For my ontological discussion see CASTAÑEDA 1977. This is an abridgment of the last two chapters of CASTAÑEDA 1982.

indexical reference to time and space. This certainty secures no specific feature of physical time, other than its being the time of the experience in question and being part of a special network of ordering relations.

The subjective and the subjective objective dimensions of certainty undergird non-reflexive consciousness. Recall the cumulative-hierarchical character of reflective consciousness. Because of it the indexicality of unreflective consciousness, together with its subjective and objective certainties, are an integral part of reflective consciousness.

The onsetting of reflective consciousness requires access to current episodes of thinking. In principle there can be awareness of one's current mental acts without awareness of oneself *qua* oneself. Thus there may be consciousness of *un*owned episodes of thinking and feeling.[8]

The highest degree of reflexive consciousness requires, besides, access to the agent, not merely as an experienced item, but as a subject, that is, as an experienced experiencer. Thus, there must be an *objective certainty* that a real entity appears as a thinking *I*. The general validity of this certainty yields an equivalence (a consubstantiation of sorts) between objective certainty and *structural intersubjective certainty*. There is, however, no certainty of any particular consubstantiation between an I and a physical embodiment of it. This is precisely the force of postulate (*I.4) above in Part I.

On the other hand, experienced *this*'s and *that*'s, which in veridical perception are the subjective tails of physical objects, lack objective certainty. They may fail to be in fact such subjective tails. They have only a general causal certainty that something causes the episodes of thinking in which they exist as such subjective tails - perhaps bereft of physical objects.

The arguments for radical skepticism about the reality of an external world bring forth a profound dimension of certainty of indexical reference. Those arguments undermine not only the local objectivity that may lie behind a given *this* or *that*, but also the general causal objectivity mentioned above. Yet, as DESCARTES argued in his celebrated *Cogito*: *Sum*, I can conceive of the world as wholly failing to exist, yet in so conceiving I secure my own existence. KANT saw perfectly well the purely structural nature of this certainty and enshrined it in his distinction between noumenon and phenomenon. In his honor we call this the noumenal certainty of first-person reference. Apparently in agreement with DESCARTES I also attribute *noumenal certainty* to our references to experienced *now*'s; but, in disagreement with him, I further attribute certainty to experienced *here*'s. As against KANT, I hold that both *now*- and *here*-references also possess noumenal certainty. I substitute a noumenon formally structured by space-like and time-like networks for KANT's wholly indivisible and holistic noumenon.[9]

8 In CASTAÑEDA (1967) a level in between unowned consciousness and full self-consciousness is recognized. It is a level that has the contrast between what is internal and what is external. Vacuous I's are posited to collect the internal. Full self-consciousness involves, besides, the contrast between oneself and other persons. Later on I realized that my two levels of self-hood correspond to some extent to MARTIN BUBER's distinction between two strands of *I*ness. One is the contrast *I-Other*, and the other is the contrast *I-Thou*. See BUBER (1984). In fact we have three strands in the concept of *I*: *I-That*[*it*], *I-That* [*He/She*], and *I-Thou*. Since the days of *Indicators and Quasi-indicators* I believe that the most complex and exciting English indicator is *you*.

9 See DESCARTES's Meditations, KANT's first Critique, Paralogisms, and CASTAÑEDA (1987b). This study complements CASTAÑEDA (1987c).

4. Fleeting Experiential Particulars and Evanescent I's

4.1 First-Person Reference and Experiential I-Equations

The many-dimensional certainty of first-person reference is part of the logic of the I's. That is, some implications are valid for first-person reference, which have no counterparts in demonstrative reference to objects. To illustrate let's return to (27). Its surface analysis is:

(27.A) I *am the same as* the author of TSM,
who feels [seems to feel]... who discusses ...

By virtue of general indexicality the experiential properties are equivalenty predicated of the *I* of the experience in the consociational form (*feels*) and in the consubstantiational form (*seems to feel*). Yet both forms of predication allow transferability of properties to the physical individual thought to be consubstantiated with that *I*. The patterns of sameness involving an *I* are communitarian. This is grounded on the objective certainty of *I*-reference. There is always a real individual that can receive whatever properties the *I* has in experience.

There are also further structural features of the *I*'s. Demonstrative reference to objects is particularized because of the plurality of objects that we may encounter at a given time. A perceptual experience presents a field which in principle can, and typically has, many *this*'s and *that*'s. Each sub-experience has a fundamental unity of consciousness, and its own I. The unity of each experience and the necessary objectivity (that is, embodiment) of the *I*'s yield together a fundamental principle in the logic of first-person reference. Let P(I) be any proposition expressed by a sentence containing any number of forms *i* of the first-person pronoun, let P(I/x) be the proposition schema or property that is predicated of what *i* denotes, and let '==>' express logical implication in the logic of the I's. Then:

(I.1*) P(I) ==> There exists an individual x such that:
I am consubstantiated with x and P(I/x).

The unitary role of each *I* is signaled here by unifying all the *I*'s that may figure in P(I) into one single *I*. The objectivity of the *I* is represented by the implied consubstantiation of the *I* with an existent individual, i.e., an individual that has a place in the causal order. Principle (I.1*) is the necessary truth underlying the equations between oneself and the persons X, discussed as (*I.3X) above in Part I.

4.2 The Fleetingness of Indexical Referents

A little reflection shows that indexical reference is perforce *personal*: one refers indexically to what one confronts in one's experiences. Indexical reference is essentially *ephemeral*: the subjective indexical items one finds in experience are different from experience to experience. Palpably, the thisnesses and thatnesses of the objects one perceives are exasperatingly fleeting. A *this* quickly turns into a *that*, and soon enough it is lost to experience and is not even a remote *that*. Nothing is intrinsically a *this*, or a *that*. One bestows this status on several very different things in succession: "This [pointing to a man] is older than this [pointing to a woman] and shorter than this ..." A *you* goes away and is replaced by another, and then there is just oneself alone fretting about something or other. Nothing is really an enduring *you*. Likewise, no moment can claim to be a *now* beyond itself - except perhaps the whole of time as confronted by God. No place has a proprietary right to be a *here* or a *there* - except perhaps the whole of the world space as confronted by God.

Is there at least an *I* that abides through the vicissitudes of its experiences? If so, which I? Mine? Well, this is the only I I can refer to singularly at this moment by using these tokens of the first-person pronoun *I*. But how enduring is it? How long can *I* exist? I believe, of course, that I *have* lived for over sixty years. Yet doesn't this believing amounts to I-now believing to have lived, i.e., to *I-now* believing that something, or, perhaps, a sequence of somethings has existed for over sixty years?

Subjective indexical particulars exist only during the experience in which they play their evanescent roles. The *I*'s are no exception.

The personal character of indexical reference raises an important problem. Having experiences is the fundamental property of a mind or person. The power to make indexical references is a basic category of a person. Hence, to think of something as a person one must be able to represent to oneself that something's indexical references. We need others to cooperate with them and to share with them the world that we all both cognize and act upon. For valuable cooperation sometimes we need to communicate transparently others' thoughts.

How can we represent to ourselves others' indexical references? The answer to this lies in the mechanism of *quasi-indexical reference*, of which we have taken some glimpses above. Quasi-indicators are pivotal mechanisms of reference in the language of other minds or persons. They capture our indexical references, ephemeral and personal though these are, into propositionally transparent, enduring, and interpersonal depictions. This of course requires a harmonious match of world, thinking, and language. It requires a comprehensive ontology that can be semantically anchored to the syntax of our language. We cannot discuss this here.[10]

4.3 The Enduring World and the Evanescent *I*'s

The ephemeral nature of indexical reference creates a serious problem. How can we refer to the same things again and again? To carry out plans we engage in we find ourselves confronting some of the same objects and persons again and again. Our plans require a diachronic unity of both the world and the agents.

10 See materials mentioned in Notes 1 and 2.

Such a unity must be established in experience. How do we do it, if the core of each experience is a manifold of evanescent particulars?

This is a profound question. It falls beyond the scope of these meditations. The answer has to lie partly in the nature of the world. But partly however the answer involves our conceptions of transubstantiation: the patterns of changes that determine the diachronic unity of substances. These conceptions are mobilized in the particular experiences of a person who posits a past reality. And this has to be done, or so it seems, by a fleeting *I* confronting a domain of evanescent particulars. Again, how? Perhaps some brief comments may not be amiss.

The world of experience is, first of all, not a Heraclitean chaos. It has some abiding hierarchical logical and causal structure. (The noumenon underlying the world and our experience is, of course, another topic.) In the second place, each *I* is the *I* of an experience. Like all indexical particulars, it is evanescent and exists only for the duration of the experience in question. An *I* exists only in the present. Third, the thread of the answer is this: An *I* is nothing but a subject and its contents are literally the contents of the experiences of which it is its subject. This opens the door to the *I* of the experience identifying itself by consubstantiation with anything in those thought-of contents.[11] Fourth, the unity and order of the world is registered in the memories of the thinker. These memories are in the doxastic pedestal that support the thinking episodes constitutive of the experience. The mobilized beliefs, assumptions, and takens-for-granted make the world with its posited past a common framework for all judgments. This mobilization yields beliefs and thinking episodes about continuant physical entities in stretches of the history of the world. These are all consubstantiations and posited instances of diachronic sameness (*transubstantiation*). The *I* of the experience appears consubstantiated with some contemporaries that have undergone those transubstantiations. Yet there is literally no enduring *I*, except for its duration in a specious present. Except perhaps God.

An *I* is intrinsically nothing but a subject of experience. It corresponds to the maximal unity of the experiences that are, at a given time, internally unified as one total experience by virtue of their being co-consciousness of a manifold of contents. An *I* is in itself the hypostastic construct of the unity of the experience of which it is its subject. Of course, as we have insisted above, behind each *I* lies a physically real, even a noumenal existent. Let's consider an example:

Friedrich's Bee Watching. At a park Friedrich is watching some bees descend on some flowers, pick up some pollen, and then fly away. He is fully aware of himself. His whole experience hinges on a succession of overlapping *I*'s existing alongside a succession of overlapping specious presents. Friedrich is enjoying several sub-experiences. He is attending to one big yellow jacket. He sees it move from a red flower to a yellow one. This seeing occupies a specious present: "From here to here." There is thus the subject of that seeing. During that interval he hears several drones from different bees. Each hearing has its own subject, an *I* that lasts less than the seeing *I*. Similarly, during the same interval he throws off several ants crawling up his legs. Each one of these seeing and throwing episodes

11 Here is a fundamental indexical premise for KANT's refutation of idealism in his first *Critique*. See also the paper by HARALD PILOT mentioned in Note 4.

has its own subject, again very short-lived. Also about the middle of Friedrich's seeing his favorite yellow jacket he feels an itching on his head; he scratches. An itching *I*, a scratching *I*, and an itching-and-scratching *I* come into existence and quickly vanish.

The itching-and-scratching *I* overlaps the other two *I*'s. During the first moment of just itching the itching *I* coincides with the itching-and-scratching *I*. Then this *I* is the subject of the integrated experiences of itching and scratching. Likewise, Friedrich's whole experience of seeing the yellow jacket fly from one flower to another pivots on one *I*. This ensues from the integration of the different sub-experiences into one comprehensive reflexive consciousness. That *I* is a unit built up from the subjects of the sub-experiences. The real *I* at a given time T is the reflexive subject of the maximal co-conscious integration of experiences at T. The specious present determined by a succession of overlapping of co-consciousness determines in the normal human cases the short-lived *I* of the interval.

Nothing so far precludes that there be one *I* unifying experiences across different persons or bodies. On the other side, the sub-experiences of a person at a given time may fail to unify into one subject of experience. In principle, for instance, Friedrich may have been mentally disorganized. Some of the experiences mentioned above may have failed to integrate at all, or may have integrated only partially. These are empirically matters that may appear in many different degrees. Psychiatric practice may have (and undoubtedly has) established many types and families of such failures of *I*-integration.

4.4 The Hierarchy Within Self-Consciousness and Psychiatric Possibilities

The reflexivity of self-consciousness, as remarked, has a internal, contentual cumulative hierarchical structure:

(1) conceptually inarticulated sensory consciousness
(2) egoless better: I-less, articulated consciousness of objects
(3) unowned consciousness of occurring mental episodes
(4) I-consciousness

At the second level a primitive relation of CO-CONSCIOUSNESS links the contents of a simple experience (or sub-experience) as the contents of *one* (sub-experience). Each experience (or sub-experience) has its own *now-here[there]* spatio-temporal framework. More or less simulataneous experiences normally combine into more comprehensive experiences. This requires an intimate organization of the different synchronous experiential spaces and times. Let's call CO-INTEGRATION the network of structural relations through which a unified total experience is built. Thus, the unity of a person's normal, fully organized total experience at a given time T is wrought out by a system of low-level instantiations of CO-CONSCIOUSNESS, and by a thorough system of instances of CO-INTEGRATION. Let's call META-INTEGRATION the relations that structure unowned reflexive experiences. Let's call SUBJECTIONS those structural relations that subordinate an experience to a subject, that is, through which an *I* is posited, or hypotstatized.

In the normal case every mechanism runs perfectly and all run in marvellous unison. In the normal case of self-consciousness all the contents of the experience are unified into sub-experiences, and these into a fully unified experience, each sub-experience is experienced as a strand of consciousness that forms part of a unified experience and is owned by an *I*. In such cases the *I* referred to is the maximally integrated and unified *I* - the *I* subsuming all the *I*'s of the unified sub-experiences. Likewise, the *now* of the total experience is the hierarchical cumulation of the *nows* of the sub-experiences.

In an abnormal case a single mechanism by itself or a combination of such mechanisms fails to work properly. Abnormal cases are data about the distinctness of strands in reality that normally go together. The closer the togetherness in question the more informative is the abnormality that breaks it. For instance, a person whose mechanisms eliciting the CO-CONSCIOUSNESS, CO-INTEGRATION, and META-INTEGRATION relations work well may yet suffer from disruption of a SUBJECTION mechanism. He may experience a sub-experience as if it were not his.

The preceding list of mechanisms engaged in the production of self-consciousness is of course nothing but a very crude armchair-philosophical schematic typology. This is precisely one juncture where psychiatry can, and should, guide the philosophy of mind.

4.5 Past Attributions to Oneself: "What a healthy child I was!"

First-person attributions always posit a present *I*. Yet consider FREUD's example (1) above:

(1) Sometimes I think what a healthy child I was!

Evidently FREUD thinks sometimes a proposition he expresses by means of a first-person past-tense sentence:

(0.I) I was such a healthy child!

On the surface the situation is of the same type as those in which we ourselves use a third-person past-tense sentence to capture (part of) what (O.I) asserts, for example:

(O.SF) Sigmund Freud was a very healthy child.

Both propositions agree on one point: that a certain individual had a certain property *in the past*. They differ dramatically concerning the utterance present, i.e., the time of utterance. Proposition (O.SF) is neutral concerning the present existence of that individual: he may very well not exist at the time of utterance. In fact, as far as (0.SF) reaches into the world, the Sigmund Freud under conideration may have died as a child, or later but before our utterance. On the ther hand, FREUD's proposition (0.I) decidedly asserts the present existence of he subject of predication. Both propositions agree only partially concerning the liachronic identity of the subject of predication. Neither posits that the past ubject is literally identical with a later subject. (0.SF) leaves it open whether the ast subject, the child, was not then a Sigmund Freud. Likewise, (0.I) leaves it pen whether the child had any experience, hence, any *I* at all. Let the child last ong enough to exist at the time of utterance. According to (0.SF) in such a case continuous biological entity exists through the whole period. Yet (0.I) does not osit a continuous entity lasting through the mentioned past through the tterance present; furthermore, it rejects any continuity of that entity as an *I*, nd leaves it undetermined whether there is a continuous biological or physical bject lasting throughout that time.

Statement (0.I) is of the logical form:

(0.I.A) There is [in a tenseless sense] an individual X such that: X *was* (consubstantiated with) such a healthy child, and X and I are [transubstantiationally] diachronically the same.

Apparently FREUD was not committing himself to the lastingness of an *I* from is childhood to the present of his statement. In the exegesized text (2) above he autiously says: "... it [= my ego = *I*] should appear, in conscious thoughts, many imes [mehrmals] and in different places or in different relations, as in statement 1)." He is not saying: "it appears in different times (Zeitungen)." Nevertheless, e does claim that one's ego lasts through many experiences, through illness and he therapeutic treatment and thereafter.

.6 Future *I*'s

irst-person future-tense statements also speak of utterance-present *I*'s. Just as tatements about one's past incorporate memories, statements about one's uture incorporate expectations. Here is, however, a serious question. One can rust the past to remain constant; but the future is not so reliable. Here lie intersting issues, which we cannot go into. Perhaps we should record only that redictions about oneself depend for their truth, *not* on the preservation of an *I*, ut on criteria of personal identity. This is another large topic.

. Conclusion

.1 The Evanescent I's, the Persons, the Ego, and the Soul

Io permanent *I* underlies the history of a person. There exist successions of phemeral *I*'s, some of which are interlocking, overlapping because specious resents are overlapping. As long as there is a continuous consciousness from me *t* to time *t*' there could be an encompassing *I* that endures from *t* to *t*'. Yet there need be no such an *I*. It all depends on the degree of organization of the experience of each moment during the interval (*t*, *t'*), and on how much overlapping and integration by co-consciousness and meta-integration the successive experiences have.

The crucial ontological point is that the *I*'s, exactly like all other indexical individuals, are ephemeral and subjective. They exist in the present. They link the person who has the experiences with the objective world. They, together with all other indexical items, provide the experience of reality, namely, the reality of the present. All of them are intrinsically simple items, and function as subjective epistemic handles of the experienced existing persons and objects.

An *I* is the creation of a process of a thinking episode that includes co-consciousness of the unity of the thinking and its contents. As we have remarked it has several dimensions of certainty. It certifies its own existence and its own role in experience. It points to the person whose thinking it is. It reveals that the person has thinking powers. But as such it reveals nothing else. The person underlying an *I* may be anything whatever. Even the underlying entity postulated as enduring in past- or future-tense statements need not be an enduring physical person, or a metaphysically transcendent substance. As KANT observed a duration of consciousness is compatible with a succession of underlying substances.[12] Each *I* indeed points to a noumenon underlying all of experience. Thus there is a strong temptation - a dialectic illusion deeply seated in the nature of the process of thinking - to equate the experienced ephemeral referent with the pointed-to experiencer in the world and with the pointed-to noumenal reality. Even KANT was not free of this temptation.

The temptation must be resisted at all levels. Nonetheless, it is of the utmost importance to fasten to three facts: (i) the evanescence of the *I*'s presupposes some underlying constant phenomenal as well as noumenal reality; (ii) that evanescence neither requires nor runs against the view that the constant element in phenomenal reality is a pattern of diachronic connections among physical individuals; (iii) likewise, neither is the lastingness of the *I*'s required for, nor does its fleetingness oppose, the thesis of a noumenal soul.

FREUD's ego is not identical with an *I*. It is an enduring set of powers to think in the first person. The sense in which an ego is the same as an *I* is at best that of consubstantiation. Hence, a person's ego is at best transubstantiated with a broken sequence of *I*'s.

Summary: This is an inquiry into the nature of what we think as "I". What does one refer to internally, *de dicto*, when one uses assertively a sentence containing an inflection of the first-person pronoun? What sort of entity that referent is? How does such a referent relate to the person calling himself or herself "I"? We shall say that a token of a form of the first-person pronoun used to make a thinking singular reference strictly or internally denotes an *I*.

No permanent *I* underlies the history of a person. There exist successions of ephemeral *I*'s, some of which are interlocking, overlapping because specious presents are overlapping. As long as there is a continuous consciousness from

12 See KANT's refutation of MENDELSOHN in the first *Critique*.

time *t* to time *t'* there could be an encompassing *I* that endures from *t* to *t'*. Yet there need be no such an *I*. It all depends on the degree of organization of the experience of each moment during the interval (*t*, *t'*), and on how much overlapping and integration by co-consciousness and meta-integration the successive experiences have.

In the normal case these mechanisms run perfectly and all run in marvellous unison. In the normal case of self-consciousness all the contents of the experience are unified into sub-experiences, and these into a fully unified experience, each sub-experience is experienced as a strand of consciousness that forms part of a unified experience and is owned by an *I*. In an abnormal case a single mechanism by itself or a combination of such mechanisms fails to work properly. For instance, a person whose mechanisms eliciting the CO-CONSCIOUSNESS (integration by simultaneous occurance within consciousness), CO-INTEGRATION (integration of diffrent contents into one unified experience), and META-INTEGRATION (structuring reflexive experience, thought) relations work well may yet suffer from disruption of a SUBJECTION mechanism (subordinating experience to a subject, thus producing the character of mine-ness of experience). He may experience a sub-experience as if it were not his. Thus psychiatry can, and should, guide the philosophy of mind in trying to delineate the diffrent types of integrating and unifying relations as structures at work in every experiencing person.

The crucial ontological point is that the *I*'s, exactly like all other indexical individuals, are ephemeral and subjective. They exist in the present. They link the person who has the experiences with the objective world. They, together with all other indexical items, provide the experience of reality, namely, the reality of the present. All of them are intrinsically simple items, and function as subjective epistemic handles of the experienced existing persons and objects.

An *I* is the creation of a process of a thinking episode that includes co-consciousness of the unity of the thinking and its contents. It has several dimensions of certainty. It certifies its own existence and its own role in experience. It points to the person whose thinking it is. It reveals that the person has thinking powers. But as such it reveals nothing else. The person underlying an *I* may be anything whatever. Even the underlying entity postulated as enduring in past- or future-tense statements need not be an enduring physical person, or a metaphysically transcendent substance.

The temptation must be resisted at all levels. Nonetheless, it is of the utmost importance to fasten to three facts: (i) the evanescence of the *I*'s presupposes some underlying constant phenomenal as well as noumenal reality; (ii) that evanescence neither requires nor runs against the view that the constant element in phenomenal reality is a pattern of diachronic connections among physical individuals; (iii) likewise, neither is the lastingness of the *I*'s required for, nor does their fleetingness oppose, the thesis of a noumenal soul.

Personen, Egos und Iche: Ihre Selbigkeitsrelationen

Zusammenfassung: Die Untersuchung betrifft die Natur dessen, was wir mit "Ich" meinen. Worauf bezieht man sich innerlich, *de dicto*, wenn man einen Satz bejahend ausspricht, der eine Flexionsform des Pronomens der ersten Person singular enthält? Auf welche Art Entität bezieht man sich dabei? In welcher Beziehung steht diese Entität zu der Person, die sich "Ich" nennt? Wir legen für das Folgende fest, daß eine einzelne sprachliche Äußerung von der Form des Pronomens der ersten Person singular, die verwendet wird, um eine gedachte singuläre Bezugnahme vorzunehmen, im strikten Sinne bzw. intern ein *Ich* bezeichnet.

Der Lebensgeschichte einer Person liegt kein dauerhaftes *Ich* zugrunde, es existieren vielmehr Abfolgen vergänglicher *Ich*e, die zum Teil ineinandergreifen oder überlappen, weil das Bewußtsein von einer Abfolge im wesentlichen Bewußtsein der unmittelbaren Vergangenheit in der Gegenwart ist. Sofern ein kontinuierlichen Bewußtsein vom Zeitpunkt *t* bis zum Zeitpunkt *t'* besteht, kann ebenso, muß aber nicht, ein umfassendes *Ich* bestehen, das von *t* bis *t'* andauert: Dies hängt vom Organisationsgrad der Erfahrung in jedem einzelnen Augenblick des Intervalls (*t,t'*) ab, d.h. davon, in welchem Ausmaß die momenthaften einzelnen Erfahrungen überlappen bzw. integriert sind dadurch, daß sie zusammen im Bewußtsein auftreten (co-consciousness) oder in Reflexionsakten strukturiert werden (meta-integration).

Im Normalfall laufen diese Mechanismen in erstaunlichem Gleichklang ab. So sind im normalen Selbstbewußtsein alle verschiedenen Erfahrungsinhalte zunächst in Untererfahrungen und diese wiederum in einer vollständigen einheitlichen Erfahrung geeint. Jede Untererfahrung wird als Bewußseinsstrang erfahren, der einen Teil der geeinten Erfahrung ausmacht und einem *Ich* angehört. Im pathologischen Fall liegt eine Fehlfunktion eines Mechanismus oder einer Kombination solcher Mechanismen vor. So können beispielsweise bei einer Person die Mechanismen CO-CONSCIOUSNESS (Integration durch gleichzeitiges Auftreten im Bewußtsein), CO-INTEGRATION (Integration unterschiedlicher Erfahrungsinhalte in eine Einheit der Erfahrung) und META-INTEGRATION (Strukturierende reflexive Erfahrung, Denken) intakt sein bei gleichzeitiger Fehlfunktion des Mechanismus der SUBJECTION (Zuordnung der Erfahrung zu einem *Ich*, d.h. Produktion der Meinhaftigkeit der Erfahrung). Eine in dieser Weise gestörte Person würde bestimmte Untererfahrungen erleben als wären sie nicht die eigenen Erfahrungen. Diese Überlegungen machen deutlich, daß die Psychiatrie für das Unternehmen der Philosophie des Geistes, derartige Strukturen jeder Erfahrung im Sinne von Relationen der Integration und Einheit aufzufinden, hilfreich sein kann und sollte.

Der entscheidende ontologisch Punkt ist hier, daß die *Ich*e, ebenso wie andere indexikalische Einzeldinge, vergänglich und subjektiv sind. Sie existieren in der Gegenwart und verbinden die erfahrende Person mit der objektiv vorhandenen Welt. Zusammen mit allen anderen Indexikalischen Ausdrücken sichern sie die Erfahrung der Realität, d.h. der Realität des Gegenwärtigen. Ihrem Wesen nach sind all diese Ausdrücke einfach und haben die Funktion, Personen und Objekte der subjektiven Erkenntnis zugänglich zu machen.

Ein *Ich* ist das Produkt eines Denkgeschehens, das zugleich das Bewußtsein der Einheit des Denkens und seiner Inhalte einschließt. Ihm kommen unterschiedliche Dimensionen der Gewißheit zu. Es garantiert seine eigene Existenz und seine Rolle in der Erfahrung. Es verweist auf die Person deren Denken es ist. Es offenbart die Fähigkeit der Person zu denken - sonst nichts. Die einem *Ich* zugrundeliegende Person bleibt hier gänzlich unbestimmt. Auch bedarf es der Postulate weder einer physischen Person noch einer metaphysischen Substanz, um die Entität zu bezeichnen, die in Sätzen der Vergangenheit, Gegenwart und Zukunft als überdauernd bzw. zugrundeliegend gedacht werden muß.

Einer entsprechenden Versuchung muß man auf allen Ebenen widerstehen. Dennoch ist es von größter Wichtigkeit, an den folgenden drei Tatbeständen festzuhalten: (i) Die Vergänglichkeit der *Ich*e setzt eine wie auch immer geartete phänomenale als auch noumenale Realität voraus; (ii) die Ansicht, daß das beständige Element in der phänomenalen Realität ein Muster zeitübergreifender Verbindungen zwischen physikalischen Einzeldingen ist, wird durch diese Vergänglichkeit weder gefordert noch spricht sie dagegen; (iii) ebenso bedarf die These einer noumenalen Seele weder unbedingt eines *beständigen Ich*, noch spricht die Flüchtigkeit der *Ich*e gegen eine solche These.

References

Austin, J.L. (1962): Sense and Sensibilia. Clarendon, Oxford.

Buber, M. (1984): I and Thou. McMillan, New York.

Burkhardt, H., Dufour, C. (1989): Zwei Prädikationsarten und ihre ontologischen Implikationen. In: Jacobi, K. and Pape, H. (eds.): Die Struktur der Welt (in print).

Castañeda, H.N. (1967): Consciousness and Behavior: Their Basic Connections. In: H.N. Castañeda (ed.): Intentionality, Minds, and perception. Wayne State University, Detroit.

Castañeda, H.N. (1967): Indicators and Quasi-Indicators. American Philosophical Quarterly **4**, pp. 85-100. (reprinted in: H.N. Castañeda, Sprache und Erfahrung, translated by Helmut Pape, Suhrkamp, Frankfurt, 1982; also reprinted in: Thinking, Language, and Experience. University of Minnesota Press, Minneapolis, 1988; cited as TLE).

Castañeda, H.N. (1974): Thinking and the Structure of the World. Philosophia **4** pp. 4-40. (reprinted in Pape 1982 and in Thinking, Language, and Experience. University of Minnesota Press, Minneapolis, 1988).

Castañeda, H.N. (1977): Perception, Belief, and the Structure of Physical Objects and Consciousness. Synthese **35**, pp. 285-351.

Castañeda, H.N. (1982): Sprache und Erfahrung (übersetzt von H. Pape). Suhrkamp, Frankfurt.

Castañeda, H.N. (1983): Reply to Plantinga. In: Tomberlin, J. E. (ed.): Agent, Language, and the Structure of the World, pp. 329-353, Hackett , Indianapolis.

Castañeda, H.N. (1986): [Replies to Rosenberg, Smith, Sicha]. In: Tomberlin, J.F. (ed.): Hector-Neri Castañeda, Profiles Vol. 6, pp. 333-398, Reidel, Dordrecht.

Castañeda, H.N. (1987a): Self-consciousness, Demonstrative Reference, and the Self-Ascription View of Believing. In: Tomberlin, J.E. (ed.): Philosophical Perspectives: 1. Metaphysics, pp. 405-450. Ridgeview, Atascadero, California.

Castañeda, H.N. (1987b): Metaphysical Internalism: Selves, and the Holistic Indivisible Noumenon: A Frego-Kantian Reflection on Descartes's Cogito. Midwest Studies in Philosophy **XII**, pp. 129-144.

CASTAÑEDA, H.N. (1987c): The self and the I-Guises, Empirical and Transcendental. In: CRAMER, K., FULDA, H.F., HORSTMANN, R.-P. AND POTHAST, U. (eds.): Theorie der Subjektivität, pp. 105-140. Suhrkamp, Frankfurt a. M.
CASTAÑEDA, H.N. (1989): [Replies to KÜNG, HECKMANN, KAPITAN, RAPP, BURKHARDT and DUFOUR, PILOT, PRAUSS, JACOBI]. In: JACOBI, K. and PAPE, H. (eds.): Die Struktur der Welt (in print).
CASTAÑEDA, H.N. (1989): Fiction, Perception, and Existence (Reply to WOLFGANG KÜNNE). In: JACOBI, K. and PAPE, H. (eds.): Die Struktur der Welt (in print).
CLARK, R. (1983): Predication Theory: Guised and Disguised. In: TOMBERLIN, J. E. (ed.): Agent, Language, and the Structure of the World, pp. 111-129, Hackett, Indianapolis.
FICHTE, J.G. (1794/1970): Science of Knowledge (translated by PETER HEATH and JOHN LACHS), Appleton-Century-Crofts, New York.
FREUD, S. (1900/1938): The Interpretation of Dreams in The Basic Writings of Sigmund Freud (translated and edited by A. A. BRILL). The Modern Library, New York.
HECKMANN, H.-D. (1989): Intentionality, Perception, and Guise Theory. In: JACOBI, K. and PAPE, H. (eds.): Die Struktur der Welt (in print).
JACOBI, K. (1989): Individuation-Prädikation. In: JACOBI, K. and PAPE, H. (eds.): Die Struktur der Welt (in print).
KAPITAN, T. (1989): Preserving a Robust Sense of reality. In: JACOBI, K. and PAPE, H. (eds.): Die Struktur der Welt (in print).
KÜNG, G. (1989): 'Guises' und Noemata. In: JACOBI, K. and PAPE, H. (eds.): Die Struktur der Welt (in print).
KÜNNE, W. (1989): Perception, Fiction, and Elliptical Speech. In: JACOBI, K. and PAPE, H. (eds.): Die Struktur der Welt (in print).
ORILIA, F. (1986): Natural Language semantics and Guise Theory. doctoral dissertation, Bloomington, Indiana.
ORILIA, F. (1988): Identity Across Frames. Topoi (forthcoming).
PILOT, H. (1989): The Executional Role of Indexical Thinking. In: JACOBI, K. and PAPE, H. (eds.): Die Struktur der Welt (in print).
PRAUSS, G. (1989): Ptolomaic and Copernican Reference. In: JACOBI, K. and PAPE, H. (eds.): Die Struktur der Welt (in print).
PLANTINGA, A. (1983): Guise Theory. In: TOMBERLIN, J. E. (ed.): Agent, Language, and the Structure of the World, pp. 43-77, Hackett, Indianapolis.
RAPAPORT, W. (1978): Meinongian Theories and a Russellian Paradox. Nous **12**, pp. 153-180.
RAPAPORT, W. (1985/86): Non-existent Objects and Epistemological Ontology. Grazer Philosophische Studien **25/26**.
RAPP, F. (1989): Ontological Perspectivity and Guise Theory. In: JACOBI, K. and PAPE, H. (eds.): Die Struktur der Welt (in print).
ROSENBERG, J.F. (1986): Castañeda's Ontology. In: TOMBERLIN, J.F. (ed.): Hector-Neri Castañeda, Profiles Vol. 6, pp. 141-186, Reidel, Dordrecht.
SARTRE, J-P. (1943): Being and Nothingness: An essay on Phenomenological Ontology (translated by Hazel Barnes). Philosophical Library, New York.
SICHA, S. (1986): Castañeda on Plato, Leibniz, and Kant. In: TOMBERLIN, J.F. (ed.): Hector-Neri Castañeda, Profiles Vol. 6, pp. 309-332, Reidel, Dordrecht.
SMITH, D.W. (1986): Mind and Guise: Castañeda's Philosophy of Mind in the World Order. In: TOMBERLIN, J.F. (ed.): Hector-Neri Castañeda, Profiles Vol. 6, pp. 167-185, Reidel, Dordrecht.
TOMBERLIN, J. E. (ed.; 1983): Knowledge and Self: A Correspondence Between ROBERT M. ADAMS and HECTOR-NERI CASTAÑEDA. In: Agent, Language, and the Structure of the World. Hackett Publishing Co., Indianapolis.

Part Four

Final Comments and Reflections

Psychopathologie und Philosophie: Synopsis und Ausblick

M. Spitzer, F.A. Uehlein, G. Oepen

1. Philosophie und empirische Psychologie

Die Heterogenität der in diesem Band zusammengefaßten Beiträge, die Tatsache, daß es keine "Schulen" interdisziplinärer Zusammenarbeit zwischen psychopathologisch interessierten Psychiatern und Philosophen gibt, sowie ein Bedürfnis, sowohl das Erreichte zu sichten als auch Problemfelder für die weitere Forschung abzustecken, fordern eine synoptische Zusammenschau geradezu heraus. Dem hierfür zunächst auf besonders allgemeine Grundzüge der Beiträge ausgerichteten Blick kann dabei folgendes nicht entgehen: Obgleich (vielleicht auch gerade weil) die Beiträge "symptomorientiert" bzw. Psychiatrie-nahe konzipiert sind, tauchen alte Fragen, wie beispielsweise (a) die nach dem psychophysischen Zusammenhang (vgl. die Beiträge von MAHER und WIEHL) oder (b) die nach der Tragweite und dem Verhältnis empirischer und nichtempirischer Theorie (vgl. die Beiträge von BLANKENBURG, EMRICH und SPITZER) bzw. (c) nach dem Verhältnis von Theorie und diese stützenden "Daten" (vgl. die Beiträge von HARRINGTON, OEPEN und SPITZER) auf.

(Ad a) Im Rahmen seiner Diskussion von Affektivität einerseits und Wahrnehmung bzw. Denken andererseits entwickelt WIEHL eine Verhältnisbestimmung beider zueinander als relativ und komplementär. Störung und Ungestörtsein, Unordnung und Ordnung gehören untrennbar zusammen, Störungen im physischen Bereich ziehen Störungen im psychischen Bereich nach sich und umgekehrt. In MAHERS Beitrag wird einmal mehr deutlich, wie Pathologie im somatischen Bereich in Psychopathologie, die zunächst "rein psychisch" bedingt scheint, umschlagen kann.

(Ad b) Die Schwierigkeiten, die sich bei der Formulierung empirisch-psychopathologischer Theorien stellen und die auf alte philosophische Probleme verweisen, lassen sich z.B. an der in EMRICHS Beitrag skizzierten Theorie der Wahrnehmung aufzeigen: Nicht nur ist das Bilden von Hypothesen zunächst eine Fähigkeit von Personen und nicht von Zellen oder Zellverbänden, auch ist unklar, was eigentlich durch diese Hypothesen "überformt" wird. Wie leicht hier einseitige Sichtweisen zu schlechterdings falschen Aussagen führen, zeigt

Watzlawicks Dictum von der "erfundenen Wirklichkeit" ebenso wie die Rede von "Sinnesdaten" oder scheinbar so schlichten und theoretisch problemlosen "aufgenommenen Informationen": Zwar wird jede Aufklärung dessen, was Objektivität ist, um eine Erörterung des Subjekts, für das diese Objektivität objektiv ist, nicht herumkommen; dennoch ist deswegen Objektivität nicht "erfunden". Auch ist der Versuch, Elemente der Wahrnehmung zu isolieren, sowohl im Rahmen empirischer Wahrnehmungsforschung als auch als Programm einer philosophischen Wahrnehmungstheorie legitim; die empirische Psychologie hat jedoch längst erkannt, daß Wahrnehmung nicht von Sinnesdaten zu Gegenständen und Bedeutungen fortschreitet, und jede Theorie der Wahrnehmung, die mit Sinnesdaten operiert, muß entweder deren aporetischen Charakter als gegeben hinnehmen oder das Konzept "Sinnesdatum" als unbrauchbar aufweisen.

Wahrnehmungstheoretikern, die gerne mit dem Begriff der Information operieren, seien zur Vorsicht die mahnenden Worte der Informationstheoretiker Bauer und Goos ans Herz gelegt: "Zu allen Zeiten hat der Mensch versucht, sich selbst im Lichte der jeweils letzten naturwissenschaftlichen Erkenntnis zu verstehen, und ist dabei im Überschwang der Begeisterung in Gefahr geraten, einen Totalitätsanspruch zu erheben." Zur "menschlichen Informationsverarbeitung" im besonderen führen die genannten Autoren das folgende an: "Wir verstehen den tatsächlichen, wirkungsmäßigen Ablauf der Informationsverarbeitung im Gehirn nur ungenügend, und wir wissen nicht, welche Schranken diesem Verständnis wesensnotwendig gesetzt sind. Voreilige Schlüsse, die naiver Weise durch (unzulässige) Umkehrung zustande kommen ('der Mensch ist physikalisch erklärbar', 'was wir an geistigen Funktionen beobachten, ist Aufnahme, Verarbeitung, Speicherung und Abgabe von Information'), sind abzulehnen: Bereits der Bereich der Sinneswahrnehmung zeigt so komplexe Vorgänge im Gehirn, daß solche Behauptungen nicht einmal als Arbeitshypothesen dienen können. Andere 'geistige Funktionen' aus dem der unmittelbaren Sinneswahrnehmung entrückten Bereich, unter Einschluß des Phänomens des Bewußtseins, lassen sich nur in rein spekulativer Weise mit der maschinellen Informationsverarbeitung in Verbindung bringen" (Bauer und Goos 1982, S. 19).

Solange sich Psychopathologen, Neuropsychologen oder Psychologen beispielsweise bei der Rede von aufgenommenen "Sinnesdaten" oder "Informationen" über die inhärente Metaphorik im klaren sind und die Rede als eine vereinfachte Sprechweise über theoretisch keinesfalls geklärte, sondern fragliche und befragte Sachverhalte verstehen, neue Hypothesen damit generieren und sinnvolle empirische Forschung treiben, ist gegen eine solche heuristische Verfahrensweise nichts einzuwenden. Wer jedoch glaubt, alte philosophische Probleme durch solche verdeckte Metaphern lösen und den Menschen kurzerhand als Personal Computer begreifen zu können (wie dies gerne die tun, die philosophische Auseinandersetzungen im Rahmen der Psychiatrie als nutzlos abtun), der täuscht sich nicht nur über sich selbst, sondern es bleiben auch die mit einer jeden Theorie von Wahrnehmen und Denken verknüpften Probleme verdeckt.

Der Beitrag von Emrich, der in spekulativer Weise den Versuch unternimmt, psychiatrische Fragestellungen im vergleichsweise wesentlich breiteren und helleren Lichtkegel der gegenwärtigen philosophischen Theoriediskussion zu sehen, ist in diesem Zusammenhang als Ausgangspunkt für weiteres Nachdenken zu begrüßen.

(Ad c) Im Beitrag von SPITZER über Ich-Störungen wird u.a. klar, daß der Psychiater nie theorielos vorgeht, wenn er die psychopathologischen Symptome eines Patienten beschreibt. Jede Aussage (Beispiel: der Patient halluziniert, äußert eine Wahnidee, verhält sich affektinadäquat etc.) enthält vielmehr notwendigerweise bereits Interpretation seitens des Psychiaters, was die Fragen nach der als Interpretament verwendeten Theorie geradezu herausfordert. Deren Beantwortung wirft nicht nur ein Licht auf das, was allgemeine Psychopathologie sein könnte, sondern macht auch deutlich, in welchem Maße psychische "Symptome" und damit das, was in der empirischen Psychopathologie gemeinhin als vortheoretische "Daten" bezeichnet wird, abhängig sind von bestimmten theoriegebundenen Vorannahmen hinsichtlich des "Wesens" des Psychischen.

Da gemeinhin die Phänomenologie als diejenige philosophische Richtung genannt wird, die am ehesten dem Überlappungsbereich zwischen Philosophie und Psychopathologie zuzuordnen ist, wird der einschlägig vorgebildete Leser nicht wenig überrascht zur Kenntnis nehmen, daß eine Zuordnung der einzelnen Beiträge nach philosophischen "Richtungen" oder deren Vertretern ein ganz anderes Bild ergibt: Neben Beiträgen, die sich selbst als in der phänomenologischen Tradition angesiedelt verstehen (BLANKENBURG, MUNDT), stehen andere Beiträge entweder in transzendentalphilosophischer Tradition bzw. beziehen sich auf entsprechende Autoren (UEHLEIN, WIEHL sowie der Beitrag von SPITZER über Ich-Störungen) oder stehen besonders der analytischen Philosophie nahe (CASTAÑEDA, EMRICH, PAPE und LEISINGER sowie der Beitrag von SPITZER zu Wahn). Daß es sich dabei um keinen Zufall handelt, sondern um eine sich immer deutlicher abzeichnende Notwendigkeit zu analytisch geklärten Begriffen einerseits und einer allgemeinen Theorie der Erfahrung andererseits zum Zwecke der Beschreibung von deren Fehlformen, ist eine These, die in der Einleitung zu dem vorliegenden Sammelband (siehe SPITZER, Einleitung) näher begründet wird. Die Phänomenologie ist damit nicht mehr *die* philosphische Theorie des Psychopathologen, sondern eine unter anderen.

2. Affekte und gestörtes Wahrnehmen und Denken

Immer wieder finden sich in der psychiatrischen Literatur, oft implizit und unerwartet, Beschreibungen von psychischer Gesundheit als einer Art "praktischer Rationalität" (EDWARDS), was selbstredend den "irrationalen" Affekten eine entsprechende Bedeutung bei der Entstehung psychischer Krankheit zuweist. Ein explizites Aufgreifen der Rolle der Affekte bei Wahrnehmungs- und Denkstörungen in mehreren Beiträgen (dies ergab sich, ohne daß eine Thematisierung des Affekts explizites Ziel war) erwies sich daher als besonders vorteilhaft. Überlegungen zum Verhältnis von Vernunft und Affekt haben eine lange Tradition und lassen sich historisch u.a. auf SPINOZA und KANT zurückführen, wie im Beitrag von WIEHL gezeigt wird. Hier wird jedoch zugleich deutlich, daß der Affekt keineswegs nur als Störung gesehen werden kann bzw. darf; vielmehr ist eine differenzierte Betrachtung erforderlich, die Affekten zwar einerseits in jedem Falle modulierende, jedoch keineswegs prinzipiell, wie oft implizit oder explizit angenommen, nachteilige Effekte auf Rationalität beimißt. Eine frühe philosophische Ausarbeitung des Verhältnisses von Affektivität und Rationalität findet sich bei LORD SHAFTESBURY (vgl. UEHLEIN 1976, S. 232-251).

Die Notwendigkeit einer differenzierten Betrachtungsweise der Affektivität ist auch eine der Schlußfolgerungen, zu der OEPEN et al. in ihren empirischen Untersuchungen zur Rolle des Affekts in der Genese von Denkstörungen gelangen. Wie deren einleitende Übersicht zur Problemlage bereits ahnen läßt, spiegelt die im Rahmen der Psychiatrie geführte Diskussion um Affektivität deren unterschiedliche Sichtweise im Rahmen der geistesgeschichtlichen Entwicklung die letzten 150 Jahre wider: War für die einen der Affekt letztlich Ursache jeder Denkstörung und nur damit das Denken zunehmend in eine Rolle lediglich epiphänomenaler Existenz gedrängt (die Ratio als Reisende in der Nußschale im stürmischen Meer wogender Affekte; Denken als nachträgliches Kohärent-Machen, Einordnen, Verbinden von (Sprach-)Handlungen, die affektiv verursacht sind), so sahen sich die anderen genötigt, der nichtssagenden These "alles ist letztlich affektiv bedingt" durch klare Abgrenzungen entgegenzuwirken. JASPERS' Diktum "nur wo gedacht und geurteilt wird, kann Wahn entstehen" ist ebenso wie die Unterscheidung zwischen primärem (dem "eigentlichen") Wahn und sekundärem (z.B. affektiv bedingtem) Wahn als Ausdruck des Versuchs zu begreifen, das Nachdenken über (patho-) psychische Sachverhalte von einem Abgleiten in die Irrationalität eines "anything goes" in Form einer "alles" begründenden Affekttheorie zu bewahren.

Wenn sich in jüngerer Zeit die Neuropsychologie als empirische Wissenschaft, mehr als ein halbes Jahrhundert nach der bereits mittels hermeneutischer Methodik erfolgten "Entthronung" der autonomen Vernunft durch den praktizierenden Neurologen und Psychiater FREUD, anschickt, mittels experimenteller Ansätze einzuholen, was geistesgeschichtlich bereits vollzogen ist, so hat dies eine klärende und damit auch korrigierende und nicht zuletzt relativierende Funktion: Was bei FREUD noch unklar bleiben mußte (um nicht den Bestand der gesamten Theorie zu gefährden) und was die FREUD-Forschung der jüngeren Vergangenheit in erhebliche Unordnung gebracht hat - z.B. die Grundannahme der Trennbarkeit von Energiegehalt und semantischem Gehalt zum Zwecke der Neukombination nach gewissen Regeln (Psycho-Dynamik damit erst ermöglichend; vgl. SPITZER 1988a, S. 203-210) -, kann jetzt auf empirischem Wege angegangen werden. Semantischer Gehalt und Affektivität (das Energie-Konzept erwies sich längst aufgrund seiner Undifferenziertheit als nicht haltbar) erscheinen neuropsychologisch nicht nur eng verknüpft, es lassen sich vielmehr die Art der Verknüpfung sowie unterschiedliche Verarbeitungsstrategien empirisch untersuchen. Die Forschung ist dabei weit von einer abschließenden einheitlichen Theorie entfernt, befindet sich aber immerhin in einem Stadium, wo sie zum einen in Teilbereichen recht plausible Erklärungen gibt und zum anderen vor allem für die Bildung neuer Hypothesen und damit für weitere empirische Forschungen sich als fruchtbar erweist.

Bedeutet dies alles für das Verhältnis von Vernunft und Affekt wirklich nur, daß mit immer rationalerer Methodik immer irrationalere Züge an der Rationalität aufgedeckt werden? - Ja und nein! Die Antwort hängt ganz von der Betrachtungsweise ab, denn in dem Maße, wie das Denken sich affektiv bedingt weiß, *weiß* das Denken; anders gewendet: Die wissenschaftliche Untersuchung von Affektivität führt programmgemäß zu deren "Rationalisierung", d.h. zu einem Verständnis von Affektivität in einem wissenschaftlichen, *rationalen* Rahmen. Dieser doppelte Aspekt kann auf die psychiatrische Sicht von Affektivität und Denkstörungen direkt übertragen werden. Die Rolle der gestörten Affektivität in der Genese von Denkstörungen wird um so deutlicher hervortreten, je klarer man *sagen* können wird, was jeweils unter Affekt *verstanden* wird, und je besser man entsprechende *funktionale Zusammenhänge* im einzelnen *begreifen* kann.

Um bei den obigen Beispielen zu bleiben: Ohne den Betrachter in der kleinen Nußschale gäbe es niemanden, der die wogende Oberfläche als solche *sähe*; Denken *konstruiert* (im nachhinein) Zusammenhänge - sogar Entitäten von der Art, daß sie sich selbst als durch diese bedingt *weiß*. Denken *setzt* sich seine Bedingungen *voraus*.

Das Verhältnis von Affekt und Denken in der Psychiatrie ist damit insgesamt ein gutes Beispiel dafür, wie alte und scheinbar abgeerntete Problemfelder durch neue Weisen des Fragens fruchtbar gemacht werden können. Daß sich hierdurch durchaus ganz praktische Konsequenzen für psychiatrische Diagnostik und Therapie ergeben, klingt im Beitrag von OEPEN et al. ebenfalls an, bedarf aber im Grunde kaum der Erwähnung.

Auch im Hinblick auf das Wahrnehmen kann die Diskussion der Rolle der Affektivität als paradigmatisch angesehen werden für die neuere Wahrnehmungsforschung überhaupt. Diese holt experimentell ein, was die philosophische Empirismus-Diskussion ganz allgemein längst gezeigt hat: Wahrnehmen ist kein passives bloßes Aufnehmen von "Daten" ("Informationen", "einfachen Ideen" etc.), vielmehr handelt es sich um eine *aktive Leistung* (vgl. die Beiträge von EMRICH und HARRINGTON sowie den Aufriß von UEHLEIN; in diesen Beiträgen auch weitere Literatur).

Sowohl die Ergebnisse der allgemeinen empirischen Psychologie als auch der Neurophysiologie (vgl. z.B. MARCEL 1983) der Forschungen zum plastischen Lernen visueller Cortex-Strukturen sowie Experimente mit unterschwelliger Reizdarbietung beim Menschen zeigen, daß Wahrnehmung ein aktiver Vorgang ist, bei dem semantische Entscheidungen in Abhängigkeit von erlerntem Material getroffen werden, ohne daß solche Entscheidungen bewußt würden. Es finden mithin beim Wahrnehmen Prozesse statt, die einerseits nicht bewußt sind, andererseits jedoch mit dem Vokabular zur Beschreibung bewußter intellektueller Vorgänge zu charakterisieren sind (Hypothesen Bilden, Entscheiden, Erkennen etc.). So macht beispielsweise der Beitrag von HARRINGTON et al. deutlich, daß das Erkennen beispielsweise von Gesichtern einen aktiven Prozeß darstellt, der - wie klinische Fälle von Prosopagnosie zeigen - bei sonst ungestörter Wahrnehmung fehlgehen bzw. ausfallen kann.[1]

Mit diesem *Einholen* nichtempirischer, aktiver, synthetischer Wahrnehmungstheorien durch die empirische Forschung stellen sich für die Philosophie aller-

1 Von besonderer Bedeutung erscheinen hier die Untersuchungen von CAMPBELL et al. an ertaubten Patienten mit Läsionen im Sehzentrum der rechten und linken Hemisphäre hinsichtlich der Fähigkeit, Gesichter zu erkennen. Es zeigte sich u.a., daß Patienten mit Läsionen in der rechten Hemisphäre Gesichter zwar wahrnehmen, aber nicht erkennen, wessen Gesicht sie sehen; Patienten mit Läsionen in der linken Hemisphäre hingegen sind hier nicht beeinträchtigt, haben jedoch im Gegensatz zu den rechtshemisphärisch beeinträchtigten Patienten Schwierigkeiten beim Von-den-Lippen-ablesen, d.h. bei sprachlichen Leistungen. Wahrnehmen ist mithin nicht gleich Wahrnehmen! Das Beispiel macht die Notwendigkeit feiner Differenzierungen innerhalb des Wahrnehmens besonders deutlich.

dings umgekehrt neue Fragen. War beispielsweise für die philosophische Wahrnehmungstheorie die Frage nach dem Subjekt der aktiven Wahrnehmungsleistung entweder überhaupt nicht thematisch oder aber rasch mit dem Schlagwort "Wahrnehmungssubjekt" beantwortet, so fordert die heutige empirische Forschung eine differenziertere Betrachtung: So scheint es z.B. bei vielen *aktiven* Wahrnehmungsprozessen angemessener zu sein, davon zu sprechen, daß sie *für* das wahrnehmende Subjekt (von Neuronen oder Neuronenverbänden) und nicht *von* ihm vollzogen werden. Ist eine solche Redeweise bei relativ einfachen Prozessen (z.B. retinale Kontrastverstärkung) noch unproblematisch, so führt sie bei semantischen Prozessen in Schwierigkeiten. Wenn beispielsweise gezeigt werden kann, daß der semantische Gehalt von subliminal dargebotenen, d.h. nicht bewußt wahrgenommenen, Worten in der Lage ist, nachfolgende Wahrnehmungen oder Verhaltensweisen zu beeinflussen[2], soll man dann sagen, daß das Subjekt dies leiste oder dies für das Subjekt geleistet werde. Wenn man andererseits im Kontext z.B. von KANT-Interpretationen davon spricht, daß das Subjekt Objektivität dadurch hervorbringt, daß das Mannigfaltige der Wahrnehmung (d.h. in der Sprache der empirischen Psychologie in erster Näherung: die Sinnesdaten) unter Maßgabe bestimmter kategorialer, d.h. semantischer Strukturen zu Gegenständen synthetisiert wird, so ist nicht klar, weshalb hier von einer Leistung des Subjekts (und nicht *für* das Subjekt) gesprochen wird. - In beiden Fällen geht es um semantische Prozesse bzw. um den Beitrag semantischer Prozesse zur Konstitution von Objekten bzw. Objektivität.

Keinesfalls kann sich der Philosoph hier durch den häufig mit Bezug auf entsprechende KANT-Kritik geäußerten Gegeneinwand, KANTS Philosophie sei *nicht* als genetische Wahrnehmungstheorie zu verstehen, aus der Affäre ziehen. Auch eine systematische Theorie des Erkennens muß die Ergebnisse empirischer Forschung dazu, *wer* (Neurone, Gehirne, Subjekte, Personen) *wie* (von der Verrechnung von Aktionspotentialen bis zur einheitsstiftenden Synthesis) erkennt, in Rechnung stellen, sofern sie sachlich und nicht rein philologisch interessiert ist.

Wird also das aktive Wahrnehmungssubjekt philosophischer Wahrnehmungstheorien durch die empirische Erforschung und damit Objektivierung seiner Aktivitäten gleichsam entsubjektiviert? Gibt es überhaupt eine Grenze zwischen Leistungen von Neuronen (-verbänden) *für* das Subjekt (Farbkonstanz, Größenkonstanz, Raumkonstanz; um nur einige Beispiele zu nennen) und Leistungen *des* Subjekts (z.B. Produktion qualitativer Bestimmtheit, Identität des Objekts mit sich selbst, d.h. Konstanz in jeder Hinsicht)? Erweist sich eine solche Frage möglicherweise als falsch gestellt? - Wenn ja, wie ist das Verhältnis von empirischer Wahrnehmungsforschung zu (transzendentaler) Erkenntnistheorie neu zu bestimmen? Einen solchen Versuch mit dem Hinweis, Inkompatibles brauche in kein Verhältnis gesetzt zu werden, abzulehnen, heißt bestenfalls, den heuristischen Wert einer Reihe interessanter Strukturähnlichkeiten (Konzepte wie Aktivität, Synthese, semantische Formung nichtsemantischen Materials etc.) zu mißachten. Im ungünstigeren Fall beraubte man sich damit eines der spannendsten Arbeitsfelder philosophischer Forschung und überließe die entsprechende

2 Für eine Übersicht vgl. DIXON 1987.

konzeptuelle Arbeit womöglich anderen, dafür nicht entsprechend ausgebildeten Personenkreisen mit entsprechendem Resultat.[3]

3. Zur Form formaler und inhaltlicher Denkstörungen

In Anlehnung an einen aus der philosophischen Tradition der Phänomenologie gewonnenen Intentionalitätsbegriff (MUNDT 1984) versucht MUNDT in seinem Beitrag, formale Denkstörungen als Ausdruck einer gestörten Intentionalität zu begreifen. Seine Analyse eines schizophasischen Textes macht deutlich, daß hinter zunächst "sinnlosen" Äußerungen durchaus ein Sinn auszumachen ist. Der Versuch, diesen Sinn zu erschließen, eröffnet einen Zugang zum Patienten, der therapeutisch nutzbar ist.

MUNDT ist sicherlich zuzustimmen, daß im Rahmen einer solchen Therapie ein Mittelweg gefunden werden muß zwischen Strukturierung und Sinngebung gleichsam "von außen" einerseits und Eingehen auf die Besonderheiten des jeweils einzelnen Individuums und seiner jeweils besonderen Sinnsetzungen andererseits. In methodischer Hinsicht birgt das Intentionalitätskonzept allerdings Schwierigkeiten, gehört doch Intentionalität zu den von der zeitgenössischen Philosophie kontrovers diskutierten Themen. Dieses Dilemma der Übernahme eines kontrovers diskutierten Konzeptes in die Psychopathologie ist sicherlich nicht allein durch eine Operationalisierung zu lösen, bleibt doch die Frage, *was* operationalisiert wurde. Umgekehrt spricht allerdings die Tatsache, daß Intentionalität kontrovers diskutiert wird, *nicht gegen* die Anwendung dieses Konzeptes im Bereich der Psychopathologie, sofern die kontroverse Diskussion entsprechend mitübernommen und heuristisch fruchtbar gemacht wird. Man könnte zudem erwarten, daß die philosophischen Probleme im Bereich der Psychopathologie nicht nur ihren jeweils spezifischen Niederschlag mit neuen Fragestellungen finden, sondern umgekehrt durch die Einbeziehung psychopathologischer Sachverhalte bereichert werden, wie dies beispielsweise CASTAÑEDA in seinem Beitrag besonders deutlich hervorhebt.

Der Versuch von HESS, das gestörte Denken Schizophrener auf ein bestimmtes Prinzip zu reduzieren, steht mittlerweile in einer ganzen Tradition solcher Ansätze. Entsprechend der gängigen Einteilung der Logik in Begriffsbildung, Urteilen und Schließen lassen sich die meisten Versuche, ein Prinzip der schizophrenen Denkstörung anzugeben, in dem Gebiet der Begriffsbildung lokalisieren: Termini wie "Schaltschwäche" oder "Assoziationsschwäche", "Gedankenverschmelzung", "Interferenz", "Overinclusion" etc. bezeichnen sämtlich Weisen einer fehlgehenden Begriffsbildung. Der bekannteste Versuch, wahnhaftes Denken auf eine Störung im Bereich des Schließens zurückzuführen, stammt von v. DOMARUS und wird beispielsweise von ARIETI (1955) als von-Domarus-Prinzip ausführlich diskutiert.

---

3 Dies mag dann den Philosophen in seiner Meinung bestärken, daß all diese experimentelle Arbeit ihn nicht zu beschäftigen braucht. (Vielleicht ist so das bei Philosophen und Psychologen nicht selten zu findende wechselseitige Belächeln der Arbeit des jeweils anderen zum gleichen Thema - Wahrnehmen, Denken - am besten zu verstehen. Sachlich ist dies in jedem Falle nicht zu rechtfertigen.)

Hess geht in seinem Beitrag davon aus, daß sich ein großer Teil der kognitiven Störungen Schizophrener formal so beschreiben läßt, daß im Verlauf der Informationsverarbeitung eine *notwendige Exklusion nicht oder mangelhaft ausgeführt* wird. Hess hofft auf diesem Wege eine Brücke schlagen zu können zwischen physiologischen Theorien über die Funktionsweise des Gehirns (es ist lange bekannt, daß man mit kleinen Neuronenverbänden sämtliche logischen Operationen modellieren kann) und psychologischen Theorien zum gestörten Denken Schizophrener. So sieht Hess in der Ambivalenz, der Unfähigkeit, die Aufmerksamkeit zu fokussieren, als auch in unangemessenen emotionalen Reaktionen letztlich einen Ausdruck der fehlgehenden Anwendung des logischen ausschließenden Oders. "Die Formulierung eines fehlerhaften 'exklusiven Oder' kann so eine lösbare Frage an die experimentelle Neurophysiologie darstellen... Die formale Analyse der schizophrenen Denkstörungen mit der Formulierung eines defekten Verknüpfungsmechanismus (im Sinne eines defekten exklusiven Oder) könnte so die Brücke schlagen zur neurophysiologischen Grundlagenwissenschaft und damit zum wechselseitigen Verständnis und zur Lösung des gemeinsamen Problems beitragen", formuliert Hess sein Programm.

Von Theorien, die auf logische Prinzipien rekurrieren, geht offenbar eine große Anziehungskraft aus. So war auch Freud fasziniert von der Möglichkeit, "alle vier bedeutenden Wahnformen" auf ein bestimmtes Urteil und vier Weisen des *Widerspruches* zurückzuführen. Arieti führt die jeglicher psychotherapeutischer Deutungsarbeit zugrundeliegende Symbolrelation auf das Von-Domarus-Prinzip zurück (!), die meisten Theorien zu einer gestörten Begriffsbildung erklären praktisch jede klinisch beobachtbare Störung, und auch das Prinzip eines gestörten ausschließenden Oder erlaubt es, praktisch jede psychopathologische Auffälligkeit zu "erklären".

Ganz allgemein muß folgender Einwand beachtet werden: Prinzipien wie das *von-Domarus-Prinzip* oder das *gestörte ausschließende Oder* (Hess) setzen allgemeinste Prinzipien der Logik (z.B. den Satz vom Widerspruch oder den Satz vom ausgeschlossenen Dritten) außer Kraft. Da jedoch aus einem angenommenen Widerspruch alles folgen kann, folgt aus derartigen Prinzipien ebenfalls "alles" bzw. läßt sich damit jedes empirische Datum vereinbaren. Damit ist nicht nur unklar, wie *zwischen* diesen Theorien entschieden werden soll; vielmehr ist mit der größtmöglichen Allgemeinheit dieser Theorien die Tatsache verbunden, daß es sich bei ihnen *nicht* um empirische Theorien handeln kann. Dies kann auch wie folgt gezeigt werden: Empirische Theorien müssen *falsifizierbar* sein, d.h. es muß angegeben werden können, welches empirische Datum bzw. welcher empirische Sachverhalt geeignet wäre, die Theorie zu widerlegen. Sowohl für die Theorie des Schlusses von akzidentieller auf substantielle Gemeinsamkeit (von-Domarus-Prinzip) als auch für die Theorie des gestörten ausschließenden Oders (Hess) lassen sich solche empirischen Fakten jedoch nicht denken. Mit ein klein wenig Interpretationskunst (die von den Autoren selbst als notwendig erachtet und durchaus positiv zugestanden wird) läßt sich vielmehr *jedes* schizophren gestörte Denken auf die genannten Prinzipien zurückführen. Wegen der extremen Allgemeingültigkeit der Prinzipien dürfte eine Applikation in der Neurophysiologie, die zu einer differenzierten Diagnose und klinischem Handeln führen könnte, ebenfalls schwierig sein.

Machen diese Einwände Theorien wie die von v. DOMARUS und die von HESS vorgestellte bereits nutzlos und überflüssig? Ja und nein! Obgleich wir zeigen konnten, daß es sich bei diesen Theorien um keine empirischen Theorien handelt, sind sie doch geeignet, die mannigfaltigen Erscheinungsweisen gestörten Denkens zu strukturieren. Die daraus resultiernde Ordnung ist als solche bereits von Wert, unabhängig davon, ob die Ordnungsgesichtspunkte zutreffend sind oder nicht, liefert sie doch die Basis für die Formulierung experimentell überprüfbarer Hypothesen in kleineren Anwendungsbereichen, d.h. bei speziellen Fragestellungen. Solange derartige Theorien nicht dogmatisch vertreten werden, sondern als ein Interpretationsversuch gestörten Denkens gesehen werden, schaden sie nicht, sondern können dem konkreten Forschungsfortschritt nutzen. Werden sie für die allein seligmachende Wahrheit gehalten und durch entsprechende Immunisierungsstrategien gegen jede Kritik abgesichert, wirken sie sich allerdings negativ aus, da sie selber ja schwerlich eine Richtschnur für Diagnose und Therapie darstellen können.

Ein gutes Beispiel für eine entsprechende Theorie ist die Theorie der Wahngenese von FREUD: Sie wurde von FREUD zunächst vorsichtig, wenig später jedoch mit Gewißheit vorgetragen, und jede weitere empirische Evidenz gegen die Theorie erfuhr eine entsprechende Interpretation, so daß sie innerhalb seiner Theorie ausgelegt werden konnte. Damit ließ sich spätestens 4 bis 5 Jahre nach der erstmaligen Formulierung von FREUDS Theorie kein empirischer Sachverhalt mehr benennen, der der Theorie zu widersprechen in der Lage gewesen wäre. Dennoch führte FREUDS Theorie zu einer Reihe interessanter empirischer Fragestellungen und entsprechender deskriptiv statistischer bzw. experimenteller Untersuchungen, wie die angloamerikanische Literatur der fünfziger und sechziger Jahre zum Wahnproblem (d.h. nach der Übersetzung von FREUDS Schriften ins Englische) zeigt (vgl. SPITZER 1988e).

Einen Brückenschlag zwischen Störungen der Wahrnehmung sowie Störungen des formalen Denkens einerseits und Störungen des inhaltlichen Denkens andererseits versucht MAHER in seinem Beitrag, der eine Erweiterung seines bereits mehrfach publizierten Ansatzes (vgl. MAHER und ROSS 1984 sowie MAHER 1988 a,b) darstellt. Sein Argument besteht letztlich in einer bestimmten Weise der Rekonstruktion der Genese von Wahn: Am Anfang stehen entweder Störungen der Wahrnehmung (z.B. Hörminderung oder Taubheit) oder eine gestörte Sprachproduktion. Als nicht beeinträchtigt werden demgegenüber die kognitiven Funktionen des Patienten angenommen, so daß es dem Patienten möglich ist, Schlüsse aus seinen veränderten Wahrnehmungen bzw. der (ebenfalls wahrgenommenen) veränderten Sprachproduktion zu ziehen. Diese Schlüsse imponieren dann klinisch als Wahn.

Im Hinblick auf die unten zu diskutierenden Ich-Störungen ist insbesondere das folgende von Bedeutung: MAHER geht nicht nur (wie derzeit in der angloamerikanischen Literatur üblich[4]) davon aus, daß Erlebnisse des "Gemachten" oder der "gestörten Meinhaftigkeit" als Wahn zu bezeichnen sind, sondern geht zusätzlich davon aus, daß es sich bei diesen Erlebnissen um einen *Erklärungswahn* handelt: Die Erlebnisse der gestörten Meinhaftigkeit bzw. des Gemachten werden als Erklärungsversuche gestörter Wahrnehmungen und gestörter Sprache interpretiert (d.h. als *sekundärer* Ausdruck anderweitiger, primärer Pathologie) und nicht als primärer Ausdruck eines ansonsten nur noch biolo-

4 Vgl. den Beitrag von SPITZER über Ich-Störungen in diesem Band.

gisch zu definierenden pathologischen Geschehens gewertet. Bedenkt man, daß Ich-Störungen im klassischen Sinne bis heute von erheblicher klinischer Bedeutung sind und ganz allgemein als psychopathologisch wegweisend für die Diagnose einer Schizophrenie angesehen werden, so wird einerseits die gesamte Tragweite von MAHERS Ansatz deutlich, entstehen andererseits jedoch auch Zweifel an dessen Allgemeingültigkeit. Der bereits von KRAEPELIN beobachtete und in den siebziger Jahren vor allem von COOPER statistisch abgesicherte Zusammenhang zwischen Wahrnehmungsstörungen und der Entwicklung von Wahn ist einerseits zwar nicht zu leugnen; andererseits jedoch werden Ich-Störungen im oben genannten Sinne häufig am Beginn von Psychosen und auch bei solchen Patienten, bei denen keine Störungen der Wahrnehmung und keine Störungen des formalen Denkens (und Sprechens) bestehen, angetroffen. Dies widerlegt MAHERS Ansatz keineswegs, sondern fordert zu genauer empirischer Erforschung des Beginns von Psychosen erneut heraus. Sollte sich dabei MAHERS Ansatz als nicht allgemeingültig erweisen, so repräsentiert er dennoch *eine* von mehreren Weisen der Wahngenese und ist von erheblichem Hypothesengenerierendem Wert für weitere empirische Untersuchungen.[5]

In GLATZELS Beitrag *Melancholie und Wahn* geht es keineswegs um eine neue genetische Theorie des Wahns aus gestörten Affekten, sondern um einen formalen Gesichtspunkt inhaltlicher Denkstörungen. GLATZEL argumentiert mit Hilfe zweier von METZGER geprägter Realitätsbegriffe dafür, daß es sich bei den Äußerungen Depressiver über sich nicht um Wahn handelt. Wenn auch die Argumentation in einigen Details kritischen Einwänden ausgesetzt ist[6], so ist seine These, Wahn liege erst dann vor, wenn auf intersubjektive Realität Bezug genommen werde, systematisch bedeutsam.

GLATZELS Argument läßt sich als gestaltpsychologische Variante des ganz allgemeinen Arguments zur Wahndefinition, das im Beitrag von SPITZER vorgestellt wird, auffassen: Ohne Rückgriff auf unterschiedliche Realitätsbegriffe wird hier zunächst gezeigt, daß subjektiv gewisse und unkorrigierbare Aussagen, d.h. Aussagen, die die ersten beiden JASPERSschen Wahnkriterien erfüllen, durchaus auch von psychisch Gesunden geäußert werden und hier den Bereich des Mentalen mit seinem epistemisch für das jeweilige Individuum priviligierten Zugang gegenüber dem Bereich des intersubjektiv Zugänglichen (Objektiven) abgrenzen. Hieraus läßt sich die zunächst sehr einfache Wahndefinition ableiten, daß es sich beim Wahn um Aussagen *über* nicht mentale Sachverhalte handelt, die mit dem Erkenntnisanspruch von Aussagen über mentale Sachverhalte

5 Angemerkt sei hier, daß es im Grunde erstaunlich ist, wie wenig über die genaue Abfolge der Ereignisse bei Psychosen bekannt ist, so daß unterschiedlichste Erklärungsansätze der letztlich resultierenden klinischen Symptomatik nach wie vor möglich sind. Mittels genauer phänomenologischer Untersuchungen, möglicherweise unterstützt durch neuropsychologische Methoden, sollte sich die Abfolge der psychischen Ereignisse (*mental events*) im Beginn einer schizophrenen Psychose klären lassen. Es sollte vor allem geklärt werden können, ob es hier eine Systematik gibt bzw. ob es möglicherweise mehrere, klar abgrenzbare Verlaufstypen solcher Ereignisse gibt. Solche Untersuchungen setzen allerdings eine komplexere Methodik (etwa im Sinne der Phänomenologie von JASPERS) voraus verglichen mit den heute üblichen "psychopathometrischen" Verfahren.

6 So haben beispielsweise die Ergebnisse transkulturell-psychiatrischer Untersuchungen zur Symptomatik der Depression gezeigt, daß das Vorhandensein der Schuldwahn-Thematik offensichtlich an den jüdisch-christlichen Kulturkreis gebunden ist und damit keineswegs die Allgemeingültigkeit beanspruchen kann, die KURT SCHNEIDER (1950) mit dieser Thematik verbindet (Urangst *des* Menschen schlechthin). Weiterhin läßt sich Religiösität von Wahn nicht durch das Moment der Kommunikation abgrenzen, enthalten doch eine Reihe von Religionen den Missionsgedanken nicht, worauf u.a. HOHLE (1977) hinweist.

vorgebracht werden. Diese Vereinfachung bildet den klinischen Begriffsgebrauch recht zwanglos ab, wie gezeigt wird, wirft jedoch ihrerseits neue Probleme der Abgrenzung von Wahn gegenüber Nichtwahn auf und zeigt deutlich die Grenzen einer jeden auf formale Gesichtspunkte rekurrierenden Wahntheorie.

4. Ich und Ich-Störungen

Daß es sich bei dem, was in der psychiatrischen Literatur mit "Ich-Störung" bezeichnet wird, um sehr heterogene Sachverhalte handelt und daß die theoretischen Überlegungen zu Ich-Störungen ebenfalls sehr heterogener Art sind, kommt im Beitrag von HERMLE et al. deutlich zum Ausdruck.[7] Der Beitrag von HERMLE et al. enthält eine Zusammenfassung von Materialien, die bei Untersuchungen zur *Meskalin-induzierten Psychose* gewonnen wurden, und ist allein bereits aufgrund der Tatsache, daß solche Daten entweder überhaupt nicht oder nur schwer zugänglich ist, von großem Wert. Wie die Diskussion der Sachverhalte in HERMLE et al. zeigt, hat man mit ganz unterschiedlichen Ansätzen versucht, sich Ich-Störungen theoretisch zu nähern.

Bei der Frage nach der Meinhaftigkeit der Gedanken und nach der Struktur erfahrender und denkender Subjektivität neigt BLANKENBURG zu der Auffassung, daß wohl ein Denken ohne Gedanken und Gedachtes nicht denkbar sei, aber keines Denkers - "Ich" genannt - bedürfe. Gedanken seien somit nicht unbedingt Gedanken einer Person, die sich als Ich/Selbst weiß und die somit alle ihre Gedanken als die ihren hat. Erlebnis- und Gedanken*inhalt* und die *formale* Struktur dieser Inhalte, daß sie eben Erlebnis und Gedanken eines Ich sind, seien nicht gegenüberzustellen. Die "dynamische Dialektik des Selbstverhältnisses" wäre "in einer *andersartigen Verschränkung* von Form und Inhalt" zu suchen. Bezeichnenderweise verwendet BLANKENBURG hier selber den Ausdruck *Selbst*verhältnis. Ohne die Struktur, die Form des Selbst scheint auch die andersartige Verschränkung nicht zu fassen. BLANKENBURGS Einwendung ist philosophisch und psychopathologisch gleichermaßen von Bedeutung.

Der Streit geht wohlgemerkt nicht um ein solipsistisches, weltloses Ich, sondern um die konkrete Person, die gerade dadurch, daß sie *auch* Ich oder Selbst ist, nicht nur in der Welt erlebend, (vorbewußt) erfahrend und agierend da ist, sondern aufgrund ihres Selbst-Bewußtseins sich denkend von anderen unterscheiden und (ineins damit) auf anderes beziehen kann. So kann sie sich ihr eigenes natürliches, leibhaftes und erlebendes Dasein ebenso zu Bewußtsein bringen, wie andere Personen gleich ihr, die Gegenstände der gemeinsamen Lebenswelt und die Welt als die umfassende Ordnung, in der alle Einzelnen da sind (UEHLEIN, in diesem Band).

Besteht BLANKENBURGS Einwand zu Recht - und hier zeigt sich die psychopathologische Bedeutung -, dann kann z.B. das "Gemachtbekommen" von Gedanken nicht mehr als Ichstörung gefaßt werden. Läßt es sich dann über-

---

7 Daß es sich hierbei um keinen Zufall handelt, sondern daß vielmehr hinsichtlich des Symptoms *Ichstörungen* ein Theoriedefizit herrscht, das zu entsprechender Unklarheit über die phänomenalen Sachverhalte führen muß, zeigt SPITZER u.a in seinem Beitrag über Ichstörungen.

haupt noch als Störung identifizieren? Das Erleben Schizophrener - so BLANKENBURG - begrenze die Gültigkeit der formalen Struktur, daß Gedanken Gedanken eines Ich seien. Hier droht der Einwand zirkulär zu werden. Wie läßt sich das Erleben Schizophrener als solches differenzieren, wenn man nicht u.a. auch von der Struktur der Meinhaftigkeit Gebrauch macht? Die Vorstellung des Gemachtwerdens, des Durchlässigwerdens der Ichgrenzen, Realitätsstörungen, Depersonalisation etc. bedürfen schon zu ihrer Identifikation/Diagnose der Voraussetzung der Meinhaftigkeit. Das gleiche gilt interessanterweise auch für die Vorstellung der Allmacht, die BLANKENBURG öfter anführt. Ohne die Voraussetzung des vereinzelten, zeitlich-endlichen Ich ist sie nicht *als Störung* zu fassen.

BLANKENBURG nennt eine Reihe von Ansichten aus der Geschichte und der Gegenwart, die seine Einwendung plausibel machen könnten. Daß er damit ebenso viele neue Fragen weckt, spricht für die Aktualität seiner Einwendung.

LICHTENBERGS "Bemerkung, statt *ich denke* könne man ebensogut sagen *es denkt* - wie man sage, *es blitzt*" (BLANKENBURG, in diesem Band), gibt sich als spielerisch leichte Widerlegung des cartesianischen ego cogito. "Ich denke" zeige nur das Vorkommen von Gedanken an und sei nichts anderes als eine unpersönliche Existenzaussage, also gleichbedeutend mit "es denkt", "es gibt Gedanken" oder "es gibt Denken". Der Satz schillert. Gelingt die Ersetzung des belasteten cartesianischen Grundsatzes (fundamentum inconcussum) durch eine unpathetische, alltägliche Anzeige von Vorkommendem? Als direkte Widerlegung kann diese Ersetzung nicht gelten, denn schon die Verneinung der Sätze zeigt, daß es sich bei dem vermeintlich *ebenso guten* Stellvertreter um keine unpersönliche Existenzaussage handelt. Existenzaussagen lassen sich sinnvoll verneinen: z.B. "es blitzt nicht", "es gibt keine(n) Blitz(e)". Die Verneinung der Existenzaussage, die "ego cogito" vertreten soll, wird selbstwidersprüchlich: "es denkt nicht", "es gibt keine(n) Gedanken, "es gibt kein Denken". Soll die Verneinung der Aussage aber sinnvoll werden, dann ist sie a) keine unpersönliche Existenzaussage mehr, nach dem Muster "es blitzt", und b) sagt der Sprecher nichts über sich aus (ego cogito), sondern über andere: "es - jenes dort - denkt nicht", "es gibt - von ihm - keine(n) Gedanken".

Die Szene, in der LICHTENBERG seine Répartie skeptisch lächelnd vorgebracht haben mag, läßt sich leicht imaginieren. Kam es ihm wirklich auf die Widerlegung von Selbst-Bewußtsein an? War sie nicht vielmehr gegen einen Cartesianer strenger Observanz gerichtet, der auch das Erleben, die vorprädikative Erfahrung, die kleinen Perzeptionen (um mit LEIBNIZ zu reden) dem Ich zuschlagen mußte, da er sie sonst unsinniger Weise der res extensa, die keine Innerlichkeit hat, hätte zuschieben müssen? LICHTENBERG widerlegt nun diese Vereinnahmung des Ich und Welt vermittelnden Mitlebens und Erlebens, indem er hingegen die res cogitans vereinnahmt und der (noch) ichlosen Erlebnisphäre zuschlägt. Eine Vereinnahmung ist so gut wie die andere.

Fr. X. v. BAADERS Satz "cogit*or*, ergo sum" könnte als Musterbeispiel eines psychopathologischen Befundes - des "Gemachtbekommens" im Sinne SCHNEIDERS - gelten, wenn BAADER nicht mit ihm ganz anderes im Sinne hätte. Er will aufmerksam machen, daß eine Person im Denken (cogito) sich nicht auch noch ins Sein bringt und sich selber die Struktur der Subjektivität gibt. "Ich werde gedacht und somit bin ich" bedeutet: ich bin von einem mir tranzendenten absolutdenkenden Sein her (cogitor), und so bin ich ein Ich (ego sum), Abbild vom Urbild. BAADERS Satz widerlegt also nicht den Sachverhalt, daß Denken "Denken eines Ich" und die Gedanken seine Gedanken sind, sondern eröffnet eine metaphysische Begründung der Person: "Als Gottes Bild und Geschöpf kann ich nicht selbständig sein, denn jedes Abbild ist dessen, von dem es Abbild ist, als spontan und frei soll ich aber doch solches sein" (BAADER 1852, S. 329).

C.G. JUNGS Traumbericht spricht gleich von zwei Träumen und dem Erwachen aus einem der Träume. C.G. JUNG träumt, daß "sein gesamtes Sein" (ebd.) von einem Jogi meditiert werde. "Ich erschrak zutiefst und erwachte an dem Gedanken: Ach so, das ist der, der mich meditiert. Er hat einen Traum, und das bin ich" (ebd.). Der springende Punkt in diesem Bericht ist nicht, daß einer an einen anderen denkt, über ihn meditiert und von ihm träumt, sondern daß der Berichtende denkt, er selber sei ein Traum, den ein anderer hat. Er wäre also, da der andere ihn träume.

Es sei einmal zugestanden, daß Meditation und Traum eine Person in 'ihrem gesamten Sein' hervorbringen können, also einen natürlichen Organismus, der lebt, agiert und sich erhält und somit anderes, ja den Horizont der Welt impliziert, einen natürlichen Organismus, der ferner Leib ist und zu einem erkennenden, denkenden Wesen gehört. Dies alles zugestanden, so ist doch auffällig, daß in diesem Bericht C.G. JUNG sich *im Denken* von dieser Traumwelt löst: "ich erschrak zutiefst und erwachte an dem Gedanken". Das Traumwesen, das geträumte Ich, das vom träumenden Jogi abhängen soll, hört im Moment des Denkens auf zu träumen. Die Gedanken und der Denkende/Berichtende gehören nicht mehr zum Traum. C.G. JUNG denkt seinen Traum, sich als Geträumten und den träumenden Jogi. Dies aber kann er, weil er erwacht ist an dem Gedanken, weil die Gedanken und der Denkende nicht mehr zum Traum gehören und weil er anderes als nur ein träumendes-geträumtes Ich ist. Nimmt man genau, was der Traumbericht sagt, so bedarf es nicht einmal seiner Implikationen - Traum und Meditation erzeugen das gesamte Sein einer Person - um zu sehen, daß er nichts gegen Denken als "Denken eines Ich" vorbringt, sondern gerade im Denken das abhängige Traumich relativiert.[8]

Die Frage schließlich, ob dem "Denken ein Ich *zugrundeliege* oder ob das Ich erst ein *Produkt* der durch das Denken (und andere Faktoren) bedingten *Zweiteilung* alles für uns Seienden in 'Ich' und 'Welt' sei - das Denken also hinter diese *Dichotomie* zurückreiche und daher nicht rein ichlicher Natur sein könne" (BLANKENBURG, in diesem Band; unsere Hervorhebungen), verschiebt das Verhältnis von Denken und Ich.

Dem Denken liegt kein Ich zugrunde und geht ihm vorher. Es wäre dann die bloße Dynamis zum Denken, die, so für sich isoliert, nicht ist. Das ursprüngliche Selbstbewußtsein ("Ich") wird als Struktur gefaßt, die Vollzug ist, nicht außer oder ohne diesen Vollzug des Denkens.

Die Alternative Ich oder Denken verstellt den Sachverhalt. Es geht weder das Ich dem Denken, noch das Denken dem Ich zuvor und läge ihm zugrunde.

Eine Person, die ursprüngliches Selbstbewußtsein ist und (ineins damit) denken kann - so unsere These -, kann sich selber unterscheiden und anderes sich unterscheiden, mit dem zusammen sie da ist. So faßt sie sich als konkretes Ich in ihren Beziehungen, im Leben mit Personen und Dingen. Hier erst tritt die Unterscheidung in *Ich und Welt* auf, eine Unterscheidung, die keine "Zweiteilung", sondern vielmehr Beziehung ist, da die Person ohne ihr anderes nicht sein könnte und dies weiß. Nicht ein irgendwie rein an sich vorkommendes Denken unterscheidet das Seiende und "produziert" somit *Ich und Welt*, sondern eine Person (die leibhaft da ist, mitlebt, erlebt und ihre Erlebnisse in Gedanken zu fassen vermag) denkt und unterscheidet sich als konkretes Ich von ihrem anderen, von den Personen und Dingen im Horizont der Welt.

Nicht das hypostasierte Denken reicht hinter die "Dichotomie" *Ich und Welt* zurück, sondern die Person, und zwar in zweifacher Weise; einmal als mitlebend-erlebende, die aus der Ungeschiedenheit ihrer Erlebnisse anderes und sich unterscheidet; zweitens als Selbst-Bewußtsein, das diese Unterscheidung denkend vollziehen kann.

Die Einwände, die BLANKENBURG vorlegt, und die zahlreichen Positionen und Lösungsvorschläge, die er zitiert, dokumentieren, wie sehr der Sachverhalt der Meinhaftigkeit der Gedanken und die Theorie der Subjektivität Gegenstand philosophischer und psychopathologischer Diskussion sind.

Wie BLANKENBURG mit Recht hervorhebt, waren Ich-Störungen in den letzten Jahren nur in geringem Umfang der Gegenstand von Diskussion und Forschung. In seinem Beitrag geht BLANKENBURG von KURT SCHNEIDERS Konzeption der "Meinhaftigkeit" des Erlebens aus und greift hierzu einen Ansatz von SPITZER (1985) auf. Diesem liegt der Gedanke zugrunde, daß eine philosophische Theorie (d.h.: Transzendentalphilosophie), die notwendige Strukturmomente einer jeden Erfahrung beschreibt, für das Verständnis von Fehlformen von Erfahrung nützlich, ja sogar unentbehrlich sei. Der Beitrag von SPITZER über Ich-Störungen verfolgt diese Überlegung weiter und präzisiert sie zugleich. Wie die Entwicklung der Konzepte im Bereich der anglo-amerikanischen Psychiatrie

8 Vgl. RODERICK M. CHISHOLM, *Questions about the Unity of Consciousness.*

zeigt, bedarf es ganz offensichtlich einer *Theorie* der Ich-Störungen - im Gegensatz zu KURT SCHNEIDER, der der Meinung war, es genüge deren pragmatisch-praktische Aufzählung -, um Ich-Störungen überhaupt als symptomatische Einheit plausibel und einer deskriptiven Erfassung zugänglich zu machen: Solange Erlebnisse der Nicht-Meinhaftigkeit von Denken oder Wollen oder Erlebnisse von bruchstückhafter Erfahrung als Wahn bezeichnet werden (und Wahn zudem als "falsche Aussage über die Realität" konzipiert wird), kann keine adäquate Bewertung des in der psychiatrischen Realität bedeutsamen Symptoms Ich-Störung stattfinden. (Auch soll niemand hoffen, daß durch ein Richtigstellen des ebenfalls falschen o.g. Wahnverständnisses bereits die Ich-Störungen wieder besser in den Blick gerieten).

Die Parallelen zwischen Psychopathologie einerseits und Philosophie andererseits sind unübersehbar bei einer Gegenüberstellung des Beitrags von SPITZER zu Ich-Störungen mit dem Beitrag von UEHLEIN, der unabhängig von jedem Gedanken an Pathologie ganz allgemein Strukturmomente des Ich in einem straffen Reflexionsgang entwirft. Wie UEHLEIN auf wenigen Seiten deutlich macht, handelt es sich bei Meinhaftigkeit, Einheit der Erfahrung oder der Unterscheidung zwischen Ich und Nicht-Ich keineswegs um lediglich klinisch brauchbare Konzepte zur Beschreibung der Pathologie Schizophrener (dies oder ähnliches hätte KURT SCHNEIDER vertreten), sondern um Strukturmomente einer jeden Erfahrungsstruktur, die sich unabhängig von jeder Pathologie entwickeln läßt.[9]

Einen verglichen mit dem Beitrag von UEHLEIN gänzlich anderen methodischen Ansatz zur Aufdeckung dessen, was wir mit "Ich" meinen, verfolgt CASTAÑEDA. Interessanterweise lassen sich auch hierdurch Implikationen für die Diskussion von Ich-Störungen gewinnen, worauf CASTAÑEDA eigens abhebt. Ein Vergleich der Zugangsweisen erscheint schwierig, wiewohl - versuchsweise - folgendes gelten könnte: Einerseits dürften sich die von CASTAÑEDA dargestellten unterschiedlich starken Identitätsrelationen für das, was wir mit "Ich", "Ego" oder "Person" meinen, als sehr hilfreich erweisen zur Klärung der oft vorhandenen Vagheit von Argumenten, die sich dieser drei Begriffe bedienen. In der psychiatrischen Literatur begegnen ebenso wie im psychiatrischen Alltag solche Fehlschlüsse immer wieder, die daraus resultieren, daß das erlebende, erfahrende Ich, das Ego (d.h. eine hypothetische, intrapsychische Entität) oder eine Person (d.h. ein leiblich-seelisches Ganzes, Einzelnes) als schlechthin identisch betrachtet wurden. Andererseits fragt es sich, ob gerade zur Aufdeckung von Ich-Störungen der Ansatz von CASTAÑEDA gleichsam weit genug trägt: Ich-Störungen bezeichnen Weisen des gestörten Erfahrens. Erfahrung liegt jedoch für CASTAÑEDA innerhalb seines Ansatzes schlichtweg vor, ist gegeben, ist nicht weiter problematisch. Ein Ich ist für ihn zwar jeweils Bezugspunkt in jeder Erfahrung, Ich als identisches, sich durchhaltendes aber wird erst aus vielen Erfahrungen und ihren jeweiligen Ichen entwickelt, d.h. ist sekundär. Dem ließe sich allerdings wiederum entgegnen, daß es CASTAÑEDAS Theorie möglicherweise

---

9 Es sei angemerkt, daß einer der Herausgeber (M.S.) diese sehr auffälligen Übereinstimmungen zwischen vermeintlich theorieloser Klinik und vermeintlich Pathologie-ferner Theorie vor Jahren zum Anlaß für eigene interdisziplinäre Untersuchungen nahm (woraus u.a. das in Freiburg im Juli 1988 stattgehabte Symposion und damit der vorliegende Sammelband resultieren).

erlaubt, unterschiedliche Weisen des Fehlgehens der Konstitution eines identischen Ich zu beschreiben analog zu unterschiedlichen Weisen der Pathologie, wie sie bei Ich-Störungen vorliegen. Es ist offen, welche Theorie sich für psychopathologische Sachverhalte und Fragestellungen als besser anwendbar erweist.

CASTAÑEDA äußert die Vermutung, daß psychopathologische Sachverhalte durchaus für philosophische Theorien über das, was wir mit Ich meinen, relevant sein können. Die Psychopathologie liefert gleichsam *Daten*, deren Interpretation einerseits philosophischer Theorie bedarf, ohne deren Interpretation andererseits jedoch diese Theorie gleichsam "leer" läuft. Liegen auch weiterführende Überlegungen hier in der Zukunft, so zeigt gerade die Problematik des Ich sehr deutlich, wie sich Psychopathologie und Philosophie gegenseitig fruchtbar ergänzen können.

Literatur

ARIETI, S. (1955): Interpretation of Schizophrenia. Brunner, New York.

BAADER, F.v. (1852): Sämtliche Werke, Bd. III, herausgegeben v. F. HOFFMANN, Herrmann Bethmann, Leipzig.

BAUER, F.L., GOOS, G. (1982): Informatik. Springer, Berlin, Heidelberg, New York.

BLANKENBURG, W. (1988): Zur Psychopathologie des Ich-Erlebens. (In diesem Band).

CAMPBELL, R., LANDIS, T., REGARD, M. (1986): Face recognition and lipreading. Brain **109**, pp. 509-521.

CASTAÑEDA, H.-N. (1988): Persons, Egos and I's: Their Sameness Relations. (In diesem Band).

CHISHOLM, R. M. (1987): Questions about the Unity of Consciousness. In: CRAMER, K. et al. (Hg.): Theorie der Subjektivität, S. 95-97.

DIXON, N.F. (1987): Subliminal Perception. In: GREGORY, R.L. (Hg.): The Oxford Companion of the Mind, S. 752-755.

DOMARUS, E.v. (1942): The specific laws of logic in schizophrenia. In: KASANIN, J.S. (Hg.): Language and Thought in Schizophrenia, S. 104-114. Norton, New York.

EDWARDS, R.B. (1981): Mental Health as Rational Autonomy. The Journal of Medicine and Philosophy **6**, pp. 309-322.

EMRICH, H.M. (1988): Die Beziehung zwischen Philosophie und Psychiatrie, vom Standpunkt einer systemtheoretischen Konzeption produktiver Psychosen aus betrachtet. (In diesem Band).

GLATZEL, J. (1988): Melancholie und Wahn. (In diesem Band).

HARRINGTON, A. OEPEN, G. SPITZER, M. HERMLE, L. (1988): Zur Psychopathologie und Neuropsychologie der Wahrnehmung von Gesichtern. (In diesem Band).

HERMLE, L. OEPEN, G. SPITZER, M. HARRINGON, A. (1988): Ichstörungen bei Modellpsychosen. (In diesem Band).

HESS, R. (1988): Dies und nicht das - dies mag das Problem sein: Formal-logische Betrachtungen der schizophrenen Denkstörungen. (In diesem Band).

HOLE, G. (1977): Der Glaube bei Depressiven. Enke, Stuttgart.

JASPERS, K. (1973): Allgemeine Psychopathologie. Springer, Berlin, Heidelberg, New York.

MAHER, B.A. (1988a): Anomalous experience and delusional thinking: The logic of explanations. In: T.F. OLTMANNS, B.A. MAHER (Hg.): Delusional Beliefs, Wiley-Interscience, New York.

MAHER, B.A. (1988b): Delusions as the product of normal cognitions. In: T.F. OLTMANNS, B.A. MAHER (Hg.): Delusional Beliefs, Wiley-Interscience, New York.

MAHER, B.A. (1988c): Language Disorders in Psychoses and Their Impact on Delusions. (In diesem Band).

MAHER, B., ROSS, J. (1984): Delusions. In: H.E. ADAMS, P.B. SUTKER (Hg.): Comprehensive Handbook of Psychopathology. Plenum, New York.

Marcel, A.J. (1983): Conscious and unconscious perception: An approach to the relations between phenomenal experience and perceptual process. Cognitive Psychology 15, S. 238-300.
Mundt, Ch. (1984): Der Begriff der Intentionalität und die Defizienzlehre von den Schizophrenien. Nervenarzt 55, S. 582-588.
Mundt, Ch. (1988): Zur Psychopathologie der schizophrenen Denkstörungen. (In diesem Band).
Oepen, G. Harrington, A. Spitzer, M. Fünfgeld, M. (1988): "Feelings" of Conviction. On the Relation of Affect and Thought Disorder. (In diesem Band).
Pape, H. Leisinger, U. (1988): Was sind Quasi-Indikatoren? Eine Einführung in Castañedas Theorie der Subjektivität. (In diesem Band).
Schneider, K. (1950): Die Aufdeckung des Daseins durch die cyclothyme Depression. Nervenarzt 21, S. 193-194.
Spitzer, M. (1985): Allgemeine Subjektivität und Psychopathologie. Hagt und Herchen, Frankfurt a.M.
Spitzer, M. (1988a): Halluzinationen. Springer, Berlin, Heidelberg, New York, London, Paris Tokyo.
Spitzer, M. (1988b): Ichstörungen: In Search of a Theory. (In diesem Band).
Spitzer, M. (1988c): Karl Jaspers, Mental States and Delusional Beliefs: A Redefinition and its Implications. (In diesem Band).
Spitzer, M. (1988d): Psychiatry, Philosophy, and the Problem of Description. (In diesem Band).
Spitzer, M. (1988e): Untersuchungen zum Wahnproblem (im Druck).
Uehlein, F.A. (1976): Kosmos und Subjektivität. Lord Shaftesburys Philosophical Regimen. Alber, Freiburg.
Uehlein, F.A. (1988): Bewußtsein und Selbstbewußtsein. (In diesem Band).
Wiehl, R. (1988): Die Affekte als Wahrnehmungs- und Denkstörungen. (In diesem Band).

Epilogue: Philosophy, Psychiatry, and Modes of Scientific Progress

M. Spitzer

1. In the year 1991 news of a discovery spread like wildfire all over the world: in the course of the landings on the moon, which were now planned on a regular basis, one had caught sight of planet which had been unknown so far. This planet was soon found to circle exactly round the earth's orbit, to be of the same size as the earth, and - seen from a distance at first - to look just like the earth. People were even more agitated when there were reports from an expedition to this planet which had been undertaken in a hurry. Everything there was said to be just the same as it is for us: there were beings just like men on earth working in factories, building houses and bombs, as well as writing poems and computer programs. Their language could be understood.

At first this world seemed to be just like ours, but on further expeditions (telecommunication was impossible because of the sun being situated between the earth and that planet) several differences were found out. On the third expedition, for instance, one of the scientists happened to strain his ankle. He went to one of the hospitals, of which there were just as many as on earth, but he was really astonished when he entered. A man with somewhat thin hair wearing a lounge suit and metal-rimmed glasses walked up to him and asked him what he wanted. He did not look like a doctor at all as he was rather awkward and dreamy. Instead of the usual stethoscope and reflex-hammer in the pocket of a white coat just a pair of dividers and a ruler were carelessly sticking out of his slightly worn jacket.

The scientist pointed to his right foot, said he felt pain and reported what had happened. Thereupon the Antiterrestrial - which is to be the name for the inhabitants of the newly discovered planet - looked at him helplessly, said there wasn't much he could do and advised him to watch his foot and not to put any strain on it for the next few days. The terrestrial, getting impatient, answered he knew that himself, asked for the X-ray department and demanded some medicine. As regards the first question the antiterrestrial could but shrug his shoulders. Regarding the second question he said (to make things easier we shall render both direct and indirect speech in translation, as even today a lot of people do not understand the antiterrestrial language): "We have several ointments, made from different kinds of earth, ground herbs, or animal components as well. But since you are describing your pain in an undifferenciated manner I don't have any criteria to treat your ailment with any of these. If I knew exacxtly what you are suffering from, things would be different.

The scientist was taken aback and said however hard he might try he couldn't say anything else but that he was in pain. But, on the other hand, for he was a scientist his curiosity was aroused and he asked the doctor what he could do for him if he were an Antiterrestrial.

"Well," the doctor replied, "if the pain is dragging, flowing, not sharp or dull" (we give a shortened version of what the Antiterrestrial said, as to the present day Antiterranian linguistics couldn't provide any adequate translations for some Antiterrestrial words, so, for instance, many terms describing pain of which there are obviously several dozens on Antiterra) "the correlation - coefficient for treatment with this ointment," he pointed to a rather large tube," is 0.74 as regards healing within three days. For the lower therapeutical aim of healing within five days it goes up to 0.82, but as regards today and tomorrow I regret having to say to you..."

It was probably a mixture of pain, helplessness and sarcasm which made the scientist say: "And what will be in three weeks' time?"

But this did not have the effect he had anticipated. The doctor took instead one of the numerous books from the shelves, flicked through it and answered: "0.96, there is no change of coefficients between the 18th and the 24th day."

More talking to himself he murmured: "Someone should really go over these tables. What is the point of having two decimal places? What about scientific precision?"

Once more completely taken aback the scientist asked him to show him the book and his curiosity seemed to have overcome the pain for good. The title was "Little Surgery", the subtitle being "SDT - 299, vol. 24", but its content reminded one more of a log table: only very rarely there were some lines of text. They obviously served to explain the figures which were listed as tables.

"Correlation coefficients," answered the doctor when he was asked what the figures meant. "Correlation coefficients, all of them. Are you a musician?"

"Yes, I play the violin." The terrestrial was dumb founded and watched the doctor who took another, slightly dusty book from the bottom corner of the shelves, blew over it murmuring "these walkmen nowadays, hardly anybody plays any music." He turned to him again: "There is a slightly better prognosis for musicians, hang on, I thought I'd read it... there we are! 0.92 - congratulations!" That seemed to have slipped out for he added at once: "These are average-figures, of course, nearly irrelevant for an individual case. Well - rub that in three times daily", he said, handed the tube to the terrestrial and disappeared through a door.

This was reason enough for the scientist to forget his pain and to have a closer look first at the books on the shelves and then all around the hospital. The following day, which was the last of the expedition, he had some further talks with several doctors and got an idea of Antiterrestrial medicine, as far as he could, being a chemist. Having returned to the earth the chemist's reports attracted much attention. What people got to know was about the following: medicine on Antiterra wasn't a business of doctors like on the earth, but of people who were like mathematicians and philosophers and whose training was also that of a mathematician or philosopher. Both sciences had a very long tradition. Already the second expedition to Antiterra had found that there were scientists of biochemistry, physiology, and anatomy but that they were of rather minor importance. There wasn't anything like connections of these sciences with medicine. By the same token the history as well as the training of this other kind of medicine was entirely different from those on the earth. On the other hand there were like with us hospitals, specialists, and GP's; also the organization of the health system was similar to ours.

2. This report made the doctors on earth curious and sceptical at the same time so that they decided on sending a group of medical doctors from all subject areas to Antiterra.

When they had arrived on Antiterra - it was lunch-time - and had been welcomed, there were at first the usual communication difficulties which they soon overcame as they were all colleagues after all. At 5 o' clock-tea both sides being driven on by immense curiosity already began to talk about subjects beyond the set phrases which had already become a habit with them when talking to visitors from the earth ("What was the flight like?" - "Just a little sunwind, nothing special."). But soon a strange phenomenon could be noticed: though they didn't have difficulties in understanding each other, communication became difficult or often impossible altogether as soon as they started talking about clinical details, because either side could not understand what the other was talking about.

In the course of this the terrestrial doctors sometimes got the impression as if they were talking to mathematicians, just as the chemist had described it, whose foot, by the way, had healed within four days. Consequently, nearly all talks with a clinical orientation didn't get beyond an initial stage.

A terrestrial psychiatrist and an internist from Antiterra, who happened to sit next to each other (already for dinner people from the same subject area were sitting together), were the only ones who had a lively discussion late into the night about important clinical parts of their subject area as they said. Both of them, however, were not taken seriously. The internist from Antiterra was notorious for showing off and acting big, and his colleagues did not take his being engrossed in talking for anything but exhibitionism. The terrestrial colleagues were not at a loss for an explanation for their communication, as psychiatrists were known for talking with everybody about everything, the less understandable the person they were talking to the better. That both of them had shown facial expressions or gestures as if they were telling each other a successful squaring of circle, of a pill against cancer or even against hypochondria did not make any difference to the other colleagues from both sides in their opinion.

After dinner they were talking nearly exclusively about general questions of medicine, its organization for instance which they found to be hardly any different. They were also talking about the training and history of medicine. Regarding the latter two issues there was again at first the situation that neither party could understand the other. But contrary to the talks in the afternoon, they gradually got closer. Instead of tracing the individual dialogues, statements, and discussions which in the course of the evening rendered a hardly comprehensible idea of the respective history of medicine and medical training, we shall give a broad outline of the picture that the doctors from the earth got and which hardly allowed them to sleep.

Antiterrestrial medicine like the terrestrial one has a long tradition. As early as two and a half milliennia ago people started thinking about medical care for the population. It was soon agreed upon that only the nation's most intelligent people should be entrusted with restoring and maintaining one's most valuable possession, health. At that time all sciences were still in their beginnings, but philosophers and mathematicians could already yield important achievements. Consequently they were intrusted with the responsibility for the business of medicine. Both philosophers and mathematicians were at first enraged and refused to do this extra work (which the doctors from the earth could understand only too well as they knew about these scientists who had nothing to do with practice and their special liking for artificially created problems which nobody can understand anyway, not to mention solve them). So they had to be beaten so as to work in the service of the sick.

Soon the scientists did out of their own free will what they had been entrusted with. They did so as they could gradually recognize parts of their former problems in their new tasks so that they could get interested in the job. (As space is limited it is not possible to give an outline of Antiterra's cultural history; it should however be mentioned that values like humanitarianism, helpfulness, and compassion came into fashion 1200 years after that). As on the earth, specialization of medicine was inevitable which, however, came about considerably earlier. It was already 2200 years ago that philosophers and mathematicians divided their common task. (Shortly afterwards beating the philosphers and mathematicians became less and less common whereas before, it had been necessary to do so every morning so as to motivate them; another 50 years later it could be given up altogether). For a long time mathematicians had been looking into statistical methods of describing complex systems; they were therefore more and more concerned with the body as the most complex system known to men at all. Soon an entire field of science, Somathematics, established itself which used elaborated mathematical-statistical methods to try and describe the behavior of the system "body" under normal and pathological conditions. The same methods could be used to evaluate certain ways of treating the sick (e.g. cold afusions or taking certain herbal teas.) The aim of the somathematicians (which had soon become the term commonly used for this group of specialists) was to develope and continually improve a medical encyclopaedia which should contain everything known about the body. The name SDT became common usage for this encyclopedia, meaning "statistical diagnosis and therapy" to which a number was added indicating the current edition. Up to the present day substantial progress has been made and the small booklet in the somathematian's pockets has developed into an edition consisting of 54 volumes proudly bearing the name SDT-299.

Somatic medicine on Antiterra did not comprise biochemistry, physiology, and anatomy. The reason for that, however, was not that these sciences did not exist. A biochemist who had taken part in former expeditions acknowledged that the colleagues on Antiterra had about the same standard as biochemists on the earth, apart from the fact that they only analysed plants and animals, herbal and animal substances and processes. On Antiterra apparently there was in fact no relation between medicine and anatomy, physiology and biochemistry.

The branch of medicine that the philosophers had taken up had undergone an entirely different development. With them statistical methods had become unimportant quite soon. The psychosophs, which had soon become the name for these specialists for the non-physical area, obviously did not need statistics to carry out their task. In the evening they tried to talk about what their branch of medicine was like and where they got their knowledge from, but the people from the earth could not make sense of it.

Around 11 p.m. all of them had become tired and their voices hoarse. As to the next day they had agreed upon looking into the practical side of things instead of continuing their theoretical discussions. They did so in the hope of mutual understanding when confronted with the sick not withstanding their different theories. Thus practice was to lead to understanding and to make things clear whereas their theories were in opposition (to be precise: not even in opposition as they could not understand their respective theory).

They arranged to meet at 9 a.m.; only the psychosophs asked their colleagues from the earth to come as early as 7.30. "We psychosophs are early birds," a young colleague said. "Unlike the somathematicians we psychosophs can really achieve something and are the real doctors. This probability-hocus-pocus really isn't satisfying in the long run." Having said that he said "good night" and disappeared.

As to the training it should be mentioned that there are huge differences between earth and Antiterra as well. On Antiterra the pre-clinical part of the medical course is completed after 4 years by taking an exam in philosophy and mathematics. Attendance of lectures in analysis, algebra, theory of games, set theory and, above all, stochastics has to be confirmed in order to be allowed to take the exam, as well as attendance of classes in metaphysics, ethics, ontology, and above all, epistemology. This is followed by two years of clinical studies which comprise descriptive statistics, statistics of inference, and special theory of probability on the one hand, and on the other hand transcendental philosophy, philosophy of mind, and general subjective ontology. Afterwards they specialize within the framework of an internship and become either a somathematician or a psychosoph. Unlike the colleagues from the earth the Antiterrestrials held their training in high esteem and valued above all its relevance to practice. This was another issue that their terrestrial colleagues could hardly understand.

3. The next morning the psychiatrists from earth met the psychosophs for "concept-discussion" which was the name this meeting had been given. Some of the people present were still tired after yesterday's short night and the younger ones had difficulties with being on time anyway. Malicious tongues said that a time that early had not been chosen because one could think clearly early in the morning but so as to have a means to control attendance. Anyway, they were sitting close together in front of a white blackboard onto which several sheets of paper of the size 50 cm x 50 cm were pinned. On these sheets one could see words, arrows, and several other symbols, partly colored.

"Anything special during the night?" asked the senior consultant having introduced the colleagues from the earth to his staff and having explained why they were there.

"Nothing" replied a voice from the left corner. "To be on the safe side I have admitted a case of someone having a personality finding problem. He can certainly become an out-patient quite soon. From next week onwards he'll come for talks three times a week."

"Is that all?"

"Round 5 a.m. there was a problem on ward C. The patient who was admitted yesterday suffering from acute disease of finiteness was pestering the other patients. Just like yesterday he thought he was God. But to make matters worse he thought he could think the thoughts of others and that his thoughts are thought by others..."

"You mean his disease tended towards mineness-disease?"

"I'm not quite sure. What we have diagnosed so far I've shown in a concept-picture, second from the right, bottom row."

The terrestrial psychiatrists practically could not understand anything so far. They might guess what a "personality-finding-problem" might be, but they had never heard of anything like "disease of finiteness" with a "tendency towards mineness-disease". The concept-picture wasn't of much help either. One could read several words, among others "I", "absolute", "boundary", "finite", "thinking", and arrows, symbolic circles and the like. Compared with the other pictures which were drawn very acurately these drawings seemed of a minor value as everything had hurriedly being drawn down in black pencil.

"Well, I think we'll need some time for diagnosis", said the senior consultant. "You should analyse other transcendental features as activity and capability to distinguish me from not-me today - just to be on the safe side. Identity and sense of time will be disturbed anyway but please look into that more closely in the following days; we have to make sure that we do not overlook anything, because otherwise in the phase of convalescence they are going to say that something has occurred again... Anything else?"

"Apart from that everything has been quiet."

"Well, then as for the pictures..."

They were now talking about the pictures in quick succession. We do not want to go into detail because the three colleagues from the earth, having tried at first just to guess what each of the pictures might mean had given up anyway. About 90 minutes later the senior consultant finished the lively discussion which some had engaged themselves in with great intent and said: "tea-time". At once the great suspense, the immense quietness that had dominated the scene so far was all over. Just one at the time had been talking, in between there had been breaks to think things over during which one could have heard a pin drop; nobody interrupted anybody else. Now a murmur arose, the four rows of chairs became a circle and they were talking leisurely. As if it had been arranged beforehand two younger colleagues left the room and re-entered shortly afterwards with a small tea-trolley. Tea was poured out and finally one of the Terrestrials picked up his courage to ask the others whether that was the daily morning-routine. The senior consultant feeling addressed before everybody else, said: "Every morning between 7.30 and 9 a.m. we discuss terminology, followed by the inevitable tea-break. Its purpose is to loosen the mind. Whereas our thinking was strictly analytical during the first 90 minutes matters are different during the tea-break. Everybody can ask whatever occurs to him - just like you did, you seem to have adopted our norms by intuition - and illogical questions and answers are accepted as well. However, during that time our thinking is much looser and more free. It would be very bad if we did the same during the discussion of terminology - if everybody was telling what occurred to him with regard to a patient we would still be sitting here at night and wouldn't have time for anything else. For us and for science, however, this break has proved very profitable, as some thoughts which seemed illogical at first glance proved, when taking a closer look, to be productive and very relevant.

4. In the meantime the internists and surgeons from the earth had met the somathematicians. After a short greeting they went to the wards and started their round. The first patient they saw was wearing a kind of cuff on his upper arm; on his bedside table there was a gauge that was connected with the cuff by two tubes. Next to it there was a sheet of paper showing several figures and a graph. One of the Antiterrestrials explained:

"This patient suffers from a headache." Pointing to the instruments he said: "If you put this cuff under pressure, the typical pulsation which can be felt on the wrist with every Antiterrestrial will disappear at a certain stage. Some months ago a physicist found out that this patients needs an especially high pressure for his upper arm cuff. The Terrestrials understood all that at once but the Antiterrestrial continued:

"But that is only of secondary importance. The patient is in hospital, as I've said, because he is suffering from a headache, but this equipment hasn't got anything to do with that. The physisist claims there is a connection between the pressure of the cuff and the headache but if you ask me, that's all nonsense." The doctors from the earth were astonished and first looking at each other than at the Antiterrestrial who continued:

"The results after examining about 1450 patients and other people are unambiguously ambiguous. There is, admittedly, an average-correlation between pressure in the cuff and frequency of headache, but there are no grounds at all for the physicist's assertion that high pressure was in itself an illness. As there are people having a headache and low pressure there are others without a headache and high pressure, which means there is nothing like a common cause, not to speak of the nosological entities the psychosophs have been able to establish."

The terrestrial colleagues hadn't expected that as in their opinion no branches of medicine could do without the notion of nosological entity, i.e. causes and clearly defined and really existing symptoms. How could any medical treatment exist without the recognition of the underlying disease? Should one be satisfied with merely curing symptoms without understanding the whole, the illness itself? In this case, however, they were cautious having themselves mainly statistical knowledge of blood pressure. They did not want to talk about statistics with their Antiterrstrial colleagues for the time being as it was practice they were interested in.

"How do you treat this patient?" they asked one of the internists.

"As in many such cases. We have about 200 drugs of which we might use about 30 for this patient. All of them have to be tried."

"But doesn't that take ages? Thirty drugs and each of them presumably for several days..."

"That is done very quickly. We give combinations of the drugs, several ones, and we watch the patient's condition carefully. If you have a balance and 12 balls one of which weighs either less or more than the others, how often will you have to weigh so as to find out this special ball without any other means?" The Antiterrestrial didn't even wait for the internist's answer who was completely taken aback. "Three times. Theory of combination, you know, theory of combination. The same is the case here. Usually we find the right drug after 4 or 5 tests."

The Terrestrials were so impressed that they didn't even think of asking problems like drug-interactions if several were taken at the same time. Instead, the Antiterrestrial proceeded:

"It may, of course, happen that pressure is lowered under the treatment of the headache, in other cases, however, the headache disappears but the pressure remains, in other cases again, just the opposite is the case. As to nosological entity - in my opinion it is high time that this idea was given up. We have wasted enough time with it. Exact observation of facts and statistics - this is our motto and we are doing quite well with that."

As if he wanted to support what he had said he continued:

"There is yet much more worth knowing. The product of consumption of porc and alcohol correlates exactly with occurence of cirrhosis of the liver; the number of smokers living in the same house with the occurence of malignant tumors; also the time of menarche correlate with the fibre content of one's food. Or with regard to this patient..."

They proceeded to the next bed in which a boy whose right forearm was swollen was lying. On the bedside table there was a small xylophone and a stop-watch and a kind of graph with some figures.

"Now this is medicine proper without any theoretical encumbrance," the Antiterrestrial said proudly. This boy fell a fortnight ago. Afterwards he had a lot of pain in his right forearm which was swollen within a short time. He could hardly move his hand. Therefore when we admitted him we made him play the song "Old Mc Donald Had a Farm" on the xylophone with his right hand and really he was playing significantly more slowly than his peers."

That was too much to take for the surgeons from the earth: "You didn't take an X-ray? No dressing? No plaster, nothing?"

Without understanding the Antiterrestrial was looking at them: "I don't know what you are talking about but above all I don't understand why you are so indignant. The idea of using a xylophone is rather new and maybe you would have preferred a recorder. Our results, however, are promising and unambiguous. The time it took to play "Old Mc Donald Had a Farm" when he was admitted correlates very well with the final result of treatment. We are likely to have found a very good means of prediction. The only problem we have to overcome now is that some patients, thank God that they are only very few of them, have some experience already. We try to overcome these difficulties on the one hand by comprising the X-positive..." "You mean the xylophone players?" "Exactly, by comprising the X-positive players in a subgroup in order to set up special correlations for them. On the other hand, we have applied for a major test, a sort of xylophone-screening. As soon as we'll have found the OMDHFPT-figure, i.e. the "Old Mc Donald Had a Farm playing time", medicine will have an instrument of excellent diagnostic value at its disposal. As to evaluating the process of healing the results are, even if only seen from a theoretical point of view, an even better reason to be optimistic: we can substract the effect of training if we measure daily and what remains is a excellent measuring instrument to evaluate the patient's condition." The Antiterrestrial's eyes were sparkling while he was saying that. They proceeded to the next patient in silence.

5. Having reached the sick-bed an Antiterrestrial who had been silent so far started speaking:

"This patient suffers from thirst, susceptibility to infections, polyuria, and occasional stomach-ache. Sometimes he is unconscious, especially after having strained himself, sometimes also after birthday parties or other parties. We treat him in a way similar to that which we have described for the first patient: we know certain drugs which have to be injected into the abdominal wall. Initially it is difficult to find the right dose but having overcome that they have a very good therapeutical result."

Once again the terrestrial internists knew everything: "Diabetes" one of them suddenly blurted out. "Have you never tried to get a clear idea of the underlying processes?"

"Of course there have been attempts every now and again to trace life back to single facts: the biochemists say that it is all a matter of biochemistry, the physiologists of physiology, and for the anatomists it's all - guess what."

"Anatomy," he was interrupted by the Terrestrial who thought this view rather strange. Before he could, however, say anything the other one continued:

"That's it. And we somathematicians neither have the time nor do we feel like getting involved in any theoretical arguments what "life" or "illness" is in the first place. We are here at the sick-bed and cannot wait until these theorists will have reached an agreement at last - in a thousand years' time, maybe. Even the best and most imaginative representative of the sciences mentioned, one who grasps the subject in the full and has made essential contributions to its progress, is utterly helpless when having to face the sick. It is for us to act and we do not have time for theories. The body's interior is so complicated anyway that even specialists are not quite clear about everything. We are doctors and it is the medic's task to see man as a whole. How then should we know more about the interior processes than the specialists? You are asking too much! We just rely on our experience - operationalized, statistically proven, and systematized."

"But didn't one try to use these sciences and their results in the particular cases to understand some illnesses - which still allows for these "last questions" to remain open?"

"Certainly there have been attempts but in my opinion - all of them useless theoretical phantasies. How could it be otherwise? What are we to think of individual results if the representatives of the sciences which yielded these results disagree on their relevance and if the basis apparently is inexplicable anyway?"

"You've said that before", said one of the Terrestrials having become curious. "Please do tell us about those who have tried it."

"Well, as we were just talking about this patient... about 20 years ago a biochemist once again tried to explain 'everything' by the fact that measuring a certain substance in the bodies of sick people yields results which differ from those of healthy people..."

"It was blood sugar, I suppose". "You may be right but this is irrelevant." The doctor from the earth looked at him in astonishment while he was proceeding: "We've often admitted theorists like that to our hospital which didn't get us anywhere; therefore some of us are rather annoyed with them and do not listen to them anymore. But the spirit and attitude of this hospital is basically to tolerate even strange theoretical ideas. That was the reason why we had taken this biochemist's assertion about the courses of the illness seriously. He was allowed to analyse the substance in all patients with the symptoms thirst, polyuria, frequent infections, and temporaly loss of consciousness. Had the theory been right there would necessarily have been a certain regularity. However, all there was were correlations, i.e. there were patients having all the symptoms mentioned before without any change of the result of measurement. But at the same time measurements of a control group yielded that there were also people who showed a change of the value. Nothing had been explained, leave alone by everything having one single cause".

"Were longitudinal sections analysed?"

"We didn't get round to doing that as we thought it was not worth the hustle. What is the use of further research if even from simple tests with cross-sections you don't get any results?"

"You would have found that those who have only an increase in blood sugar at first, later fall ill with the same symptoms as the others," was the Terrestrial's reply.

"And how about the cases where it is the other way round?"

"Well, of course, there are coincidences which, however, do not contradict the theory that there is a certain illness caused by increase in the value of blood sugar."

"You don't mean to say that on the one hand there is a nosological entity comprising the patients' symptoms and on the other hand someone having all the symptoms does not suffer from this illness?"

"Just that," the Terrestrial assured his astonished colleague from Antiterra.

He objected: "that is nothing but a stratey of immunization. We have had that before: first a simple hypothesis about the causes of the illness is set up which is then falsified straight away," the Antiterrestrial's voice became higher and louder and it was obvious that he was getting agitated. "Instead of admitting that biochemistry isn't any good for medicine a succession of supplementary hypotheses is added, everything is getting more and more complicated and in the end none of us has got a clue what the theorist is on about."

"Well, life is complicated."

"Certainly but we clinicians need simple concepts, things which are practical, no theoretical hocus-pocus... I am sorry about getting so agitated ... but, you know, it is always the same: some smart-aleck comes along who has not the faintest idea about the patients. But then he claims to know the final cause of everything. We've really been tolerant again and again and let them carry on but we've given up taking that seriously. Tests like that I've just been describing have been rather frequent in the past and have always ended similarly. To come back to our example: at first there were high correlations. Initially everybody was enthusiastic but this mood soon died away. Too many wrong positive and wrong negative results were found when measuring this substance which, by the way, really may have been blood sugar. Long-term studies would have taken too much effort and did not seem to lead to any new results. If only the positive results of measuring had been wrong, one might have decided to make further tests a year later whether some people might not possibly have fallen ill. But as there were wrong negative results as well one didn't even try that. It is just that we have patients with all the symptoms, admittedly rarely, and normal blood sugar value."

"May I repeat what I've suggested before?"

"You think one should assume that it is another illness?"

"Precisely".

"Well, I've said it before: strategy of immunization. Look... what we've got is our experience and nothing else. We manage quite well with that. Why then should we let ourselves in for pure theory, phantasies?"

"Has no-one ever found the causes of certain illnesses by using these connections between biochemistry and medicine?"

"Never." The Terrestrial could hardly believe that. But it was soon dawning on him what the reason might be:

"You've always calculated correlations?"

"Always."

"And you've always got correlations."

"Precisely."

"Which is to say that for you progress of discovery means to find correlations between symptoms that the patients show which can either have occurred spontaneously or may have been provoked artificially and then to confirm them statistically?"

"We not only correlate symptoms but also symptoms with outcome measures, with therapeutic efficacy of certain drugs, and - a quite new branch - with symptoms occuring in relatives of the patient. We would certainly like to have clearly defined nosological entities like the Psychosophs, for instance. But they are better off than we are. There is a lot which can be said clearly about thinking as there are directly discernible, necessary relations which it would be stupid to try and either confirm or falsify by means of statistics. Life, however, is something unfathomable, final. We'll never be able to entirely understand it." The Antiterrestrial had spoken these last words as if it was his creed. As if stimulated by that one of the internists from the earth asked him:

"So in your opinion scientific theorems consist either in a statements about things directly experienced or in logical, that is to say statistical statements?"

"Precisely that."

"And how about that theory itself?" The Antiterrestrial became thoughtful. He hesitated for a long time and all he said then was: "Well, we assume that... that is how things are."

"Another theorem which does not belong to either group of scientific theorems which you accept is the following: "Life can not be understood". Your idea of science is obviously determined by certain assumptions which do not fall within the scope of science."

"That's all above my head. I don't really know theorems except those relating to facts of experience and logical-statistical ones. And life - that is just inexplicable," answered the Antiterrestrial angrily.

"You might be wrong there."

"Here on Antiterra the sciences which deal with that problem certainly don't give any reason to be hopeful. They totally disagree and there are controversies even within the individual approaches. The sciences look at things from different aspects within a different framework."

"They look at totally different matters - shapes of bones and organs, functions, molecules and get entirely diffrent results."

"They look at different aspects of one thing - life."

"Why then do they disagree? What they do we just call the sport of arguing."

"There could be many totally different reasons. I don't know your biochemists, physicists, and anatomists. They might put a different value on the relevance of the particular subjects for finally deciding issue; any profession also involves a certain degree of organisational blindness. Possibly something totally different might be the reason: scientists are only human so they might be concerned with influence, prestige, power, politics... let's leave that." All of them were nodding in agreement and all of them were silent for a short time.

"Anyway, I know now why you've never got anything but correlation-coefficients." The Antiterrestrial looked at the Terrestrial in astonishment who continued: "The final authority of justification are correlations and not knowledge of the interrelations of life as it is on earth."

"Do you know then what life is in the end?"

"We know a lot of details. Your question tends towards the wrong direction. You expect too much at the time. Your motto is "everything or nothing". I guess the reasons why we are more modest in this respect are historical. When was calculation of correlations invented?"

"About 2700 years ago."

"There we go! So you've always taken correlations as your yardstick when the points at issue were complex and animated natural processes."

"What else? I don't see how it could be otherwise?"

"You've, however, just mentioned briefly that things were different with psychiatry, I mean psychosophy, but I don't know anything about that and therefore..."

"Neither do I..."

"And therefore I would like to try to explain to you in how far our idea of medicine differs from yours by using a model."

"You are really making me curious."

"I've understood there is a long tradition of mathematics and logic on Antiterra ..."

"... I don't exactly know for how long they've been in existence but you are certainly right - it might be 2 or 3 milliennia."

"Right. Regarding the statement '2 x 5 = 10', what would you think of someone trying to prove that statistically?"

"That's nonsense."

"And what would you say if, for instance, I had to deal with five pairs of things which I had to count every day and if I then found that on some days there are only nine of them?"

"Well, that wouldn't mean disproving the term '2 x 5 = 10'. One would set up supplementary hypotheses to explain these irregularities, for example, that there were sometimes not 5 pairs of things or that one might have been lost during the counting or that 2 have joined together or that one has counted wrongly ..."

"All strategies of immunization," the internist from the earth was smiling.

"Nonsense," the outraged Antiterrestrial interrupted him.

"You think the best thing to do is to accept as an explanation an empirical hypothesis which corresponds in the best way with the proven facts."

"That is what you have to do, as by no means the following would be accepted: that the product of 2 and 5 isn't always 10. By the way, to use statistics to prove or disprove this asertion isn't possible in the first place because statistics have to refer to exact mathematics. One would hopelessly get caught in a vicious circle and everything would be lost, you couln't even state that 1 = 1."

"We agree on that" said the Terrestrial.

"Of course, but what has that got to do with our patients here?"

"There is a nosological entity called "Diabetes mellitus" on the earth of which an increase in blood sugar content of certain body fluids is characteristic. This effects several molecules, functions and organs which in the end leads to exactly those symptoms that this patient shows. By understanding the molecules functions and organs as a whole we get a rough idea of the processes. We don't know everything, above all we haven't solved the "secret of life" but we know a certain amount, especially things which are relevant to therapeutics."

"What about those who show the symptoms, whose body fluids have the normal blood sugar content, i.e. those that are in your opinion 'false negative'?"

"They suffer from a different disease."

"You mean the same is the case as for the term "2 x 5 = 10"

"Not quite. The mathematical term is necessarily true. Science's terms about 'the animated', however, have been found empirically ..."

"I'm beginning to understand what you're getting at with your example: what matters is what you assume as irrefutable or at least fundamental. That is obvious for mathematics - you wouldn't get anywhere if you tried to prove its axioms, let alone by statistical means. For science matters are more complicated. Because - let me think ..."

"Because you on Antiterra have started from the assumption that human life finally is incomprehensible, progress of knowledge in your medicine ..."

"... at least as far as the somathematicians are concerned ..."

"... is determined by the idea of finding better correlations within the area empirical knowledge. This is why clearly defined nosological entities could never develop; we would say: as there is always the possibility of someone having lice and fleas at the same time you could never find correlations of 1.0. But at the same time correlations of 1.0. were, in your opinion, the only right way to find distinct nosological entities and thus to the present day you could not get anything beyond correlations. You've been looking for correlations and found them."

"It is apparently in the nature of the matter that we've never found anything beyond that, i.e. other than correlations."

"Surely you've tried a lot and collected a vast amount of empirical data, also with regard to therapeutics?"

"Precisely. The new SDT-300, which is to appear soon, is said to consist of more than 100 volumes," said the Antiterrestrial.

"But for the individual case this knowledge will be rather useless," replied the internist from the earth.

"Unfortunately yes. But we have come to terms with that. It is only later that final statements can be made. This patient here...," he pointed at the poor Antiterrestrial who had fallen asleep in the meantime, because in the course of the discussion he had probably noticed that it was not him they were talking about but general issues which he could not understand, "his chances, for instance, are good if he gets a certain injection of a certain drug in the abdominal wall daily."

"How did you find this drug?"

"By chance - like all great discoveries of medicine."

The internist could hardly believe that, but he could understand it to a certain degree as he had only recently read a report on Semmelweis and Flemming ...

"We know even more, however: if, for example, the patient's lymphatic glands are very swollen and he is having pain in the area of his flank and he is a heavy smoker ..."

"Then he suffers from another illness or maybe three illnesses at a time ..."

"Then he doesn't stand a good chance and will probably die very soon."

"Exactly! He is suffering from a different illness."

"We would say: the correlations are different."

"That isn't enough for us on earth. In this case I would suppose that the body fluids' sugar content is fine (unless he had fleas and bugs) and that the similarity of the symptoms is due to the accidental co-orrurrence of two or three illnesses. One of them (that one which, among other things, causes the swelling of the lymphatic glands and susceptibility to infections) has a bad prognosis."

"What do you mean by speaking of "bad prognosis"? You should be able to say exactly for how many days the patient shall live if you really know the cause of the illness."

"Not quite, I have said it before: we on the earth know a lot but not everything. We also use statistical methods, for the prognosis, for example. We regard statistical results, however, as something provisional, which only points to the fact that we do not yet have any other means to get exact information. Since we assume that animated nature ist comprehensible on principle, although we postpone 'last questions' and do not yet know a lot of things in detail, we also use other methods to get insight into the matter. Furthermore we regard these as "more fundamental" as they really enable us to see relations and as they are often relevant to the individual case."

"I cannot really believe that."

"I suppose so."

"You mean there is really the possibility of showing relations without statistics?"

"Precisely." The Antiterrestrial didn't really want to take that, although he was well aware that he would probably have to do so, which also meant accepting all the consequences for his everyday work and science in general. But he did not yet admit defeat: "Isn't it unscientific to refer to some theories and not to empirical knowledge and nothing else?"

But the Terrestrial replied calmly: "Is it unscientific to state that '2 x 5 =10'?" Now his colleague gave in. "And your theory ..."

"Unfortunately we have rather too many theories so far. Often there are very elaborated theories about certain interrelations the results of which, however, haven't been taken advantage of inpractice. On the other hand there are also cases where unfortunately we have to rely on statistics. As to these cases, however, we assume that we don't yet know everything..."

"Whereas on principle we have started from the assumption that there is nothing to be known."

"That's it." They proceeded to the next bed.

6. The psychiatrists and Psychosophs had finished their tea-time as well - as they used to call this break which they were careful not to extend any longer than 30 minutes. Afterwards they had started their round.

The next patient claimed that his thoughts were not his own thoughts, sometimes were made by others, and that sometimes others could hear them. He complained that his feelings, impulses, thoughts, and actions were not his own but imposed by some external force. He also complained that he had difficulties with reality in the way, that sometimes things did feel somehow unreal, and that sometimes he felt an immediate relationship between certain objects or events and him. Having been questioned, he admitted that when his illness was worst, he had the immediate experience that the world depended on his breath. He had to breathe constantly and hardly to prevent the world from stopping to go. This was a hard burden for him.

This time, a terrestrial psychiatrist tried to give to the others a lesson how one would describe and diagnose the patients statements on earth: "In this case the symptoms are perfectly clear: the patient mentioned some delusions that are quite common in an illness we call schizophrenia. He mentioned the delusion that his thoughts were broadcasted, and the delusion that his thoughts were withdrawn, and also spoke about the delusion of thought control."

"I cannot understand" was the reply of the Antiterrestrial, "what do you mean with 'delusion'?"

"Oh, that's easy," the Terrestrial felt quite sure "a delusion is a false personal belief based on incorrect inference about external reality..."

"But this patient is not talking about external reality at all. Neither does he talk about inferences he made, but apparently he talks about his immediate experience, I mean about the ways his immediate experience has changed. What he says I do not regard as false at all and he is not talking about the outside world but about his experience."

"But he speaks about broadcasting..."

"He is not trained in transcendental philosophy and is not a psychosoph at all. He has to use some metaphor to talk about his experience because the structure of experience is so basic, so principal ... Therefore ordinary people do not know anything about it."

"I do not understand. When there really is a structure - I have not heard about something like that - of experience, which is, let us say, represented in each terrestrial or antiterrestrial subject which makes experience, why don't we know? Shouldn't we know? And isn't the fact that we do not know a prove that there is no such structure?" A murmur went through the antiterrestrial psychiatrists.

"The opposite is true!" was the reply of the Antiterrestrial. "First of all, we all know how to speak but perhaps none of us would be able to write down the principles of how we do it, which would amount to a comprehensive grammar book. Even the people who deal with language scientifically would have difficulties in doing it, and there are still a lot of unresolved questions. So being able to do something doesn't imply any knowledge about its principles."

"But experience is so basic that we should know at least a little bit..."

"Not at all! Look: sometimes we see an elephant and sometimes we do not. The result is, that an elephant, when present, is noticed. The point: if you always saw elephants you'd probably not noticed them. I mean, if there is no difference, noticing is really difficult." The Terrestrial, mouth and eyes a bit more open than usual, hardly understood.

"Transcendental structures, I mean structures regarding the conditions of the possibility of experience, have been recognized by the psychosophs very early. You can think about them without referring to patients, but if you look at the patients, you can almost grasp them with your hands. You suddenly have the difference you lack when you simply think about them. Patients indeed do vary with respect to some of these structures and these structures become evident to every observer, who tries to make sense out of statements like these we've just heared of that patient. The patient clearly uses metaphores. He cannot use the language of perception which would be useful if he wanted to describe hallucinations, neither can he use his language of emotion which would be useful to describe emotional disorders. He has a disturbance of experience and for him there is no language to describe this disturbance at all because he is not a transcendental philosopher or a psychosoph. But his utterances make perfect sense in the framework of transcendental philosophy. His account is not false at all. Certainly, when his disturbance lasts longer, he will develop some kind of explanation and these explanations will refer to the broadcasting of thought or to some technical gadgets or demons or something else. When this has happened, we speak of a deluded patient. But you have to differentiate delusions from metaphorical talk about disturbances of immediate experience." The

Terrestrial somehow got an idea of what the Antiterrestrial was talking about. "Is it always possible to tell what is a metaphor and what is a delusion?"

"Sometimes it is indeed not easy to tell, but in most cases things are quite obvious. Indeed, if you do have the referencial frame of transcendental philosophy, you can always ask about some other transcendental structures and if the patients' utterances are metaphors for pathological changes in transcendental structures, they always make sense in this framework. Delusions do not make sense in this framework at all."

There was a little pause. The Antiterrestrial thought about what the Terrestrial had said and suddenly came up with a question:

"I would predict that your patients quite often do complain about what you call 'false believes' referring to being controlled, thought broadcasting or insertion and the like."

"You are perfectly right".

"Then - how do you explain this phenomenon?"

The Terrestrial felt uneasy. Indeed, he had never thought about that question. The Antiterrestrial didn't wait for the answer.

"Delusions with regard to their contents, at least in our sense, do refer to the person's idiosyncratic history and to the cultural background. So the content of delusions varies in a broad range. In these cases, however," he pointed to the bed (the patient actually had left the room), "patients always do mention the same things. This should have been the first hint for you, that this kind of disorder cannot just be a matter of content. Secondly, the patient is not interfering at all. He's just talking about his experience. Didn't you notice that? I mean, the first mental event of that disease is not a disturbance in perception or behavior, but a disturbance in experiencing the world, and that's what these patients are talking about just when they get ill. In later states of the illness delusions will probably be developed, especially by the more intelligent patients..."

"But how do you explain, that only about 70 % of our patients do have that kind of delusions?" The Terrestrial was quite upset.

"Either you interpret the metaphors of the other 30 % of the patients in a wrong way or they simply do have another disease," was the simple answer of the Antiterrestrial.

While approaching the next bed the senior psychosoph started talking once again:

"I see, that's last night's patient who suffers from this personality-finding-problem. You must have that on the earth as well. The essential feature is severe subjective distress regarding inability to reconcile aspects of the self into a relatively coherent and acceptable sense of self. There is uncertainty about a variety of issues relating to personal identity, including long-term goals, career choice, friendship patterns, sexual orientation and behavior, religious identification, moral values, and group loyalities. These symptoms last at least three months and result in impairment in social or occupational (including academic) functioning. Frequently, the disturbance is epitomized by the individual's asking the question: 'Who am I?'"

"We on the earth call that 'identity disorder'."

"That seems to me quite a confusion of terms," said the Antiterrestrial. "Identity is for us the unity of the person experiencing and acting in time. Identity disorders are serious mental disturbances which affect the unity of the experiencing and acting subject. We psychosophs have done intensive research on that field for a long time. We would need a lot of explanations to show you in detail what we have found out about these disturbances. There are some inevitable connections with the experience of time, production of reality and mine-ness. But we shall better leave that. All this is not the case with this patient. All he has is a personality-finding problem. An identity disorder, an identitosis, as we would call it, is, here anyway, an altogether different matter."

The colleagues from the earth were rather impressed with the Antiterrestrial psychosoph's subtle terminological differentiations. Obviously they had in fact done quite a lot of research on the different aspects of the Antiterrestrial psyche and the terrestrial psychiatrists somehow had the feeling that their term "identity" was in fact rather clumsy. By the same token they realized that they themselves not only spoke of "disturbed identity" for the problems that this youth obviously had only, but also for schizophrenia. Something must be wrong there.

They left the room and went into the corridor where the senior psychosoph suddenly stopped and turned to the psychiatrist from the earth: "What I really want to know now is whether you don't have any concept-discussion or anything similar. As the Terrestrials shook their heads he proceeded:

"How about diagnostics? What criteria do you use to asign the occurrence of certain symptoms to a nosological entity and how are they classified?"

"Well, it might be best to begin with your last question," began one of the earth's psychiatrists, "for classifying the sick we rely entirely on experience and nothing but experience..."

A murmur went through the people in the corridor - to rely on experience - how should that be possible for psychosophy and psychopathosophy...

"That is to say, we also have nosological entities, of course, certain notions and terms. They are, however, defined statistically, i.e., they are finally the result of experience." The murmur was increasing: statistics - that had been given up 2000 years ago: just empirical data and statistics - they did not want to believe that. How should that be possible? Suddenly one of the Antiterrestrial colleagues started talking who had been rather quiet so far and had just been shuffeling along in the nearly endless train of doctors on their round:

"Would you mind me trying to put that more clearly?" All at once everybody was silent, but then one of the Terrestrials said quickly: "Please do so."

"Before I started my training in psychosophy I had done an internship at a somathematic hospital. As you've been talking of statistics I might be the one who is most likely to be able to clarify that. A psychosoph forgets rather quickly what he has learnt about that during his studies." The others nodded. "I assume that if you deal with statistics you do not only statistically analyse the daily data that you get without any effort from your bedside, but that you also use certain, let me call them, methods of provocation so as to aim at deliberately getting certain data."

"Exactly. We use certain methods of testing, above all questionnaires for diagnosis and differenciated diagnosis of the cases. We have a group of patients and a group of items or tests and try to find common features in the patients' reactions to certain items which enable us to develop instruments that may clearly and unambiguously classify illnesses and diagnoses."

"But how do you get the clearly defined illnesses that you need to set up a questionnaire in such a way that you can clearly distinguish whether the case tested shows occurrence of the illness or not?"

"That is a very difficult problem indeed," said one of the Terrestrials. "You are right in saying that we should first decide whether we have a case of the respective illness or not. Only then it will be possible to devise and valuate a questionnaire so as to record the respective illness as simply and exactly as possible." It was obvious that the Antiterrestrial had a commanding knowledge of statistics for he replied:

"So the difficulty is that you have to measure your measuring instruments itself by something else and surely you will agree that the measuring instrument cannot by any means be any better than that which it is measured by. How do you measure your measuring instruments?"

"When we validate a new method of testing or a new questionnaire, the experts' opinion, i.e., the opinion of experienced psychosophs, as you would call them, is the final authority for us."

"And they have a good idea of the illness, the terms which belong to it etc.?"

"Well it is, at any rate, these experts who have the greatest experience."

"But no theory?"

"Theories are useless without practice, but maybe not for you. We, however, have a great many theories about the psyche and its disturbances - in fact, so many that one gets the impression that there are none at all as so much is contradictory and inconsistant. This is why we've completely broken away from theory and rely on nothing but empirical knowledge and its "improvement" by statistics."

"Fair enough, but doesn't that imply then that validating tests and questionnaires goes back to nothing but empirical knowledge again?"

"Of course - what else?"

"Are your experts' judgements without any theories, concepts - I'd nearly said without thoughts?"

"Of course not. Each of them will not only have a great deal of empirical but also of theoretical knowledge, i.e., we'll be well aquainted with current theories of the psyche and psychopathology."

"So their personal preferences as regards theory will also influence their empirical knowledge?"

"I cannot see how that could be avoided."

"But that implies that the measuring instruments which have been judged according to these opinions can finally never be anything but projections of an expert's opinion. That, however, means that even very elaborate calculations can never get beyond the way things are as represented by current expert's opinions."

"If you want to put it like that." The psychiatrists from the earth had begun to feel rather uneasy during this discussion.

"Are there no objective, which is to say, theoretical criteria, to prove the quality of the statistical methods? Is that what you have described really all, on principle I mean?" insisted the Antiterrestrial.

"Yes, but how could it be otherwise?" Everybody had been listening attentively and thinking hard, above all the Antiterrestrial who obviously had an idea:

"Maybe an analogy might help us along."

"Let's try it - if it helps to clarify what you are trying to say".

The Antiterrestrial went to a white blackboard hanging in the corridor, took some concept-pictures down which were pinned onto it and started drawing:

"Imagine straight, convex, concave, and s-shaped rulers which are made in such a way that only one of their edges can be used for drawing a line. Furthermore they have a handle formed like a ball so that you cannot turn them upside down. We shall call straight rulers normal, the bent ones ill. Could you then imagine that you cannot tell from looking at the rulers whether they are straight or bent, which is to say that 'straight' and 'bent' are qualities which are, so to speak, hidden. They show, however, in the rulers' 'behavior'. Behavior is to be that you use them to draw triangles - always using one ruler at a time and in such a way that you start with drawing the base, that you then move the ruler in a parallel way and displace it clockwise by an angle between 0° and 180°, you then draw the next side and proceed in the same way for drawing the third side. You only use one ruler at a time for drawing one triangle."

"You'll get strange triangles: some shall be Euclidian, others shall have sides which are totally bent which probably will imply that they will also have strange geometrical qualities." The Antiterrestrial was drawing some triangles on the board: some had sides which were curved outward, others inward. Other triangles had S-shaped sides.

"Exactly. Let us assume we didn't know anything of geometry, but would like to understand these rulers and their funny behavior by analysing their behavior, i.e. the triangles."

"We could, for instance, use a protractor and measure the angles. That would make it easy to tell "ill" from "healthy" rulers on grounds of their behavior, which is to say on grounds of the triangles they produce."

"You've forgotten that we assume not to know any geometry. We don't know any connections, which includes the theory that the sum of the angles in a triangle is 180°. Even worse: as we do not know whether certain lines are straight or bent we are not able to divide an angle into two equal parts. There are, therefore, no protractors or, if you want to put it like that, many, all of which have a different gradation such for instance..." He was drawing some protractors on the blackboard some of which had a regular gradation, others an irregular one. So the same angle might be measured as having 30° with one protractor, 32° degree with the next one and 28,5° with the third one. So the angle was the same but the measuring instrument different.

"We have to assume, of course, that you cannot tell whether a protractor has a regular or irregular gradation by looking at it. I admit that my theoretical experiment takes some trouble. But I think what we can realize from it will be worth the mental effort."

"Just carry on," the Terrestrial encouraged him, "protractors having a gradation that you can read but of which you cannot tell whether they are regular or irregular are nothing compared with the theories of some of our colleagues as regards our psyche's inner life."

"I'm very pleased that you are so open-minded - we psychosophs regard it as one of the highest virtues to be willing to have a good look at new thoughts," said he and finished his drawing.

"Taken together all your assumptions, we shall never be able to tell 'healthy' from 'ill' angles, shall we?" one of the doctors from the earth said with resignation.

"That depends on your method! We should first try and realize why empirical knowledge and statistics alone can never be sufficient means to get a result, i.e., a definite statement on the basic disorder of the rulers..."

"You mean as regards their being bent which shows their strange behavior..."

"Right, eh, to get these results."

"Would you allow me to think out loud?"

"Please."

"We could draw many triangles with many rulers and then measure and add up the angles. On the condition that the rulers are unsystematically bent and the protractors unsystematically irregular, we would probably get the well-known Gaussian bell-graph-correlation if we had the angles round 180° on the X-axis, and the frequence of triangles with a certain sum of their three angles on the Y-axis."

"But of course we wouldn't get the geometrical theory." In the meantime the Antiterrestrial was roughly drawing the Gaussian distribution curve on the blackboard. At its highest point on the horizontal axis one could read the gradation 180° , to its left 170°, to its right 190°. The vertical axes showed frequency of triangles. They all agreed that the curve could only look that nice and regular if one drew and calculated several thousand triangles in this way.

"You cannot really expect to get any results by merely calculating the arithmetical mean which is the most simple of all statistical operations known. We could also conduct more complicated operations. We could, for instance, draw curves where all the triangles had been measured with one protractor." The Antiterrestrial was again drawing graphs with the horizontal axis being the same, the graphs, however, rather resembling histograms. The highest columns were to the left of 180°, then to the right and the third time just at 180°. To their left and right there were other columns of various height. They were, however, decreasing in height towards the left and right respectively.

"If several healthy rulers shall be among them, one will be able to somehow tell a healthy behavior from any other behavior."

"Precisely" the Antiterrestrial replied. "The only disadvantage is that the direction of deviation from the point 180° is always a different one depending on the protractor used. If, on the other hand, we measured one single triangle with all the protractors, we would get about the following graph, assuming that the degree of being bent statistically varies, and that there are also some protractors which are not bent." He was again drawing a histogram. This time the highest column was at about 175°.

"For this curve we assume, of course, that what we see is an ill behavior, i.e., a triangle having bent sides which are slightly curved inwards. The class of protractors which are not bent stands out from all the others."

"On earth we have had multivariated statistics for over 20 years. We could use that to statistically prepare matrices of the sums of angles formed by behavior and items, or rather angles and protractors, in such a way that you get a group of triangles the sum of whose angles measured with a group of protractors will always come to 180°. The snag, however, is that also the sum of the angles of triangles having S-shaped sides if measured with regular protractors comes to a sum of angles of 180°, although they are bent. On the other hand by using bent protractors straight angles will be classified as ill, maybe even statistically significant..."

"What I've been using this analogy for so far," the Antiterrestrial was explaining, "has been to show the following: in this way we can never get any knowledge of angles and their laws. You cannot get the axiom: 'the sum of all angles in a triangle is always 180°'. All you can get is the statement: 'the mean of the sum of the angles of all triangles measured with all protractors is 179,333°' or something like that."

"What you're saying is very interesting. I suppose I understand you rightly if I assume that it should be possible to differenciate quite well between, let us say, two different ways of being bent by using some protractors which are, however, irregular, namely the convex or concave ones."

"Precisely".

... "And a - eh, schizoaffective, eh - a ruler having both basic disorders - it produces triangles having S-shaped sides - would, depending on the respective theory, be likely to..."

... "You mean depending on the respective protractor..."

"Precisely, it would be likely to be classified once as this and a second time as that..."

"Especially because its behavior would also vary a lot. If you use such a ruler to draw smaller triangles it will surely be possible to get "conspicious behavior" only as regards one of the basic disorders. Only after analysing more subtly many different reactions of the ruler, i.e. many angles drawn, one could realize that it shows both basic disorders, being bent concavely and convexly. But we'll better leave that. Let us get to the crucial point."

They were all listening attentively to what the Antiterrestrial was saying.

"As soon as I do not only have my bent measuring instruments and rulers but also a theory of the rulers' behavior, for which I can show essential interrelations without really existing rulers, as soon, or rather, only if I have that, I can come to any knowledge. Merely relying on empirical knowledge and statistics doesn't by any means enable me to get out of the 'sog of multivariation', i.e., under no circumstances to get anything but statistical statements. Would you consider that we've been talking of things as simple as rulers and triangles. As regards healthy and sick people you cannot get far by 'analysing the data' and statistics. One might be able to say some commonplaces and to give the status of a scientific statement to some trivialities that are nothing but common knowledge anyway by stating a certain level of significance. You don't get anything else, you can't get anything else! To get back to our analogy: it is only after I know what the sum of the angles of a triangle necessarily is that I can validate my measuring instruments by this criterion and then use these objectively validated instruments for further operations of measuring. In this way you would probably understand the characteristics of the several groups of triangles and the several groups of rulers which leads us to the issue of realizing the basic disorder..."

"I know what you're getting at: as soon as one has a fixed point one can proceed from that," one of the psychiatrists said.

"... And without this point you get nothing but statements of probability." There was a short silence. Then as if he had suddenly realized what it was all about the same psychiatrist asked full of excitement:

"Are you saying that there are necessary conditions similar to those of geometry..."

"Analogous. And even that might be a confusing term," the Antiterrestrial interrupted him.

"... that there are necessary conditions in the field of psychiatry or, as you say, psychosophy, as well?"

"Psychosophy and psychopathosophy are nothing but the sciences of such conditions or rather relations."

"But psyche, mind, thinking - each of them is incomprehensible, they are the greatest secrets and the human mind is far too limited to make any scientific and unambiguous statements about them." The Terrestrial was getting more and more agitated. "As far as I know, our philosophers on earth do not know anything - they are just arguing all the time."

"You're asking too much! We psychosophs know quite a lot, but not everything. Your question on the final essence of being or the question why it is that the world really exists and does not not exist or, for instance, the question why we are thinking and have a mind, what that goes back to, these are questions all of which we postpone. It is, however, possible to show several interrelations, for example between the concept "I" and the concept "object". These considerations help towards a better understanding and better classification of the occurence of illnesses. It is our conviction, you know, that whoever deals with mental disturbances has to understand the mind."

"You mean that there is really something to be understood, real insights into real, objective relations?" the Terrestrial could hardly believe that.

"Certainly. The psychosophs have been investigating that for 2000 years. The discipline of psychopathosophy is somewhat younger. But it has gained a lot from its connections with psychosophy."

"And you think that this is the only way to get beyond correlations, statements of probabilities, factors and variance?"

"If you really want to penetrate and understand the area of mental illnesses, how could it be otherwise? But if you take a broader look at what you do everyday when you describe things, there is nothing special at all about it!"

"I do not understand," was the confused reply of the Terrestrial.

"Look: whenever you describe something, you need to have some theory ..."

"I always thought, first description (without theory) and then theory ..."

"That's impossible, as we just have seen ..."

"I haven't seen anything ..."

"Think of the triangles! The best description of their behavior is the theory of geometry. Without such a theory and without an attempt to create one (as the statistical approach can be understood), you would not even know what to look at and perhaps describe the colors of the triangles or their smell ..."

"... Eh...?"

"The point: there are just no such things as 'mere data'! Everything is and has to be interpreted. Interpretation is inevitable. The consequence: do not try to avoid it but think about it."

"But a patient who just says that he is hearing voices ..."

"... That's a good example! How would you describe what he or she is experiencing?"

"I would call that a hallucination."

"That's it! But that's in no way 'just a datum'!"

"The hell, why?"

"Look: You just have defined delusions. Why don't you call the patient's experience a delusion? Isn't it a false personal belief based on incorrect inference about external reality and firmly sustained in spite of what almost everyone else believes and in spite of what constitutes incontrovertible and obvious proof or evidence to the contrary?"

"Of course. But the patient talks about perception."

"So you have a theory that allows you to distinguish crazy talk about perception and about everything else ..."

"You could say so, but what's the matter ...? Perception is something different ..."

"First I could question the fact that the patient really is perceiving: at least our patients, if carefully investigated, are almost always able to distinguish their real hearing and their hearing of voices by some quality, even if they are (what mostly is the case) not able to say what quality that is."

"Its the same with our patients."

"Well, why then do you speak of perception? - The answer: If you do not only want to say that somebody is 'crazy', but if you want to say more, you have to have a theory. Only by means of a theory you will be able to distinguish certain aspects of what the patients say, only by applying a theory you will get different 'symptoms' of an illness. Without a theory, there is no progress in science because the theory tells you what to look at, in short: facts do not create a theory but are defined within the context of a theory. There is no such thing as pure data."

The terrestrial psychiatrist was really confused. Data for him have always been the most a-theoretical kind of things. Theory had to be eliminated, especially when describing a patient: "We always tried to minimize inference by interpretation ..."

"But nevertheless you interpreted - I bet not as good as we did, because we always knew, that interpretation and inferrence are inevitable. Think again of the triangles! Minimizing inference by not using any theory to describe them may be superficially attracive but really has very little to offer as a scientific goal, even on the basic observational level. Observation without inference is impossible, and there is nothing minimal about the inferences characterizing much of basic observation in our paragon of science - physics. Hydrogen atoms were inferred from complex patterns of scintillations on zinc sulfide screens. Inferrences regarding subatomic particles are even more complex and abstract. Are physicists performing bad science? In short: You have to have a theory ... even a false one is better than none."

"False?"

"False! A pendulum has always been regarded as something regular and something well understood, and the laws that had been used to describe its behavior have been very successful - just think of clocks and their importance to science, navigation or even everyday life and its structure. Nevertheless, a pendulum may exhibit chaotic behavior that has, at least on our planet, been discovered only in the recent twenty to thirty years... Even false theories are helpful, they allow our experience to be structured... Think of all the false theories in science, heliocentrism, phlogiston, ether, vitalism etc. What we believe to know now, we do so with the help of the observations and thoughts that were generated to some extend by these theories. False theories are much better than none... and to try get rid of theories at all is just to forget that simple fact: if you do, you will either continue to use theories but will not know it and thus become dogmatic or you will not be able to gain any knowledge - I don't know what is worse..."

They proceeded to the next ward.

The round of both the somathematicians and the psychosophs took a very long time on that day. It was the same on the following days and the time that the expedition was to spend on Antiterra was far too short for all those who were taking part in it. After the expedition had arrived on the earth again their colleagues could hardly believe what they told them about their experiences on Antiterra. For the psychiatrists it was most difficult to explain their experiences. They met with a lack of understanding on the part of most of their colleagues. They did not give up hope, however, as one had planned further contacts with the psychosophs. Maybe soon one would have a better understanding of things on the earth as well.[1]

1 This is the translated and slightly different version of the seventh chapter of M. SPITZER: *Allgemeine Subjektivität und Psychopathologie* [General Subjectivity and Psychopathology], Frankfurt a.M. (1985). As the reader will have suspected not everything which seems to be fictitious, is really fiction. The Diagnostic and Statistical Manual of Mental Disorders (DSM-III) now is used widely all over the world. Whoever has smokers among his relatives or likes porc and alcohol or even likes to have some unusual knowledge about acceleration (premature sexual maturity) which has not yet been explained, should look for information in the February and March editions of *The Lancet*, in *Annuals of Human Biology* **12**, or the 1985 edition of *New Scientist* (03/07/85, p. 7; 03/28/85, p. 5; 11/21/85, p. 31). Correlations of the time it takes to play well-known folk-song with psychiatric diseases have been subject to psychiatric research. The relevant books on the history of medicine will give information about SEMMELWEIS and FLEMMING, i.e. on the conditions how penicillin and childbed-fever respectively had been discovered. There is a solution to the ball-balance-problem (not to be tried by means of combination-theory, but by mere thinking), and as for *Chaos in the swing of a pendulum* have a look at an article with the respective title in *New Scientist* (07/24/86, p. 37-40). We did not indicate our sources, but among others cf. A.J. AYER, *Language, Truth and Logic* (1940), D. FAUST, R.A. MINER (Am J. Psychiat **143**, pp. 962-967, 1986), G. PATZIG, *Nachword zu R. CARNAP, Scheinprobleme der Philosophie* (1976), R. RORTY, *Philosophy and the Mirror of Nature* (1979), A.N. WHITEHEAD, *Process and Reality* (1978), J. ZUTT, *Anthropologische Psychiatrie* (1963), as well as the *DSM-III*.

Author Index/Personenregister

Subject Index

Sachregister

MIX
Papier aus verantwortungsvollen Quellen
Paper from responsible sources
FSC® C105338

If you have any concerns about our products,
you can contact us on
ProductSafety@springernature.com

In case Publisher is established outside the EU,
the EU authorized representative is:
Springer Nature Customer Service Center GmbH
Europaplatz 3, 69115 Heidelberg, Germany

Printed by Libri Plureos GmbH
in Hamburg, Germany